Eat Better, Feel Better

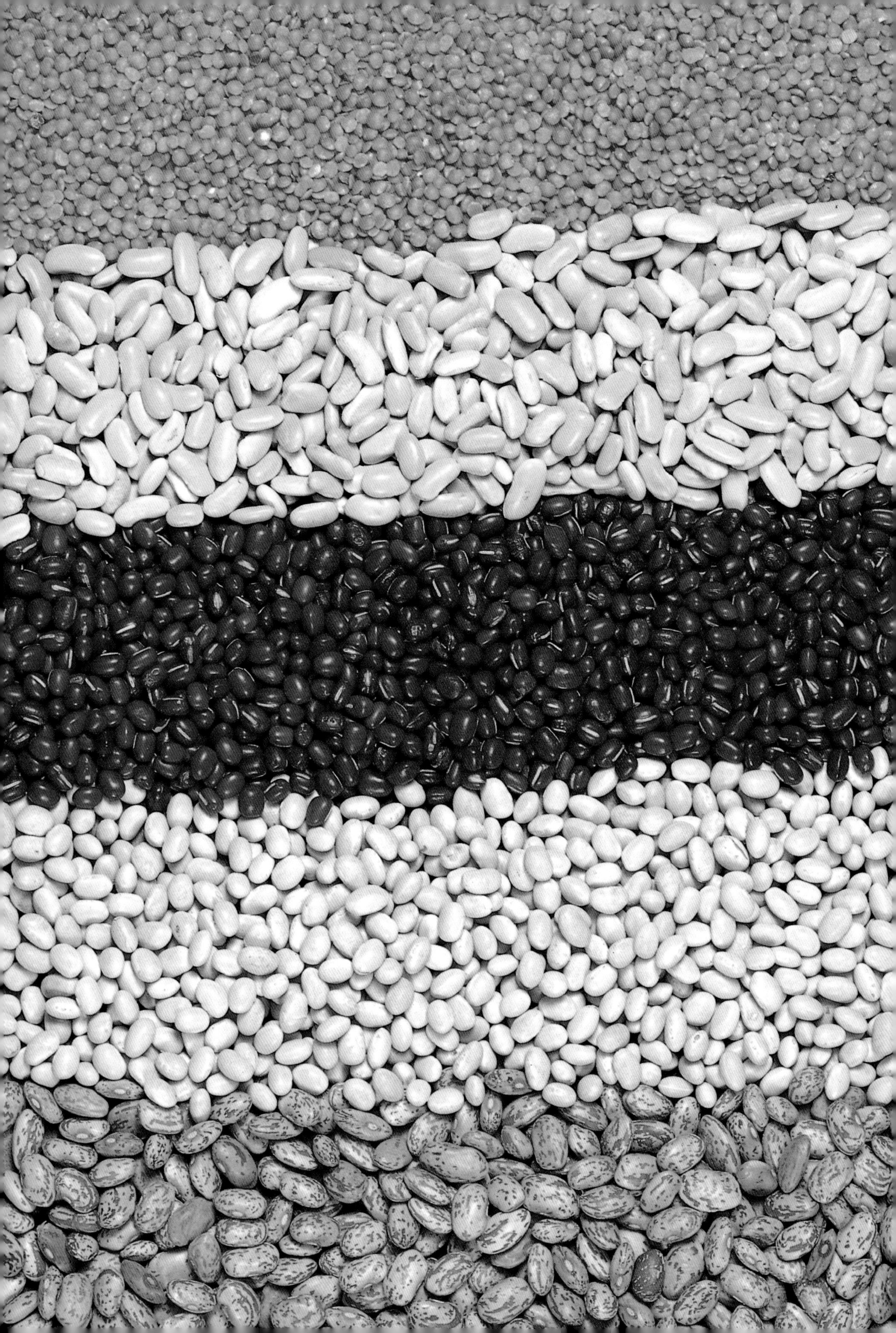

Eat Better, Feel Better

MARY DEIRDRE DONOVAN

TODTRI

A QUANTUM BOOK

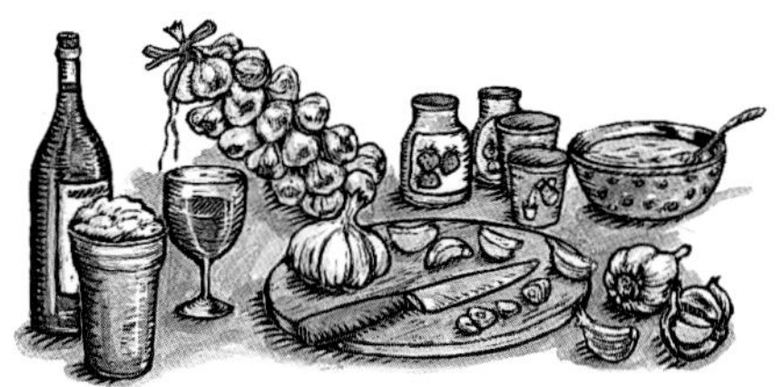

Published in the United States by
TODTRI Book Publishers
254 West 31st Street
New York, NY 10001-2813
Fax: (212) 695-6984
E-mail: info@todtri.com

Visit us on the web!
www.todtri.com

This edition printed 2002

ISBN 1-57717-253-1

QUMNUT

This book is produced by
Quantum Publishing Ltd
6 Blundell Street
London N7 9BH

Printed in China by
Leefung Asco Printers Ltd

CONTENTS

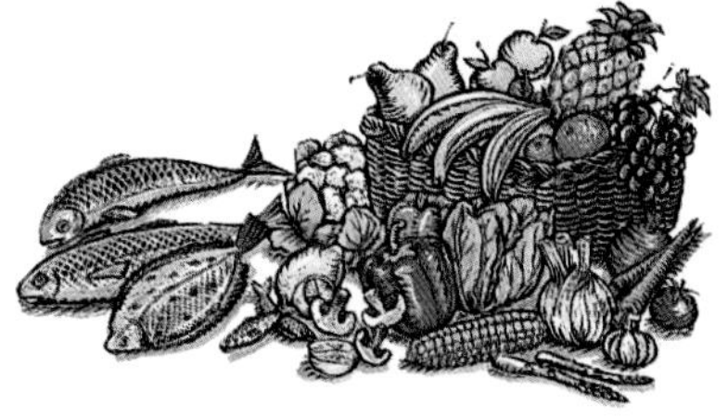

INTRODUCTION
8 – 21

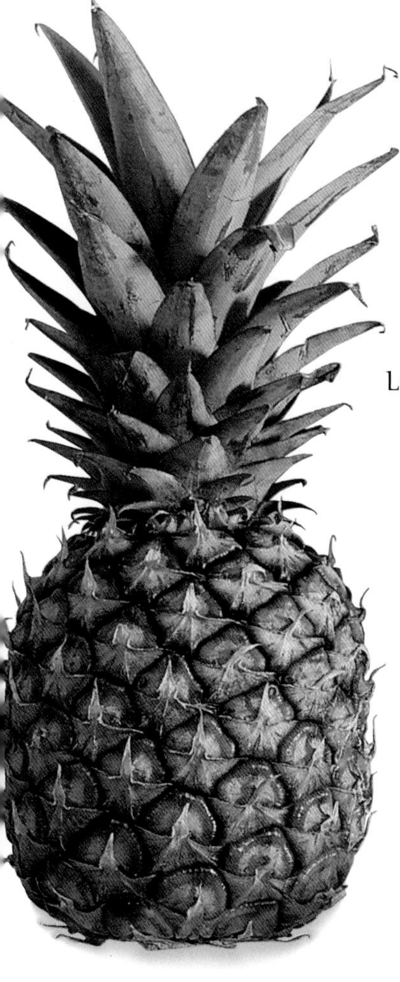

FOODS
22 – 103

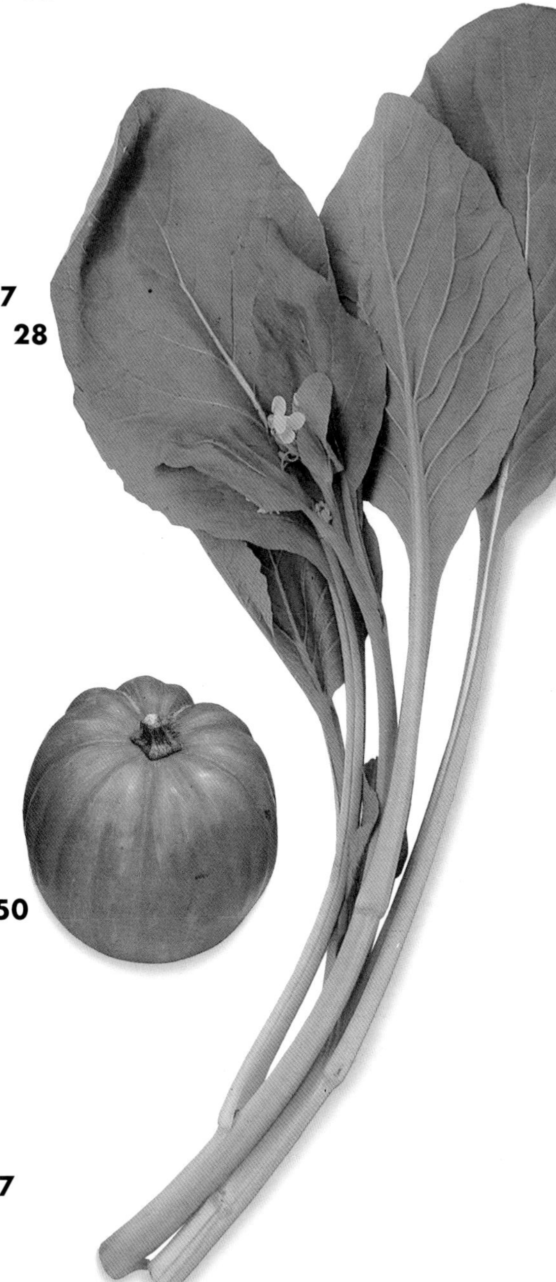

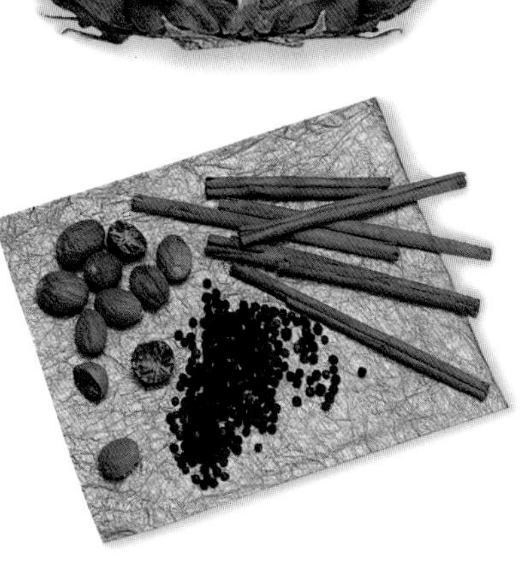

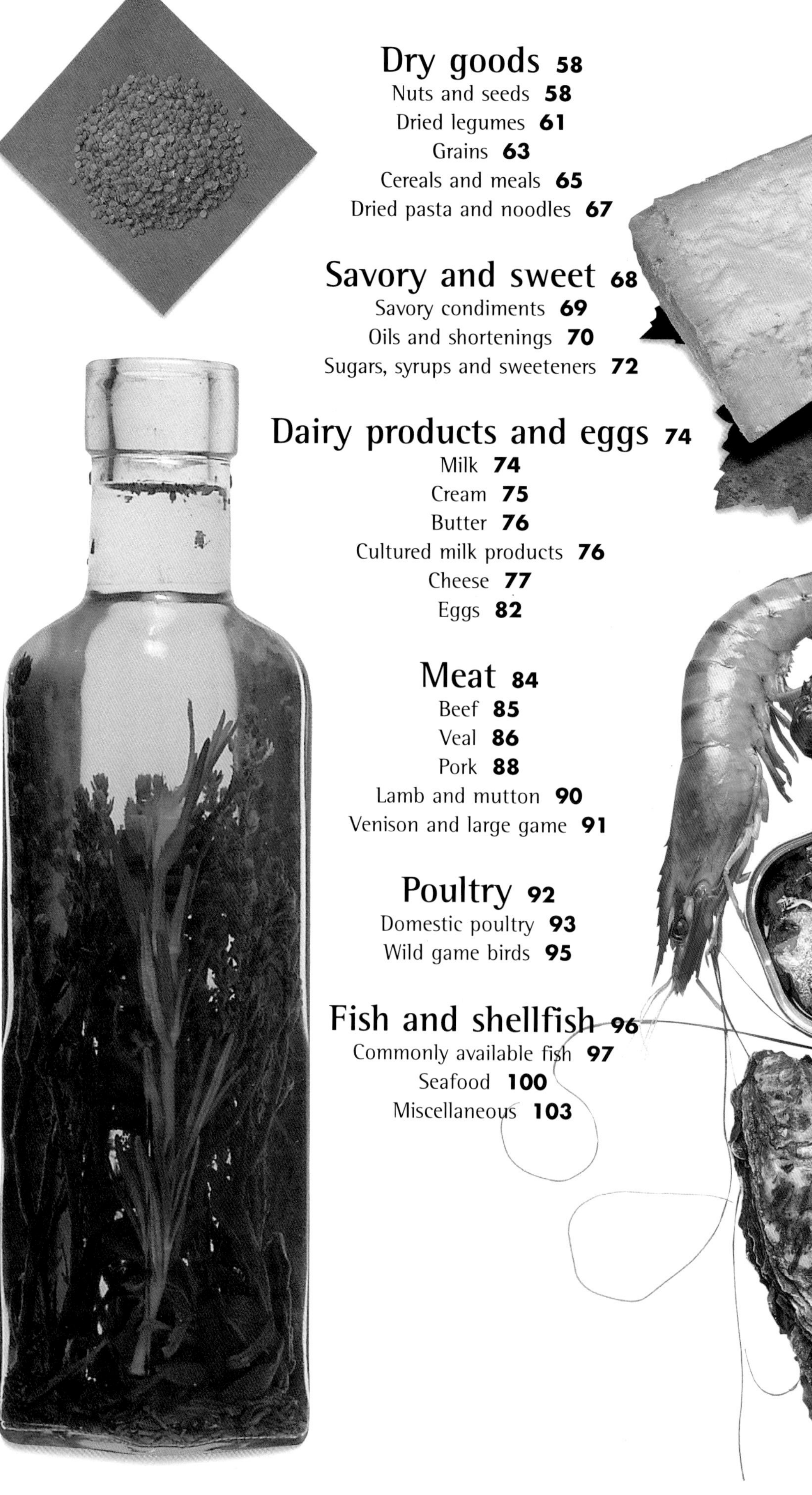

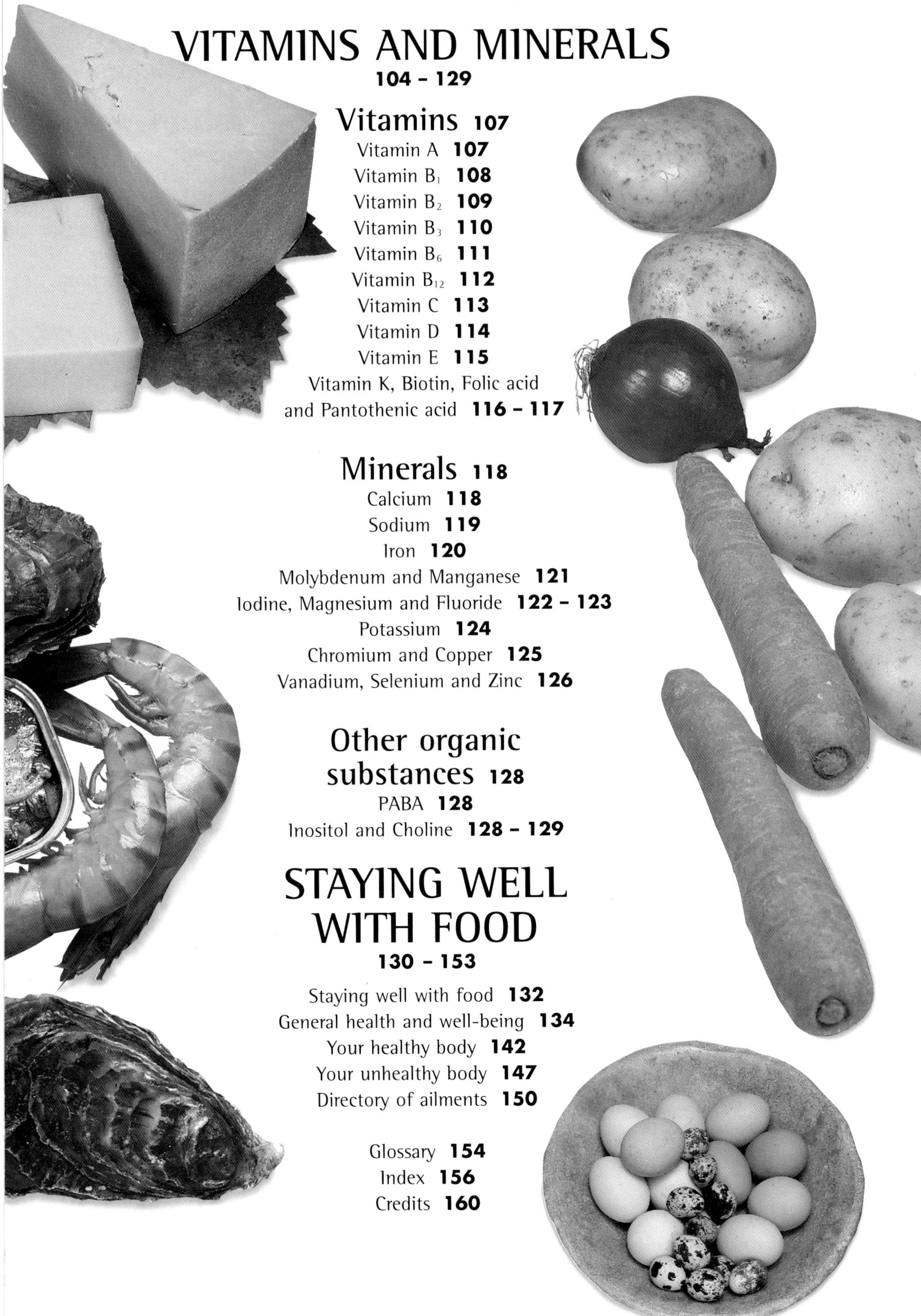

VITAMINS AND MINERALS

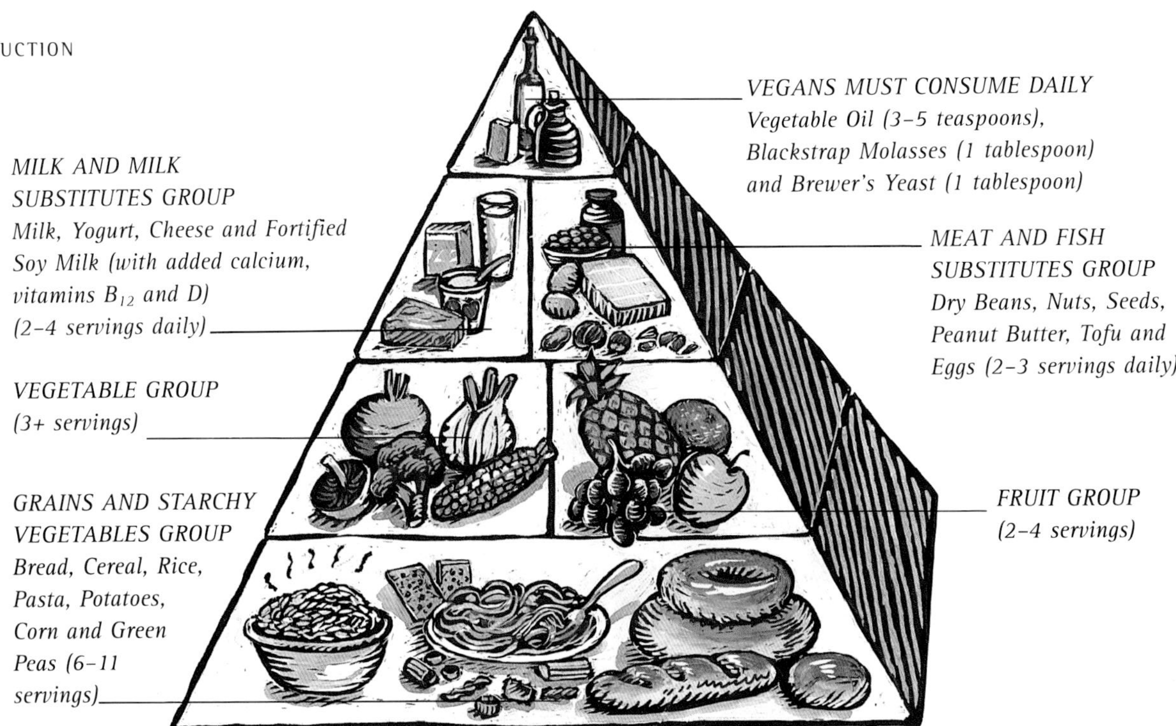

VEGETARIAN FOOD PYRAMID

GRAINS AND STARCHY VEGETABLES GROUP
Bread, Cereal and Potatoes (5–11 servings [e.g., a slice of bread] daily)
FRUIT AND VEGETABLE GROUP
(5 servings daily)
MILK AND DAIRY FOODS
Milk, Cheese and Yogurt (2–3 servings daily)
MEAT, FISH AND ALTERNATIVES
Poultry, Meat, Fish, Eggs, Beans, Legumes and Nuts (2–3 servings per day)
SUGAR, SWEETS AND CAKES
(use sparingly)

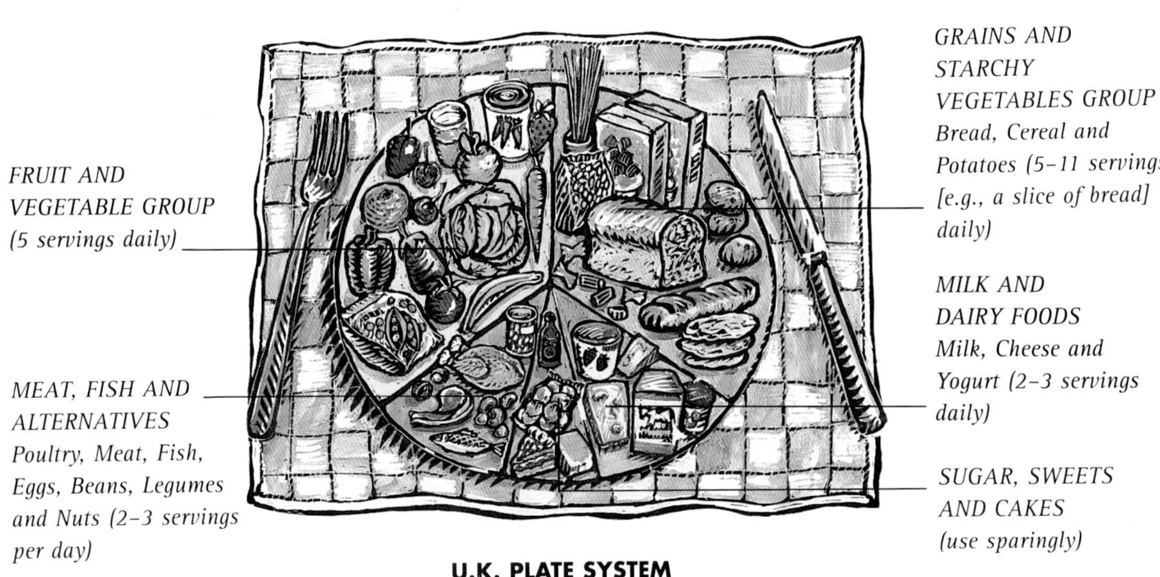

U.K. PLATE SYSTEM

The Vegetarian Food Pyramid gives the vegan option of replacing dairy products with milk substitutes such as soy or nut milks but suggests that they be fortified with calcium and vitamins B_{12} and D. (A vegan is a strict vegetarian who does not consume animal food or dairy products.) For those following a vegetarian diet meats, poultry, and fish can be replaced with dry beans, nuts, seeds, tofu, nut butters and eggs. The apex of this pyramid includes some foods that vegans must consume daily to maintain optimal levels of specific nutrients.

In the United Kingdom (U.K.) the "Balance of Good Health" uses a plate system rather than a pyramid, but the principle is the same. Two-thirds of the diet should be composed of fruit and vegetables (five servings a day), bread, other cereals and potatoes. The remaining third comprises milk and dairy foods, preferably low-fat; meat, fish and alternatives, also preferably low-fat versions; a small amount of foods containing fat, and a small amount of sugar.

WHAT THE FOOD GROUPS HAVE IN COMMON

Each food grouping model supports some basic principles. These are:

- **maintaining a healthy body weight through a combination of a healthy diet and exercise**
- **thinking of a balanced diet as something to be achieved over the course of a day or week, rather than in each dish or meal**
- **keeping total fat intake at or below about 30 to 35 percent of the day's total calories**
- **replacing saturated fats with monounsaturated fats from sources such as olive oil**
- **drinking sufficient water throughout the day**
- **eating more fruits, vegetables and starchy foods, and selecting a good variety to produce energy and assure adequate levels of vitamins, minerals and fiber**
- **reducing the quantity of and frequency with which fatty meats, poultry, fish, eggs and whole milk cheeses are included in the diet**
- **reducing the amount of refined sugars consumed**
- **avoiding highly processed or refined foods**
- **keeping sodium consumption within a range of approximately 1,600 to 3,300 milligrams per day**
- **keeping alcohol consumption at moderate levels. (For women one or two glasses of wine a day, with one to two alcohol free days; for men slightly more.)***
- **reducing the amount of dietary cholesterol in the diet (suggested by some models)**
- **For some people reducing total calorie intake**

***Not all dietary recommendations condone alcohol or suggest that it is important or beneficial. This is an optional part of any diet.**

What We Drink

Like vitamins and minerals, water is a noncalorific essential nutrient. It is needed to keep your body running properly. Our bodies are made primarily of water. Drinking the recommended eight glasses of water (53 fl oz/ 1.5 litres) per day keeps joints properly cushioned, helps to get the necessary nutrients to the spot where you need them and cleans out toxins from your system.

In moderation tea, coffee and other caffeinated beverages (especially colas) may not be harmful to most individuals; except for pregnant and breast- feeding women, three to five cups of coffee per day appear to have no adverse effects. However, those who become nervous or jittery or who have trouble sleeping should cut back or eliminate caffeine. Another option is to have only one caffeinated beverage, early in the day.

Alcoholic beverages are also deemed admissible in most healthy eating plans as long as there are no health indications such as liver conditions, diabetes, alcoholism and pregnancy that would make alcohol a problem. In fact, many studies have pointed to a correlation between moderate consumption of alcohol (and in particular wine) and a decreased incidence of heart disease.

Juices made from whole fruit and vegetables are usually calculated as part of your daily serving of vegetables. Juice drinks, as well as other soft drinks, on the other hand, are generally nothing more than sweetened, flavored water. Beware of any claims on the label maintaining that the beverage has 100 percent of the day's requirement for various vitamins and minerals anyway. If you are eating properly, you should be getting adequate supplies of vitamins and minerals anyway. If you aren't, the quantity of refined sugar you will be ingesting along with those calories makes their nutritional value suspect.

▼ *It's important to drink plenty throughout the day. Around eight glasses of fluid is the ideal to aim for, but avoid too many sugary drinks.*

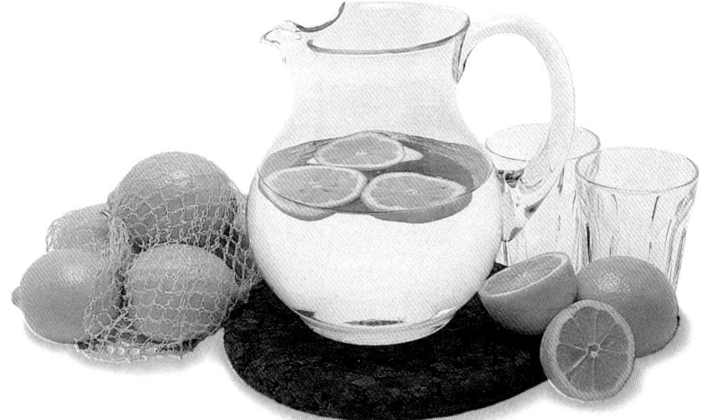

The Role of Exercise

A sedentary lifestyle is in part accountable for the huge increase in the numbers of people who are overweight and obese. It also affects the way many people feel at the end of the day. Instead of being physically tired, ready to enjoy a deep, rejuvenating sleep, we are left anxious, fretful and mentally tired. Our bodies are suffering from lack of aerobic, anaerobic and stretching exercise.

Exercise cannot be ignored as part of a daily routine. The many benefits include:

- weight loss
- improved muscle tone
- increased endurance
- freedom from insomnia
- prevention or delay in onset of osteoporosis
- reduction of severity of PMS and menstrual discomfort
- clearer thinking and better memory
- improved outlook on life in general

▼ *Exercises that work muscles through improving their strength (anaerobic exercise) and improving their flexibility (stretching) are as important as aerobic exercises.*

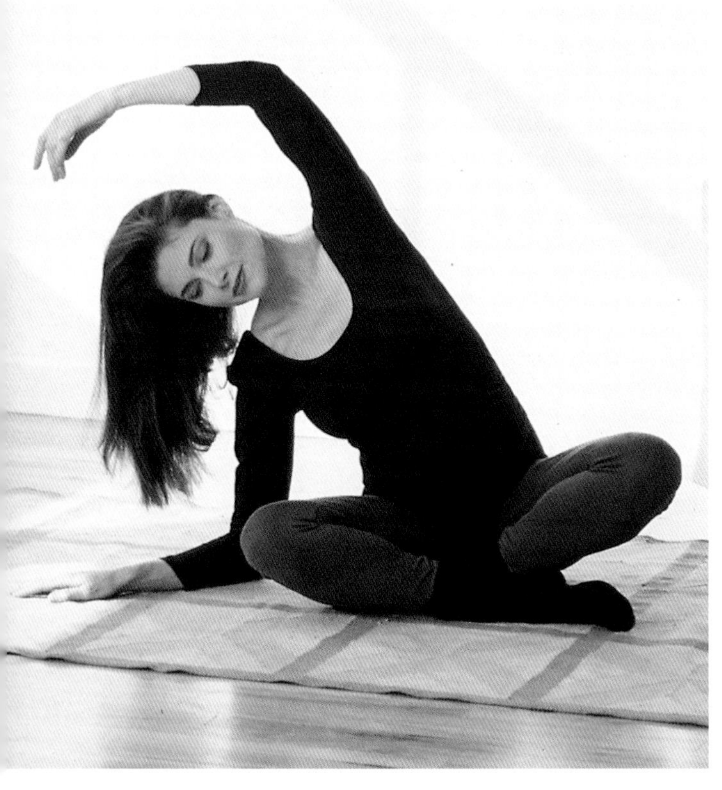

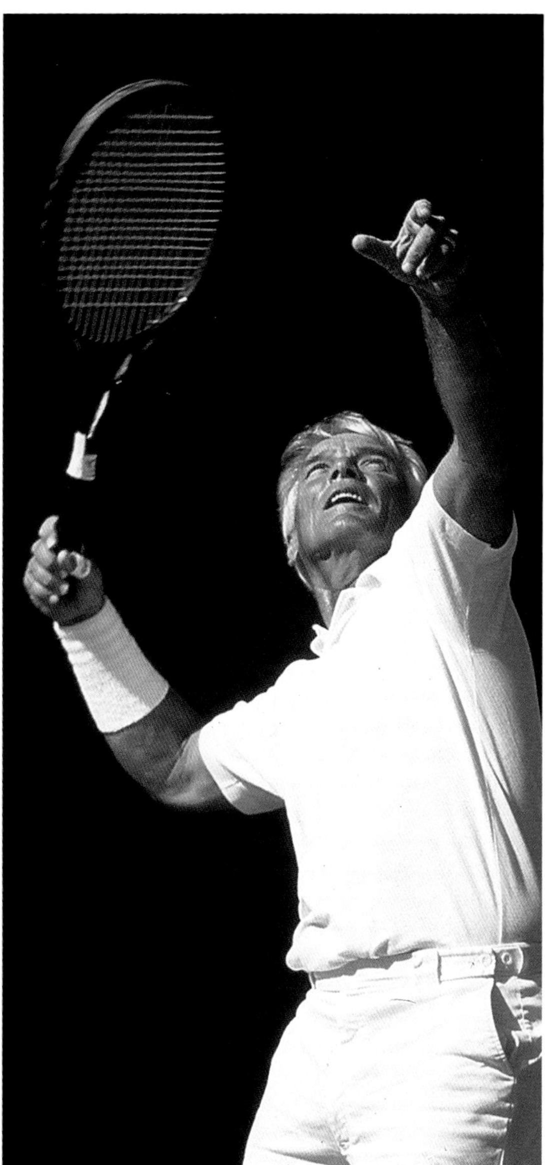

▲ *Including regular aerobic exercise in your weekly schedule is an important way to maintain a healthy heart and lungs. Choose whichever activity you enjoy most.*

Aerobic activities are those that increase oxygen consumption and cause our cardiovascular system to work harder. Jogging, running, walking, tennis, soccer and swimming are all excellent options. Anaerobic activities do not increase oxygen consumption and mainly use large muscles. The types of exercise in this category include calisthenics, strength training, weight-lifting and resistance exercise. Stretching exercises include yoga and t'ai chi. The most effective exercise routines incorporate all three types of exercise over the course of a week.

What's In The Food We Eat?

All food provides us with energy, which is usually measured in calories (cal) or kilojoules (kJ). Energy is provided by carbohydrates and protein (4 cal per gram), fat (9 cal per gram) and alcohol (7 cal per gram). Although carbohydrates and protein both provide the same amount of calories, the body tends to use carbohydrates and fat for its main supply of energy. Because fat also makes food very palatable, it is easy to eat too much fat. Starchy foods such as bread, potatoes, rice and pasta contain little fat but lots of carbohydrates, so this is why we are encouraged to fill up on these sorts of foods.

Without energy we could not maintain life, but we need to balance the amount of energy we need against the amount we consume. If we eat a lot but don't exercise enough to use up the excess calories, then energy will be stored in the body as fat. Conversely, fat stores are used up when the amount of energy supplied in the diet doesn't match the amount required to maintain all the body processes and activity.

Some people count calories in order to help them maintain their weight, but it can be unhelpful to become too obsessive about counting every calorie.

With increasing numbers of people becoming overweight and obese, it is important to recognize the dual role of diet and exercise. Obesity leads to many chronic disease states including hypertension, heart disease, some cancers, diabetes and arthritis. Some emotional and psychological disorders are also linked to being overweight.

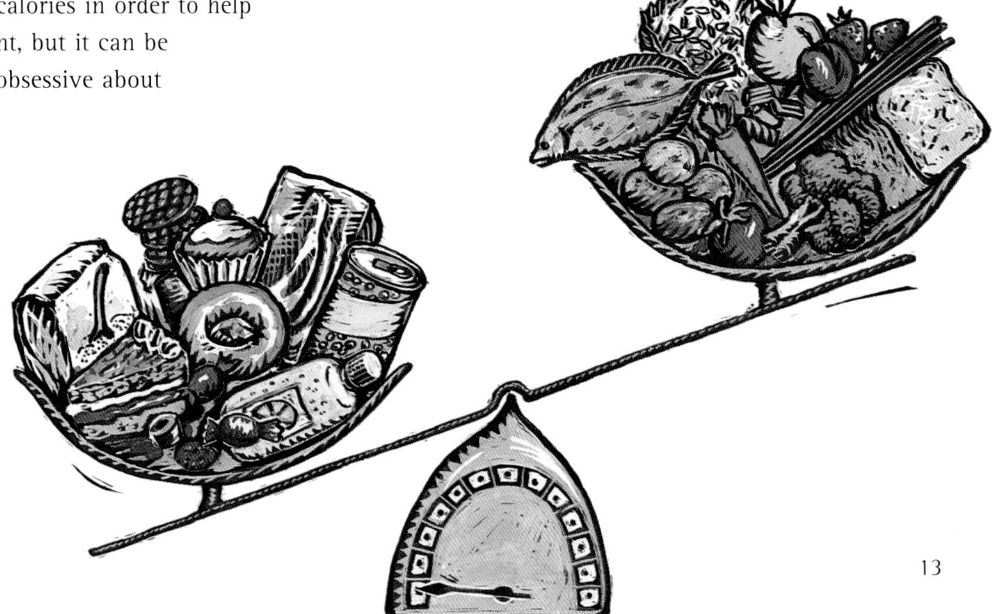

▶ *The key to a healthy diet is achieving balance. Cereals, fruit and vegetables should be eaten often, while high fat, high-sugar foods should only be eaten occasionally.*

MACRO NUTRIENTS

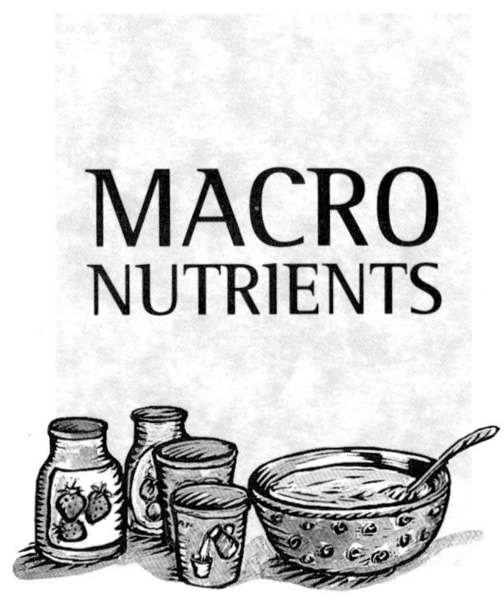

Proteins, carbohydrates and fats are the major, or macro, nutrients in food.

Proteins

Few people ever suffer from protein deficiencies. Instead, our diets tend to include too much protein, especially meats. This has the effect of increasing the quantity of saturated fats in our diets, leading to high blood cholesterol levels.

Shifting toward leaner cuts of meat, and using more skinless poultry, fish and foods such as dried beans and tofu, will provide protein without too much fat.

Proteins are composed of smaller groups known as amino acids. Some can be made in the body while others must be provided in the diet. These are essential (or indispensable) amino acids (EAAs or IAAs).

Foods such as meat, milk, cheese and eggs are "complete" proteins. This means that these foods supply the essential amino acids in the correct amounts. In general, a single 6-ounce (175-gram) portion of meat, poultry or fish coupled with one to three servings of a low-fat dairy food throughout the day will meet an individual's requirements. For a vegetarian, about 10 ounces (250 grams) of beans or legumes are needed daily. Plant-based foods contain protein but may lack one or more EAAs (IAAs). This deficiency is usually overcome by eating different plant foods together; for example, legumes and grains, nuts and grains.

Most classic vegetarian meals rely on balanced food combinations such as rice and beans that provide all of the essential amino acids (EAAs or IAAs) in good balance.

For a vegan more care is required, and nuts, and legumes should be eaten regularly.

▼ "Simple" sugars found in foods such as honey, jams, table sugar and fruit juice can cause tooth decay if eaten to excess.

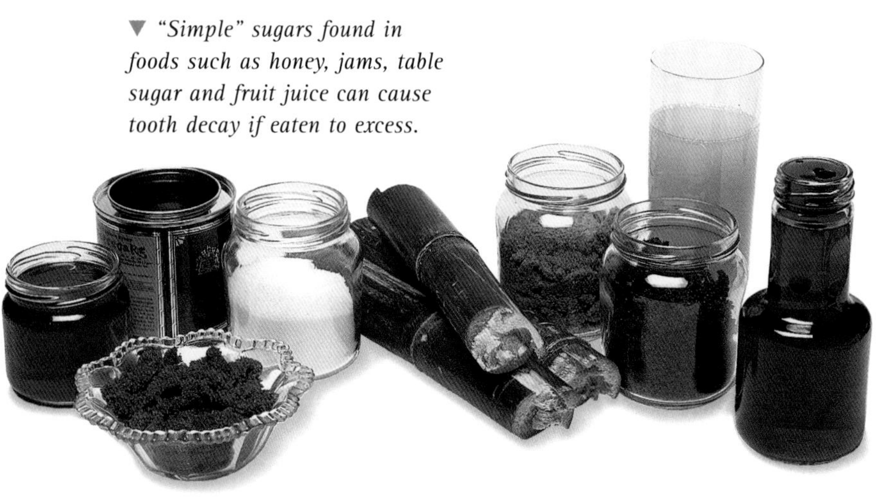

Carbohydrates

There are two types of carbohydrates: starches and sugars. Complex carbohydrates contribute to a healthy diet by providing an energy source that is released in an even, gradual manner. Your body can use fats and protein to provide energy, but these nutrients must first be altered into a form that your body can use. Complex carbohydrates are the body's preferred energy source.

Starchy foods such as potatoes, bread, rice, pasta, noodles, corn and dried legumes provide not only carbohydrates but also fiber, protein, vitamins and minerals.

Sugars are found in milk as lactose and in fruits, vegetables and honey as fructose. Sucrose is usually obtained by extraction from sugar cane or beet and is the table sugar we know.

Sugars vary in their ability to cause dental decay, but all except lactose can be fermented by bacteria in the mouth, yielding acid that attacks the tooth enamel.

REFINED SUGARS

Food manufacturers sometimes use alternative names for sugars. These can include invert sugar or syrup, honey, raw sugar, brown sugar, cane sugar, muscavado sugar, molasses, concentrated fruit juice and maple syrup.

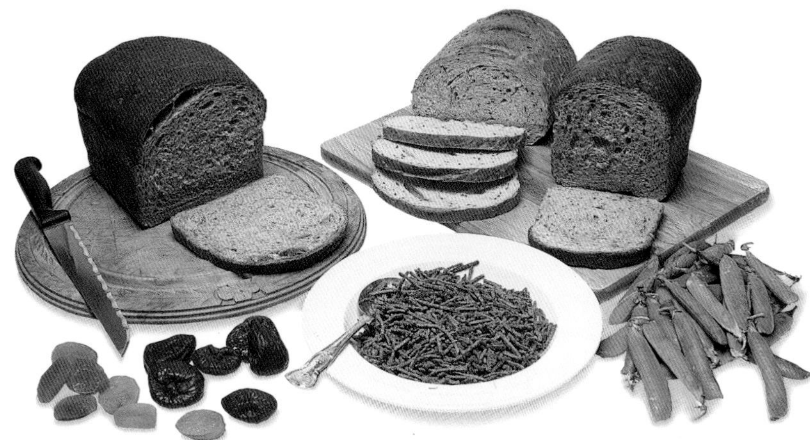

▲ *Carbohydrates are vital energy foods in our diets. Good sources include bread, cereals, legumes, fruits and vegetables.*

Glucose, dextrose, maltose and fructose are commonly used and are no different to sucrose sugar in their effect on the teeth.

Sugar can boost the caloric level of foods without offering any other nutritional benefit.

FIBER

Dietary fiber or nonstarch polysaccharides are only found in plant foods. Some are soluble and some insoluble but both play an important role in regulating the functioning of the intestines.

Fiber can hinder the absorption of some minerals from foods, but this may only be a significant problem to vegans who eat large quantities of beans and whole-grain cereals.

Some fiber is fermented in the large intestine and this provides a small amount of energy. There is evidence that diets rich in fiber help with diabetic control, and soluble fiber from oats, legumes and guar gum has also been shown to help lower blood cholesterol levels. High-fiber diets are bulky, and this can aid calorie-controlled weight loss, constipation and some forms of irritable bowel syndrome.

Some sources of fiber include:

- **Good sources:** peas; beans; dried apricots and figs; whole wheat, grain, and rye breads; bran-based breakfast cereals
- **Fair sources:** fruits, vegetables and nuts; pasta

Meeting Carbohydrate and Fiber Requirements

Most dietary guidelines recommend that at least 50 percent of your day's total calories should come from carbohydrates, with as few of those calories as possible derived from refined sugars found in sweeteners, candies, pastries and carbonated beverages.

Fiber is another important part of a healthy diet. Most people don't include the correct level of fiber-rich foods in their diets. Four portions of fruits and vegetables and two cereal-based dishes will meet most people's requirements.

Fats and Oils

Fat is needed by the body to build cells, provide energy and to protect organs from damage. Vitamins A, D, E and K are dissolved in fat, and fat is needed for their absorption.

Fat is made up of two compounds, fatty acids and glycerol. The fatty acids may be saturated, monounsaturated or polyunsaturated, and different foods contain a mixture of each. Foods that contain a lot of saturated fatty acids include butter, cream, fatty meats, bacon fat, poultry skin and lard.

Saturated fatty acids raise the levels of undesirable low-density lipoprotein (LDL) cholesterol in the blood, and dietary recommendations are that no more than 10 percent of total calories should be provided by saturated fatty acids.

Conversely, monounsaturated fatty acids have a tendency to lower the levels of undesirable cholesterol in the blood and raise the level of more beneficial forms. The net result is that individuals whose diets rely upon monounsaturated fatty acids, rather than saturated fats, are less likely to develop hardening of the arteries (atherosclerosis). Olive and canola (rapeseed) oil contain mostly monounsaturated fatty acids, although nuts, avocado, meat and dairy products contain some too.

Polyunsaturated fats and oils are still preferred to saturated fats but do not have the same benefits as monounsaturated fats. Polyunsaturated fats are found mainly in sunflower and corn oils and in some vegetables.

Vegetable oils are often used in the preparation of shortening and margarine. Part of the process is known as hydrogenation, which changes the overall structure of the fat. Substances called trans fatty acids are produced, and they are believed to behave in a similar way to saturated fatty acids.

Oily fish contain fatty acids called long chain polyunsaturates. People such as Inuits who eat a lot of oily fish are far less prone to heart disease and strokes. This is because the fatty acids make the blood "thinner" and less likely to clot.

Some people use supplements of these beneficial fatty acids. EPA (ecosapentaenoic acid) and DHA (docasahexaenoic acid) are the chief constituents.

CHOLESTEROL

Cholesterol is another type of fat. Dietary cholesterol is found in foods, particularly animal products. Blood or serum cholesterol is that which is found in your bloodstream and made in the liver.

Dietary cholesterol has a smaller effect on blood cholesterol than saturated fat. In most people the liver can alter the amount of blood cholesterol it makes according to how much dietary cholesterol is eaten.

Plant-based foods, even those high in saturated fats, do not contain cholesterol. This means that peanut butter, almonds, olives, beans and sesame seeds are all cholesterol-free.

Keeping Dietary Fat at a Healthy Level

The problem facing most people is that they consume too much fat; often 40 percent and more of the calories they eat comes from fat. It appears that as an individual's fat intake goes up, so does the risk of developing heart disease, stroke and hardening of the arteries.

Most nutritionists suggest that fat calories should be kept between 30 and 35 percent of the day's total calories.

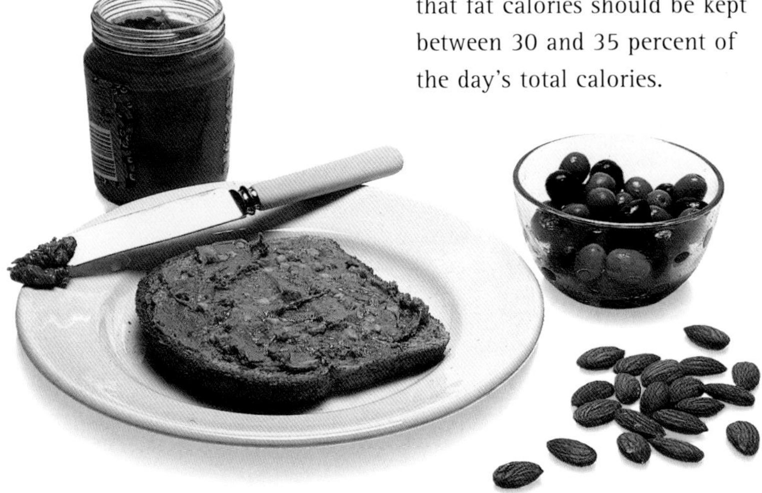

▲ *Some fat (for example, from vegetable oil and nuts) is essential in the diet, but too much—especially saturated fat—is undesirable.*

MICRO NUTRIENTS

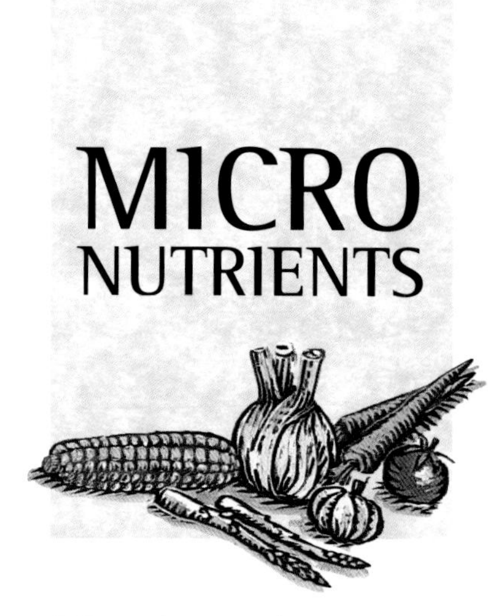

Vitamins and Minerals

These micronutrients are vital for various functions in the human body.

Many folk cures were based on the fact that a specific food could replenish the missing nutrient. Around the turn of the twentieth century, chemists were able to isolate these compounds. They were initially identified by letters and later given more specific names. Deficiency diseases were also identified. National dietary recommendations for vitamins and minerals have been based on the levels required to prevent those diseases. (See pages 106–129 for more information about specific vitamins and minerals and their relationship to health and well-being.)

WATER-SOLUBLE VITAMINS

Vitamin C (ascorbic acid) and the B vitamins can be dissolved in water. This means that you need to replenish these vitamins daily, since they are readily lost from the body in waste fluids. They are also sensitive to prolonged exposure to heat, air and light. Cooking foods to retain maximum levels of the water-soluble vitamins is a challenge, but one that can be accomplished as long as you are careful not to overcook foods, prepare or cook them too far in advance or leave them in water.

FAT-SOLUBLE VITAMINS

Vitamins A, D, E and K are fat-soluble. This means that they are stored in fat, which is far less simple to remove from the body than water. *Megadoses* of vitamin supplements can easily cause toxic levels to build up, leading to serious disease, even death. Unlike water-soluble vitamins, these vitamins are usually stable during cooking.

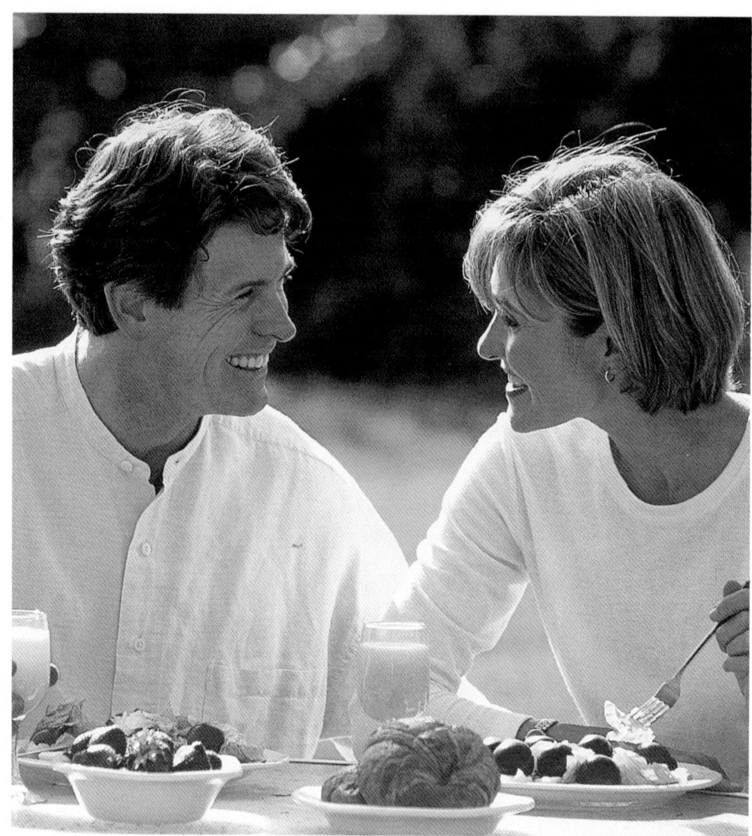

▲ *Micronutrients (vitamins and minerals needed only in small amounts by the body) are essential for good health and can be obtained by eating a diet rich in fresh foods.*

ANTIOXIDANTS

Carotenes, including beta-carotene, as well as vitamin C and vitamin E and selenium, have antioxidant properties. This means they mop up free radicals that are produced by the body and that can attack important molecules such as DNA and proteins. If the DNA in a cell is damaged, the cell is more likely to become cancerous. Free radicals can also oxidize polyunsaturates in foods and cells and may alter the undesirable LDL blood cholesterol, leading to atherosclerosis, or hardening of the arteries.

Foods rich in carotenes, vitamin C and vitamin E appear to protect against this damage and include yellow and orange fruits and orange and dark-green vegetables.

MAJOR MINERALS

Calcium, potassium, phosphorus, chloride, magnesium, zinc, iron and sodium are required by your body in significant quantities and need to be part of your daily diet.

TRACE MINERALS

Fluoride, copper, selenium, iodine, manganese, chromium and cobalt are also required but in tiny quantities.

Meeting Dietary Requirements for Vitamins and Minerals

Today, as we continue to learn more about the role of vitamins and minerals in maintaining health, questions about the value of supplementation are cropping up. Many people use vitamin and mineral supplements to bolster their immune systems and help prevent micronutrient deficiencies. Modest supplementation is perfectly safe, but self-medication can have serious consequences if an individual takes megadoses, especially of the fat-soluble vitamins and some minerals. (See also *Vitamins and Minerals* on pages 106–129.)

Vitamin and mineral supplementation should not be necessary if you don't have any special needs and follow a varied daily diet rich in whole grains, fruits, vegetables and low-fat dairy foods.

Creating a "Healthy" Diet Plan

Choosing foods from the various tiers of the relevant pyramid to make up our daily diet is a good way to be sure that we are getting a balanced assortment of all the nutrients we need. Relearning about food and adjusting our expectations and attitudes may take a while but are important in developing a successful "healthy" diet plan.

A variety of foods is one way to ensure that your meals are appealing, both in their appearance and their overall flavor. After all, if food does not look good and taste good, you are not going to want to eat it day in and day out. The goal of overhauling your personal eating patterns should not be simply to lose a few pounds. It will be far easier to maintain your improved, healthier lifestyle if you view it as a whole new way of eating that you can and want to maintain without feeling deprived or cheated.

Modifying Recipes

Recipe modification is one of the simplest ways to introduce good nutritional cooking practices into your repertoire of dishes. You will soon find

COOK BETTER, FEEL BETTER

The following suggestions can help introduce healthy cooking practices into any cooking style, whether you are preparing meals for a young family or for just yourself, whether you are a strict vegetarian or are a confirmed "meat-and-potato" person. You will undoubtedly begin to see a change for the better on your plate and in your overall well-being as healthy practices start to become the rule.

- **First look at what you are currently eating and write down all the foods and drinks you eat over three days.** Then look at one of the food models and compare your diet with it. Which groups do you eat too much of, and which too little?

  Decide on the changes needed and introduce them gradually. You don't need to do it all at once, but set realistic goals and try to achieve them. You are more likely to succeed by making adjustments fairly gradually.
- **Place a greater emphasis on grains, legumes, vegetables and fruits, rather than relying on meats, fish or poultry as the "center of the plate".** Many ethnic cuisines popular today have traditionally relied on this practice, and it ensures the inclusion of plenty of complex carbohydrates including fiber, vitamins and minerals. Top a steaming mound of couscous with a savory vegetable stew, for example, or serve curries over a steaming rice pilaf. Polenta or grits can be broiled (grilled) and topped with ragouts of mushrooms or eggplant (aubergine). If you are serving animal-based

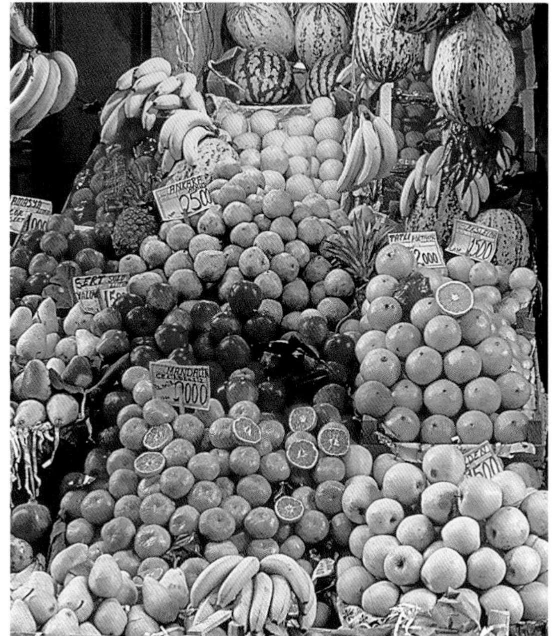

▲ *Fresh produce provides a wide selection of nutrients essential for good health.*

many ways to modify and adapt your current, comfortable cooking style to meet your new expectations for overall health and well-being through better eating. You can make some simple adaptations by broiling (grilling) a piece of chicken instead of sautéing it or replacing a fatty cut of meat with a leaner one.

Stuff vegetables with mixtures of rice and vegetables rather than meats. Replace the ricotta and eggs in your lasagne filling with steamed spinach and mushrooms seasoned with plenty of herbs and garlic.

Purchasing for Nutrition

Making the right choices at the market can make a great difference to your diet. It is also the best means of assuring yourself all the richest sources of the nutrients. The following suggestions are a good way to begin.

PRODUCE

If you have the time, space and inclination, there is no better way to assure yourself of fresh vegetables, fruits and herbs than to grow them yourself. Even if you live in an apartment, you can grow some varieties in window boxes or as potted plants. Failing that, search out greengrocers, farmer's markets, orchards and farms that offer cooperative growing programs or

---

foods (which are excellent sources of iron and zinc), use smaller portions.

- **Use monounsaturated or polyunsaturated fats and oils whenever possible and reduce the use of saturated fats.** Not only does the total amount of fat in your diet have an effect on your overall health, but the kind of fats and oils you use also play a role. If a recipe calls for butter, lard or shortening (margarine), which are all saturated fats, you may be able to replace those ingredients with an oil such as olive, canola (rapeseed), corn, safflower or peanut. Use the smallest possible amount of these oils when you sauté or pan-fry because even though they are less saturated than butter or shortening, they are still high in calories.
- **Use high-calorie and high-fat foods (eggs, cream, butter, cheeses and refined sugars) sparingly.** This step often presents the greatest challenge to anyone who has grown accustomed to relying on rich foods to act as the major carriers of flavor on a plate.

  Cutting calories should always include cutting fats. Cream, cheese, butter and oils add more calories, weight for weight, than other foods. When you do add them to a dish, use them sparingly. Use smaller quantities of strongly flavored cheese or grate a little cheese over your pasta, in place of a cheese sauce. Use low-fat versions of dairy products when you can and substitute low-fat yogurt or fromage frais for cream in soups and flans.
- **Learn a variety of seasoning and flavoring techniques to help reduce a reliance on salt.** Salt is relied upon as a seasoning and flavor enhancer in many dishes. If you are used to seasoning foods generously with salt, you may need to take the time to measure salt, instead of adding it "to taste". Gradually, you will lose your tolerance for lots of salt.

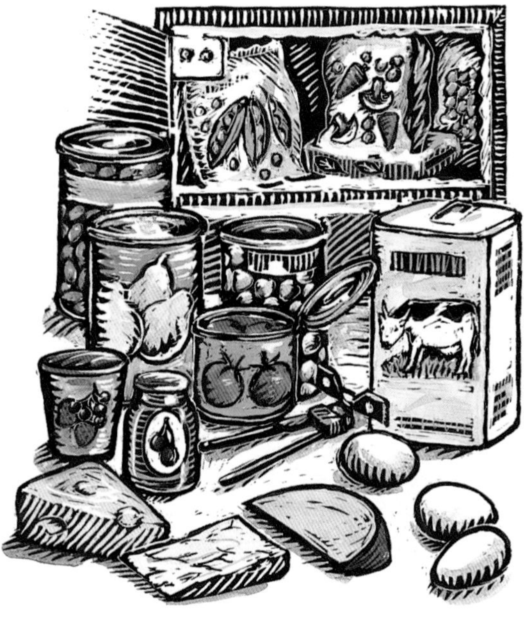

"pick-your-own" operations. Stores that feature natural or organic foods are also a good source of high-quality produce.

The fresher the produce is, the better choice it is. When fresh fruits and vegetables are difficult to find or are too expensive, frozen or even canned versions are frequently good substitutes. Canned tomatoes, beans and other fruits and vegetables are also good choices. Be sure to read the labels and opt for reduced-sodium, reduced-sugar or lower-calorie versions whenever you can.

DAIRY PRODUCTS

Instead of whole milk products, look for products prepared with skim milk or part-skim milk. Reduced-fat types of yogurt, cheeses and sour cream are widely available.

MEATS, POULTRY AND FISH

Concerns about the quality and wholesomeness of meats, fish and poultry seem to grow each day. Many people have grown increasingly wary about where they purchase these items, as well as how often they eat them, if they still include them in their diets. If you follow the suggestions of eating pyramids, your overall consumption of animal foods will drop and be in smaller quantities. In that case, it might make sense to invest a little extra time and effort in finding the best possible purveyor and looking for organically raised meats.

There are many other ways to add flavor to foods. Wines, vinegars, citrus juices, spices, fresh herbs and low-sodium soy sauces can all be used.

Some ingredients, such as capers, bacon, olives, hard grating cheeses, processed and canned or frozen foods, may already be high in salt or sodium. Choose low-sodium options when you can and/or cut back on the added salt if you are including these types of ingredients.

- **Know what a "healthy" standard serving of the foods you eat looks like.** Portion control is one of the most effective ways to help improve the nutritional profile of a meal. By removing the skin from chicken, trimming visible meat fat and omitting the cream, you will considerably reduce the amount of fat, cholesterol and calories. Reduce portion sizes of meat, fish, poultry, dairy foods and fatty foods.

Increase portions of fruits and vegetables and make starchy foods—whether bread, potatoes, grains or pasta—the bulk of the meal. This will increase antioxidant vitamins, minerals and fiber levels.

- **Prepare and cook all foods carefully to preserve their nutritional value, flavor, texture and appeal.** Chopping foods early, overcooking them, keeping them warm for too long or stewing them in water can destroy or cause essential nutrients to leach out. It will also affect the taste. Match the cooking method you select to the food you are preparing. Use methods that do not introduce additional fats and oils whenever possible. Broiling (grilling), dry roasting, boiling, microwave cooking and steaming are good examples.

Cook foods as close as possible to the time you plan to serve them. This will minimize nutrient loss, as well as ensure that the food is at its best when you put it on the table.

Some cuts of meats and poultry are naturally leaner than others. Skinless chicken breast, for instance, is a leaner option than chicken thighs with the skin on. Beef that has relatively little marbling or that has been trimmed to remove all visible fat is also a good choice.

White fish such as sole or flounder are typically lower in calories and fat than oily fish such as salmon, trout or mackerel. However, experts feel that oily fish are beneficial to one's health and should be included in the diet once or twice a week.

Smoked, cured or processed meats such as bacon or sausage can still be used, as long as you exercise care and moderation. Look for reduced-sodium-and-fat versions. Serve them once or twice a month or in very small amounts a few times a week, if you like.

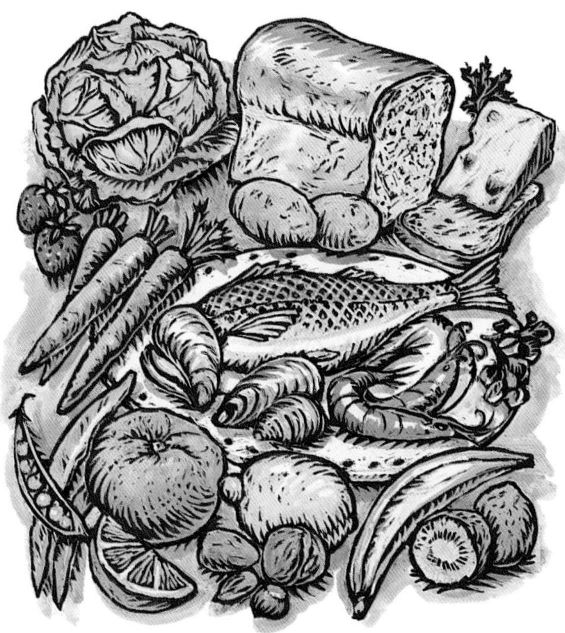

GRAINS AND CEREALS

Rice, millet, corn and other grains are widely available. Try other grains, too, and do not forget that pasta, potatoes, bread and noodles are all starchy nutritious foods—just remember not to add too much high-fat sauces and spreads.

Look for whole-grain or minimally processed versions of these items for the best nutritional value. They often contain a greater quantity of vitamins, minerals and fiber than refined versions.

- **Select foods that can do the most to help you meet your personal goals.** The foods you eat affect your sense of well-being in many ways. Pay attention to which foods make you feel vibrant and alive and which ones make you feel de-energized. Use the various charts and tables in this and other books to find the specific foods that offer the greatest nutritional benefit. If weight loss is part of your overall plan to feel better, choose foods with a high vitamin and mineral content but with few calories provided by fat.

  In general, the closer a food is to its natural state, the higher its nutritional value. Locally picked fruits and vegetables, for example, do not travel as far or as long to get to the market, which means that they will retain more of their nutrients than those that have been picked for a few days. Whole grains are a better source of a wider variety of nutrients than polished, refined or quick-cooking varieties.
- **Make your diet fit in with your lifestyle.** If you need to use a few processed foods, select low-fat versions or limit the number of times a week you consume them. Processed foods can be useful and the fact that they are processed doesn't necessarily mean they are not nutritious. Frozen vegetables often contain more vitamins than so-called "fresh" ones, but if salt, sugar and fat have been added, the food may not fit in with your nutritional goals. Be sure to read any nutritional information on the label. Make comparisons to be sure that you are getting the most flavor, the best quality and the least unwanted additives possible.

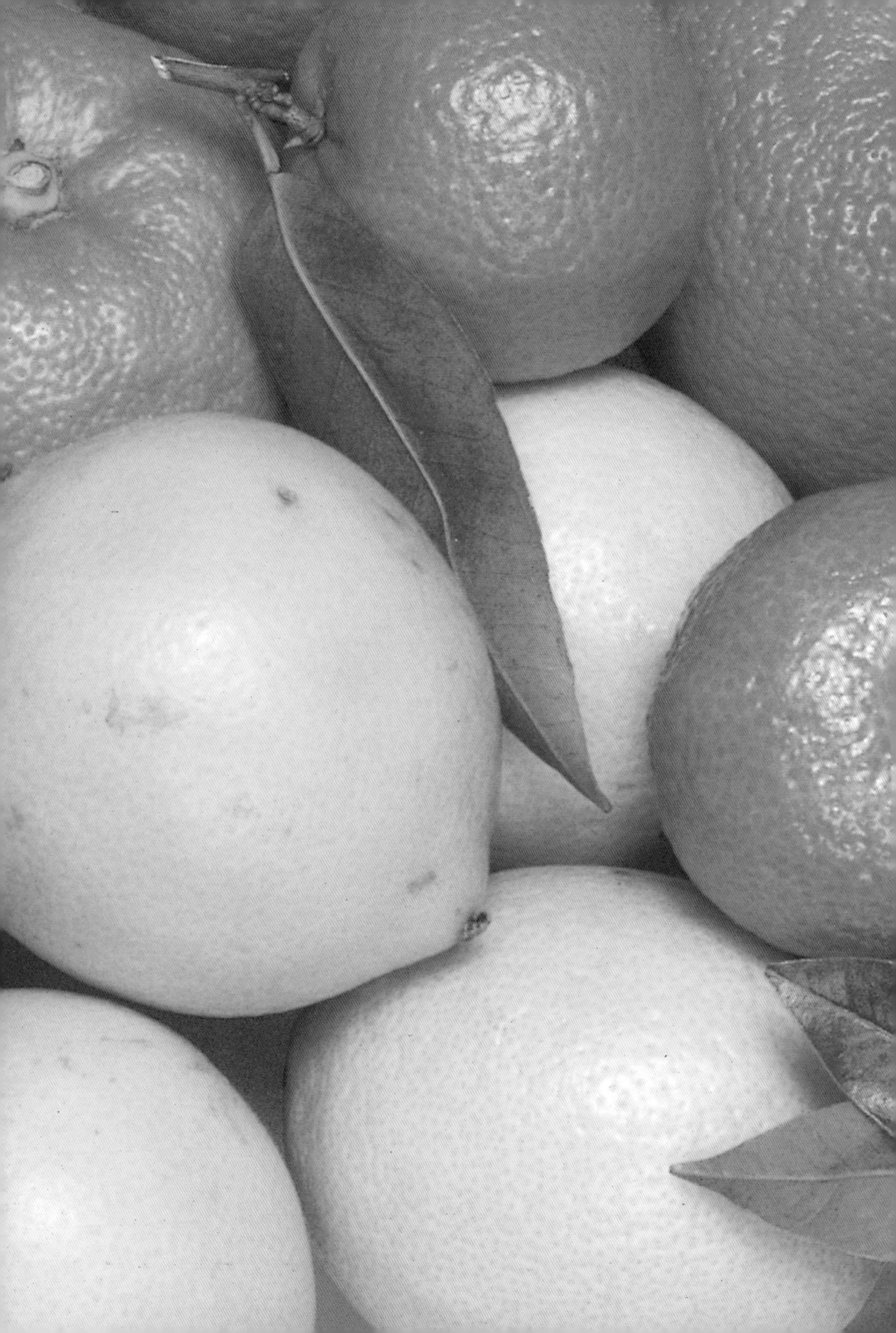

FOODS

Food is the currency of life. None of us can live very long without food to nourish us, and even a day or two without it makes us feel weak and unwell. But food is more than just a passport to life; it is our key to well-being, and a tremendous source of enjoyment.

This section includes analysis charts to help you compare relevant nutrient content for selected items from each group of foods.

For details of the source for this information please see page 107.

Cooking Greens

Cooks are beginning to make use of the wide variety of cooking greens such as spinach, Swiss chard, kale, escarole and dandelion greens. Also popular are collards and mustard greens. This is partly due to the potent vitamin and mineral "cocktails" they deliver.

Cooking greens have rather limited shelf lives and should be used as soon after they are purchased as possible. Tender young greens can be eaten raw and are perfect for stir-frying, which retains the nutrients well.

Kale, collards and other leafy green vegetables are an excellent source of particular carotenoids which help prevent against age-related eye disease.

COLLARDS

Popular in the U.S., collards have large, flat, rounded leaves. They are available year-round, especially from summer into fall.

SPINACH

Spinach leaves may be thickly veined or flat, depending upon the variety. Deep green in color, this vegetable is available year-round. It is traditionally thought of as a rich source of iron, but binding agents called oxulates inhibit absorption of the mineral. Spinach may be steamed, sautéd, braised or served raw in salads. Adding a little butter or oil helps improve absorption of the rich supply of carotenoids in spinach.

SWISS CHARD

Swiss chard has deeply lobed, dark green, glossy leaves; stems and ribs may be white or deep ruby. Available in fall, it may be steamed, sautéd or braised.

KALE

Kale has ruffled leaves and is available in late fall. It may be steamed, sautéd (especially with garlic), braised, or used in soups.

ESCAROLE

Escarole is a heading green with scalloped edges on its leaves. The flavor varies from slightly bitter to very bitter; it is often served in soups and casseroles.

DANDELION AND MUSTARD GREENS

Dandelion greens have narrow leaves with deep teeth along the edges, and are available in spring. They have cleansing and diuretic properties (helping to flush out toxins). Mustard greens have deeply scalloped, narrow leaves and are available in summer.

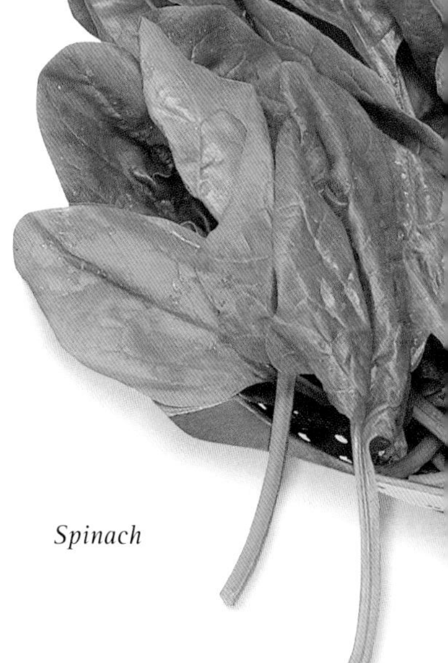

Spinach

Asparagus

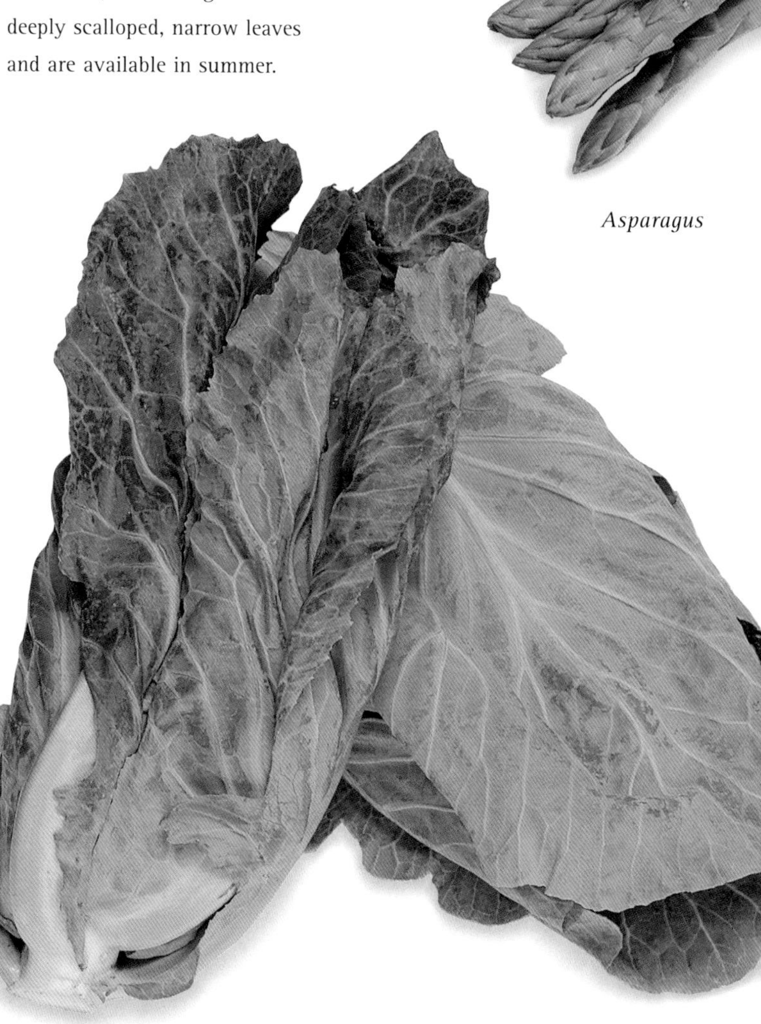

Collards

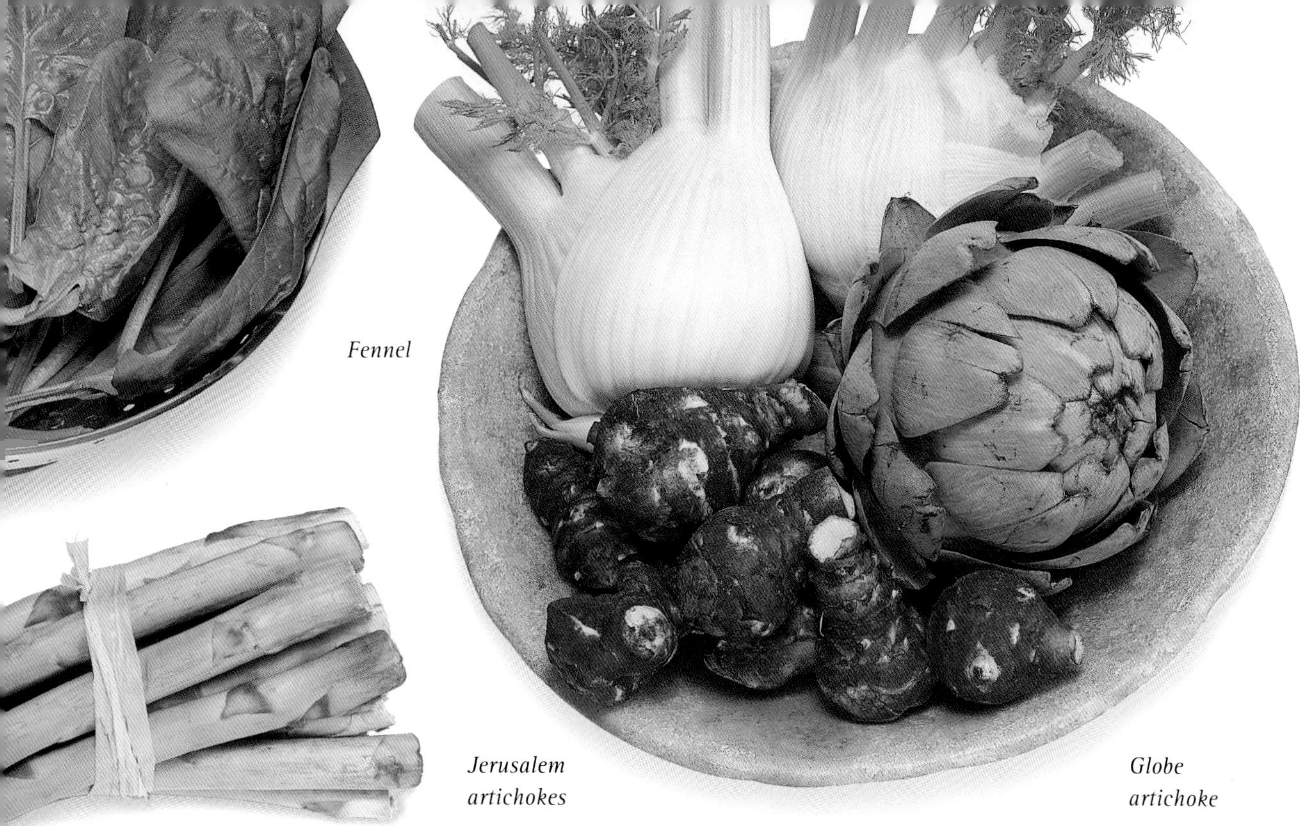

Fennel

Jerusalem artichokes

Globe artichoke

Buds, Shoots and Stems

This family consists of plants that produce shoots and stalks used as vegetables. Globe artichokes, asparagus, bamboo shoots, celery and fennel are examples.

ASPARAGUS

Asparagus is part of the growth cycle of a fern. Green asparagus is harvested as the stalks shoot up above the ground. White asparagus is grown by mounding soil over the vegetable as it emerges from the ground in order to keep it away from sunlight. The stalks should be firm, fleshy and full and should have no evidence of browning or wilting. Asparagus is an excellent source of folic acid, which is required for proper fetal development and healthy red blood cells.

FENNEL

Fennel is a bulb with long stalks and feathery tops. It has a light anise or licorice flavor.

COOKING GREENS, BUDS, SHOOTS AND STEMS

	NSP(g)	*Vit C(mg)*	*NAeq(mg)*	*B_1(mg)*
Artichoke, globe, boiled in unsalted water *9 calories (portion 50g)*	–	0.50	0.75	–
Asparagus, boiled in salted water *33 calories (portion 125g)*	1.75	12.50	1.75	0.15
Fennel, Florence, boiled in salted water *6 calories (portion 50g)*	1.20	2.50	–	0.03
Celery, raw *2 calories (portion 30g)*	0.33	2.40	0.12	0.02
Spinach, boiled in unsalted water *17 calories (portion 90g)*	1.89	7.20	–	–

GLOBE ARTICHOKES

Globe artichokes are members of the thistle family. The artichoke itself is the bud of the plant and grows on a stem. The Jerusalem artichoke (a completely different vegetable) is actually a tuber and is a member of the sunflower family.

BAMBOO SHOOTS

Bamboo shoots are taken from an edible bamboo. They are occasionally available fresh in some markets. They can also be found canned, packed in water and are featured in Asian cooking.

CELERY

Celery was once used exclusively as a medicinal herb. (In traditional Chinese medicine, for example, it was used to treat high blood pressure.) This vegetable grows in a bunch that consists of ribbed stalks surrounding a paler, more delicately flavored heart.

Lettuces and Other Salad Greens

Eating salads is one of the easiest ways to ensure that you are getting a good range of vegetables. In addition to the lettuces and greens suggested here, add grated, diced or sliced raw or cooked vegetables, grains or lean meats to make a good one-dish meal that is satisfying, healthy and quick to prepare.

While iceburg lettuce is a nutritional low scorer, other salad greens do much better. Darker green salad vegetables tend to provide a better supply of vitamins and minerals than paler ones.

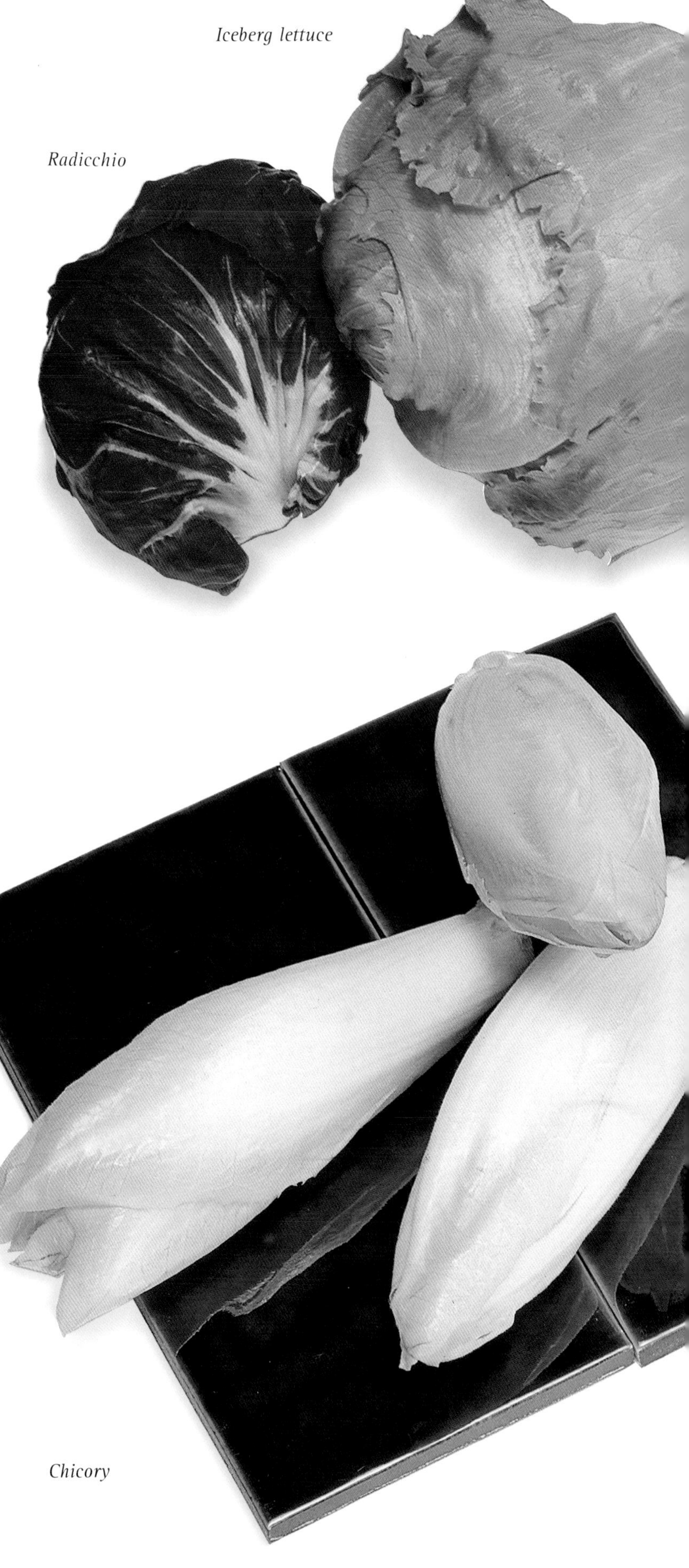

Iceberg lettuce

Radicchio

Chicory

HEADING TYPE LETTUCES

Iceberg, Boston, Butterhead (round) Bibb

Bibb, Boston and butterhead (round) lettuces are heading salad greens. They have soft, tender leaves with a mild, delicate flavor. These lettuces may also be prepared as braised vegetables.

Iceberg lettuce is a tight heading lettuce with pale green leaves that are very mild in flavor. The color varies, depending upon the time of year it is harvested.

BUNCHING TYPE LETTUCES

Belgian endive (chicory), Radicchio, Chicory (curly endive), Watercress

Belgian endive (chicory) is a tight, oblong heading vegetable with a slightly bitter flavor. In addition to its use raw in salads, it is also often prepared as a braised vegetable. It may also be known as witloof chicory.

Radicchio is a heading form of endive (chicory in the U.K.), with deep red to purple leaves and white veining. The flavor is sharp or bitter.

Chicory (called curly endive in the U.K.) has sharp "teeth" on curly leaves.

Watercress is a bunching green, often used as a garnish, with rounded scallops on deep green, glossy leaves. It has a pungent, peppery flavor and, eaten in generous amounts, supplies good quantities of vitamin C, beta-carotene, calcium and iron.

LETTUCE AND SALAD GREENS	*NSP(g)*	*Fe(mg)*	*Vit C(mg)*	*Vit A(mcg)*
Lettuce, iceberg, raw *10 calories (portion 80g)*	0.48	0.32	2.40	6.67
Chicory, raw *3 calories (portion 28g)*	0.25	0.11	1.40	5.60
Watercress, raw *4 calories (portion 20g)*	0.30	0.44	12.40	84.00
Alfalfa sprouts, raw *1 calories (portion 5g)*	0.09	0.05	0.10	0.80
Radicchio, raw *4 calories (portion 30g)*	0.54	0.09	1.50	–
Bean sprouts, mung, raw *6 calories (portion 20g)*	0.30	–	–	–

Pods and Beans

These vegetables include fresh legumes, such as peas, beans and bean sprouts, as well as corn and okra. All are best eaten young and fresh, when they are at their sweetest and most tender. Once picked, they begin to convert their natural sugars into starch. Garden peas and sweet corn are especially prone to flavor loss.

Some fresh peas and beans are eaten whole, when the pods are still fleshy and tender. Other peas and beans are removed from their inedible pods.

SPROUTS

Alfalfa, Mustard, Bean sprouts, Radish

Sprouts can be produced from a variety of grains, beans and vegetables and are a good addition to salads. (Avoid potato sprouts because these contain a toxin.) They range in flavor from very milky (alfalfa or bean sprouts) to spicy (radish or mustard) and provide digestible protein, B vitamins and vitamin C.

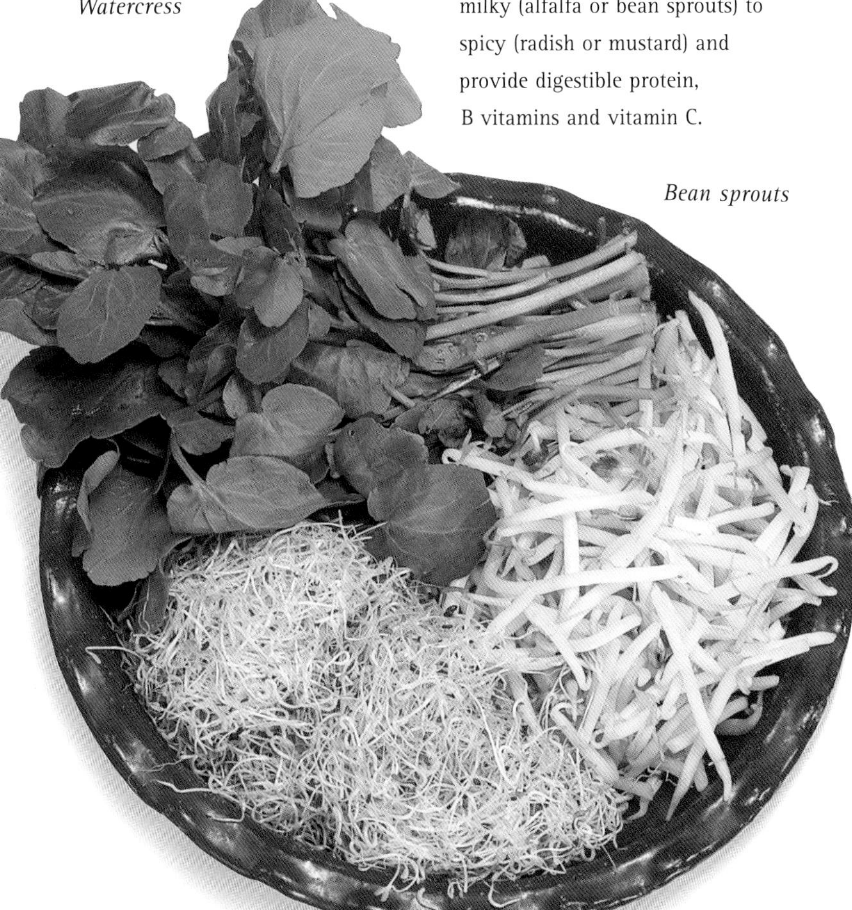

Watercress

Bean sprouts

Alfalfa

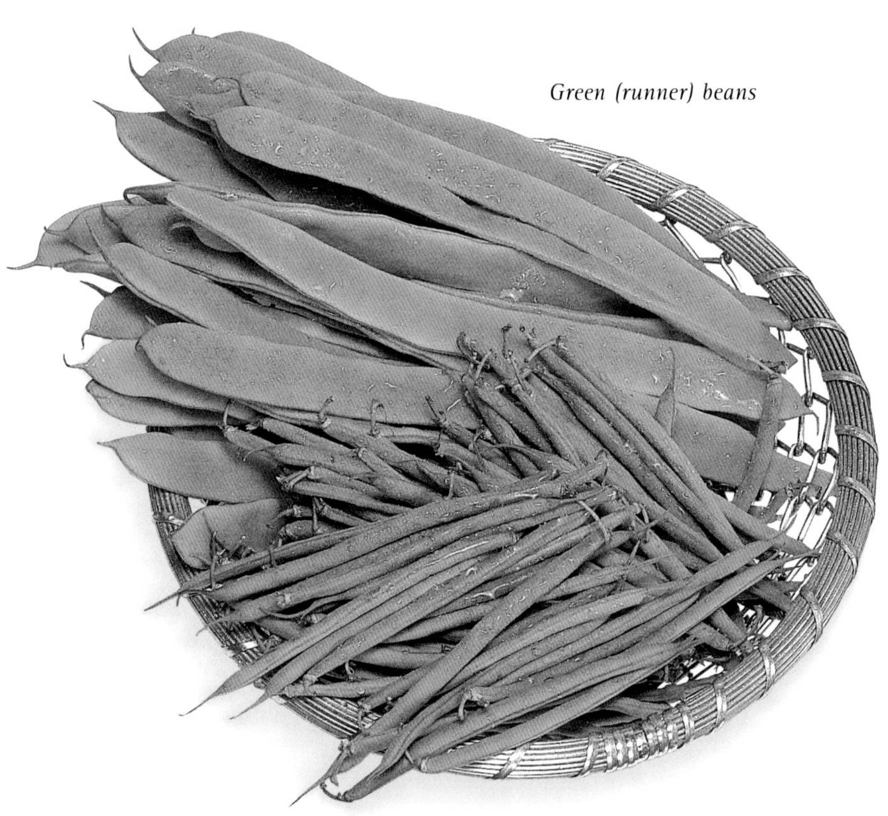

Green (runner) beans

Bobby (French) beans

BEANS, EDIBLE PODS

Green (runner), Burgundy/purple, French

Green (runner) beans are long, slender and flat. Available in mid- to late-summer, they are usually sliced, boiled and served as a side dish.

Burgundy/purple beans are similar in shape to green beans but have deep purple to maroon skin that turns green when cooked.

French beans are smaller and thinner than green beans and have velvety skin. They are usually served as a side dish.

OKRA

This pod is the fruit of an annual plant of the cotton family. It is widely used in Indian cooking and dishes from the southern U.S. It may be used to thicken soups and stews, or eaten as a vegetable. It provides valuable amounts of fiber.

BEANS, INEDIBLE PODS

Black-eyed peas, Fava (broad) beans pods, Flageolot pods

All beans in this section are available both fresh and dried. They are good sources of protein and soluble fiber, which may help reduce cholesterol levels.

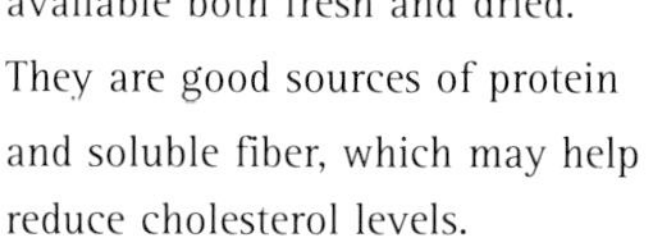

Black-eyed peas grow in green pods often mottled with brown; the beans are round and tan with a black "eye." They are available throughout summer and into fall.

Fava (broad) bean pods are long, large and light green; the beans are a delicate green color, almost kidney shaped. They may be cooked and eaten cold; large beans must be peeled before they are eaten.

Flageolet pods are green; they contain light green beans. Available in mid-summer, they may be cooked, puréed, braised or used in soups.

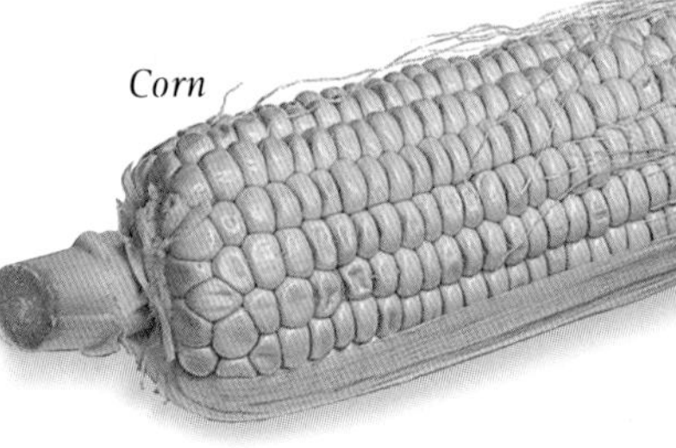

Corn

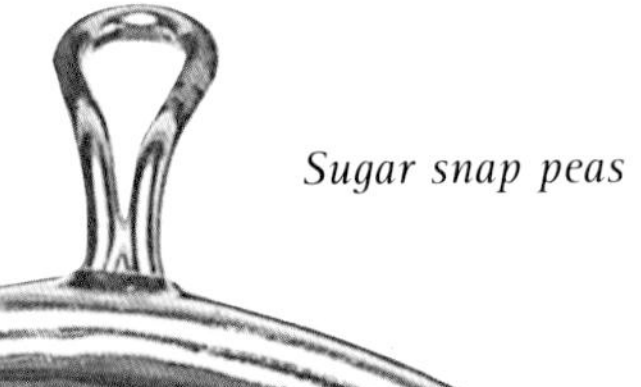

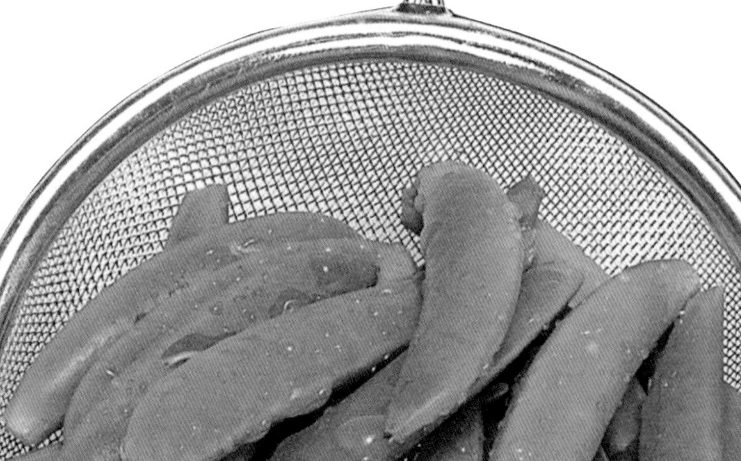

Sugar snap peas

PEAS

Garden (Petits pois), Snow (mange-tout), Sugar snap

Garden pea (petits pois) pods are tapered and rounded and should "squeak" when rubbed between the fingers. The peas are round and pale green when raw. They may be steamed, stewed, chilled, puréed or used in soups. Frozen peas may actually be a better source of vitamin C than fresh ones.

Snow pea pods (mange-tout) are flat and dull green when raw. Available in early spring to summer, they are steamed or stir-fried.

Sugar snap pods are deeper green than those of garden or snow peas. They may be steamed or stir-fried.

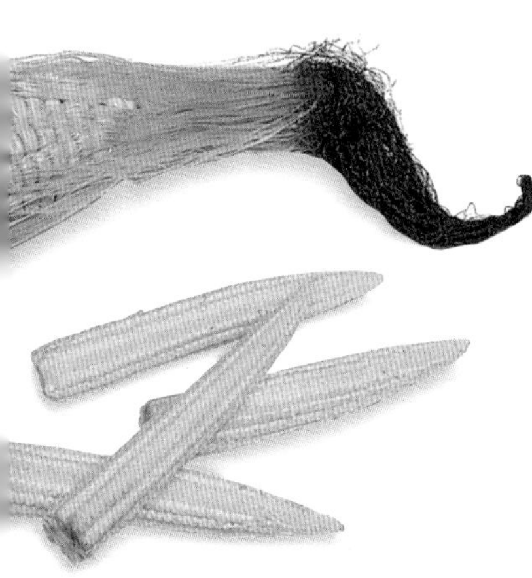

CORN

When served fresh, this vegetable is known as sweet or green corn. Fresh corn should be husked and plunged into boiling water or steamed until just tender. Other methods of preparation include roasting, baking and grilling.

Corn is a good source of energy and fiber and also provides the more unusual carotenoid zeaxanthin.

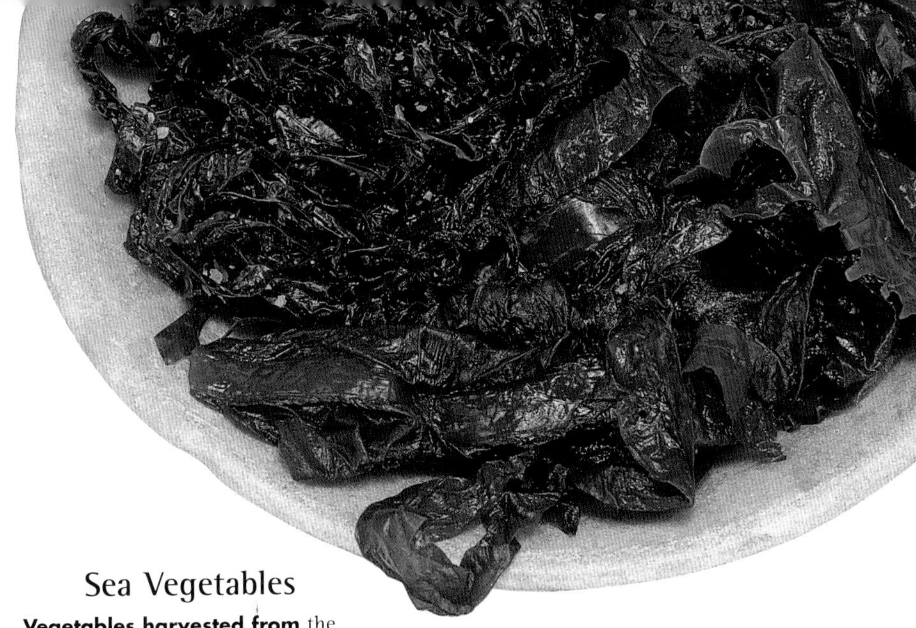

Laver (Nori) and Wakame

Sea Vegetables

Vegetables harvested from the sea are fairly common in the cuisines of coastal areas but are inevitably less familiar in landlocked places. The following seaweed and sea vegetable varieties are often available fresh or dried. They are an extremely rich source of iodine (which helps regulate the metabolic rate) and can be very valuable in the diet of vegans, who may not otherwise consume iodine.

Some sea products are eaten as vegetables or used as edible vegetable wrappers. The only drawback is their high sodium content.

LAVER

Laver (also known as nori) is usually used as a wrapper for sushi (cold rice balls). It is sold in squares or circles and should be kept airtight and crisped briefly in a flame before use.

KELP

Kelp (also known as kombu) is a deep olive green with a distinctive sea flavor and fragrance.

WAKAME

Wakame may be green or brown. The former is used as a vegetable; the brown variety is usually minced and added to rice and vegetable dishes.

PEAS, BEANS AND SEA VEGETABLES	PROT(g)	NSP(g)	I(mcg)	FOLAT(mcg)
Peas, frozen, boiled in unsalted water *48 calories (portion 70g)*	4.20	3.57	1.40	32.90
Snow peas (mange-tout), boiled in salted water *23 calories (portion 90g)*	2.88	1.98	–	5.40
Fava (broad) beans, boiled in unsalted water *58 calories (portion 120g)*	6.12	6.48	4.80	38.40
Green beans/French beans, boiled in unsalted water *20 calories (portion 90g)*	1.62	2.16	–	51.30
Seaweed, wakame, dried, raw *35 calories (portion 50g)*	6.20	23.55	8,415.00	–
Corn, whole cob, boiled in unsalted water *132 calories (portion 200g)*	–	2.60	–	–

"Fruit" Vegetables

"Fruit" vegetables are so called because they are technically fruits, even though in the culinary sense they are more often thought of as vegetables.

AVOCADOS

These pear-shaped vegetables come in two main varieties, one with dark green skin and the other with warty, black skin. The flesh is smooth and delicately flavored. Cut surfaces must be treated with lemon or lime juice to prevent browning.

If avocados are not ripe when you purchase them, store them at room temperature (around 70°F/21°C) until they soften.

In comparison with other vegetables, avocados are high in fat and calories, but they contain mostly monounsaturated fats, which help protect against heart disease. They are also rich in vitamin E, which is an important antioxidant in the human body.

Green- and black-skinned avocados

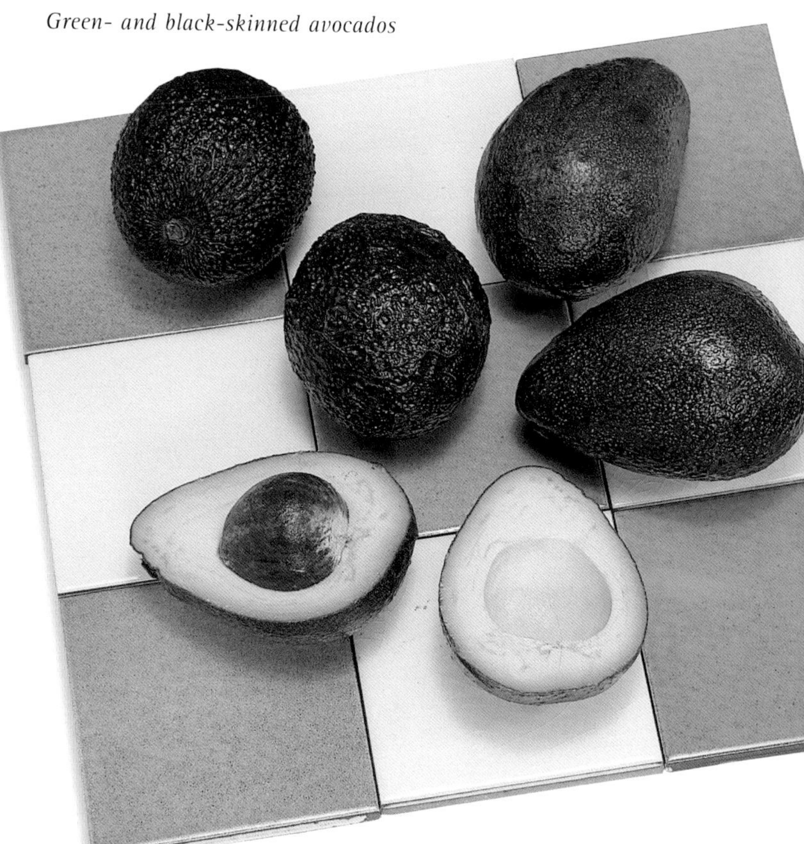

TOMATOES

Beefsteak, Cherry, Plum, Tomatillos, Yellow slicing

These succulent "vegetables" are actually berries. They are grown in hundreds of varieties, in colors from green to yellow to bright red. All have smooth, shiny skin, juicy flesh and small, edible seeds. Most tomatoes grown commercially are picked young and allowed to ripen in transit. They are a good source of a carotenoid called lycopene, which is associated with lower risks of prostate and lung cancer. Processed tomatoes (for example, puréed or paste) actually provide more readily absorbed lycopene than fresh tomatoes.

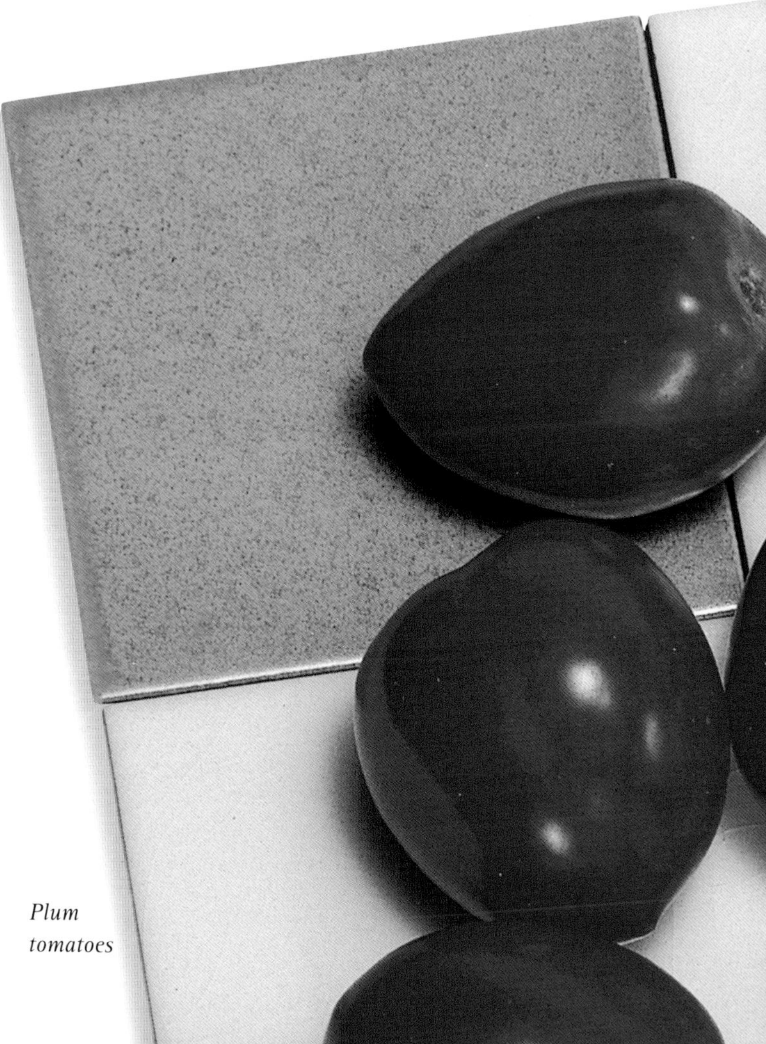

Plum tomatoes

Slicing tomatoes, including the deeply ridged beefsteak variety, are favored for use in salads and other uncooked preparations.

Cherry tomatoes are small red or yellow tomatoes that grow in clusters; the yellow version is low in acid. They are also suitable for salads and crudités.

Plum tomatoes are egg-shaped and red, with a relatively greater proportion of flesh. They are used for sauces, purées, soups and other cooked dishes.

Tomatillos are small, green round berries with a light green to brown papery husk that taste like green tomatoes. Available in mid- to late summer, they are usually cooked before use in sauces.

Yellow slicing tomatoes are a smooth-skinned, low-acid variety. They are available in summer.

"FRUIT" VEGETABLES

	NSP(g)	*FAT(g)*	*Vit C(mg)*	*Vit E(mg)*
Tomatoes, raw *14 calories (portion 85g)*	0.85	0.25	14.45	1.04
Avocado, Haas *330 calories (portion 173g)*	5.88	34.08	12.11	5.54
Plantain, boiled in unsalted water *224 calories (portion 200g)*	2.40	0.40	18.00	0.40

Avocado is a rich source of vitamin E. Other good sources include foods fried in corn or sunflower oil, sunflower seeds (6.0 mg per 16-g portion), sweet potato (5.7 mg per 130-g portion), mayonnaise (5.7 mg per 30 g) almonds (3.2 mg per 13-g portion).

PLANTAIN

A type of cooking banana, plantains have a lower sugar content than eating bananas. They are cooked in a wide range of savory West Indian dishes.

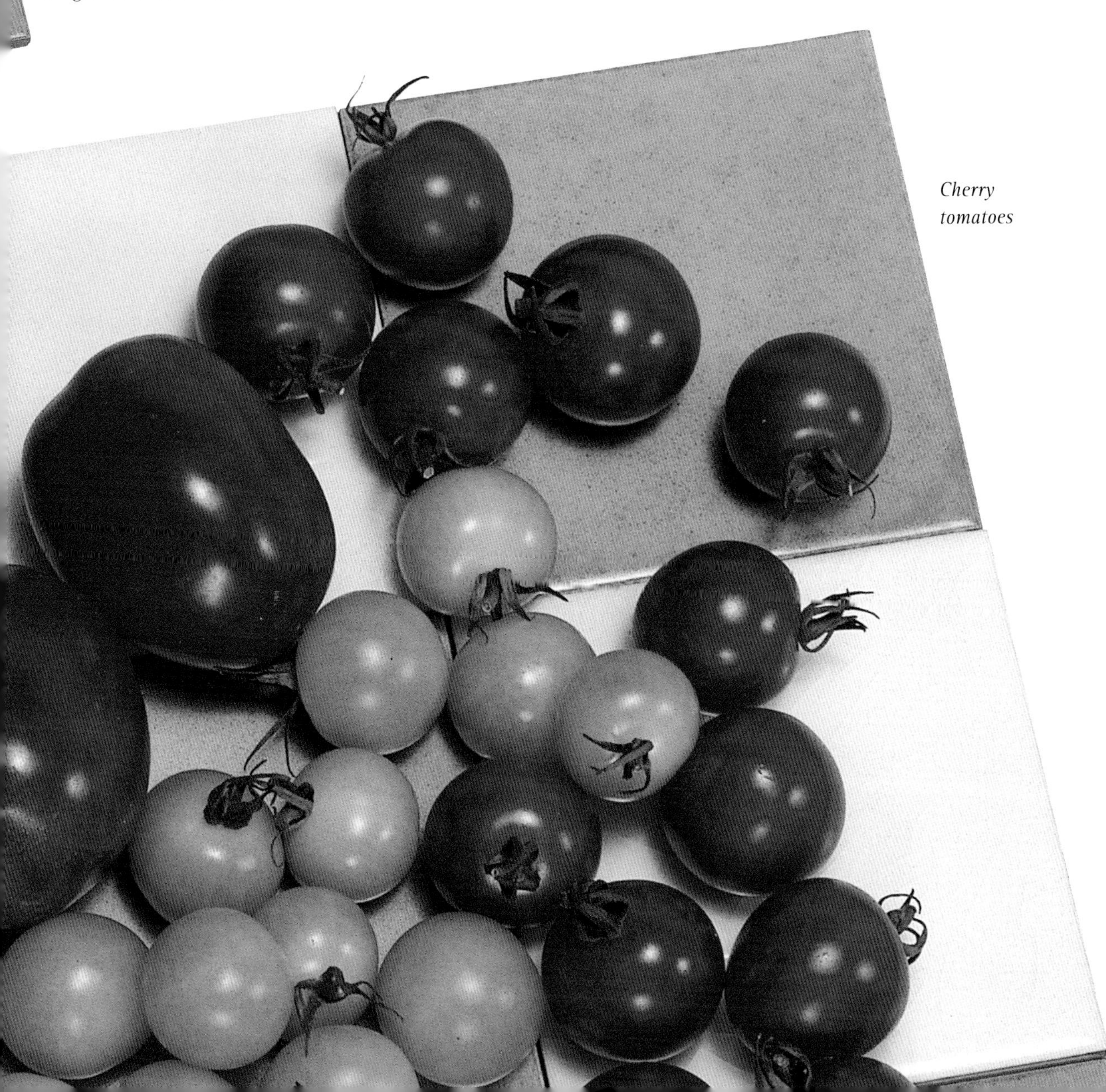

Cherry tomatoes

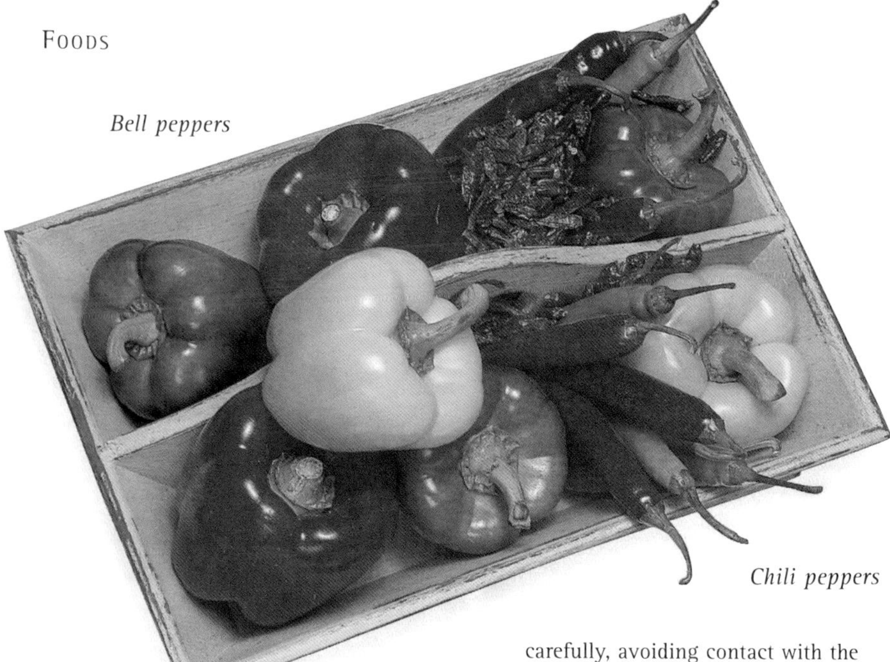
Bell peppers

Chili peppers

BELL PEPPERS

Bell, or sweet, peppers are named for their shape and come in several colors—green, red, yellow, even creamy white and purple. All peppers start out green, but special varieties will ripen into rich, vibrant colors. Sweet peppers have similar flavors, though red and yellow varieties tend to be sweeter than green peppers.

Bell peppers are hollow, except for whitish ribs and a core with a cluster of small seeds. Generally, both ribs and core are removed before use.

Peppers are one of the best sources of vitamin C (twice as rich as oranges).

CHILI PEPPERS

Chili peppers are related to bell peppers but are usually smaller and contain spicy, volatile oils. A host of fresh and dried chilies is widely available. They may be bought whole, canned, flaked and ground. The hotter the peppers, the more important it is to handle them carefully, avoiding contact with the eyes and delicate skin and washing the hands thoroughly after contact. Far from damaging the stomach, chilies can actually protect against stomach ulcers, but do go easy if they obviously upset you.

There are several varieties of chili, but generally, the redder and smaller the pepper, the hotter it is.

Banana peppers (also known as Hungarian wax peppers) and habañeros (also known as Scotch bonnets) are considered the hottest peppers.

Compact, tapered chilies, jalapeños may be deep green or red. They may be pickled or canned (whole or chopped).

Gourd Vegetables

Cucumbers, eggplants (aubergines) and the many squash varieties are all members of the gourd family. They have fairly tough rinds, thick flesh and flat, oval seeds. Summer squashes are picked when they are immature to ensure delicate flesh, tender seeds and thin skins. Winter squashes are characterized by their hard rind and seeds.

Cucumbers are a common ingredient in salads and crudités and as part of uncooked sauces or soups such as salsa or gazpacho. They have little nutritional value but are refreshing and low in calories.

CUCUMBERS
English/Burpless, Kirby

Cucumbers are used in salads, pickles, relishes and uncooked sauces.

English/burpless cucumbers are long, even cylinders with some ridging; they have no seeds and are used in salads and crudités.

Kirby is a short, chubby variety with green skin, deep ridges and warts; it is often used in pickles.

SUMMER SQUASH
Pattypan, Zucchini (courgettes)

Summer squashes have relatively subtle flavors, which make them popular for use in vegetable stews or soups as a vehicle for other flavors. Zucchini (courgettes) are probably the most familiar of the summer squashes, and

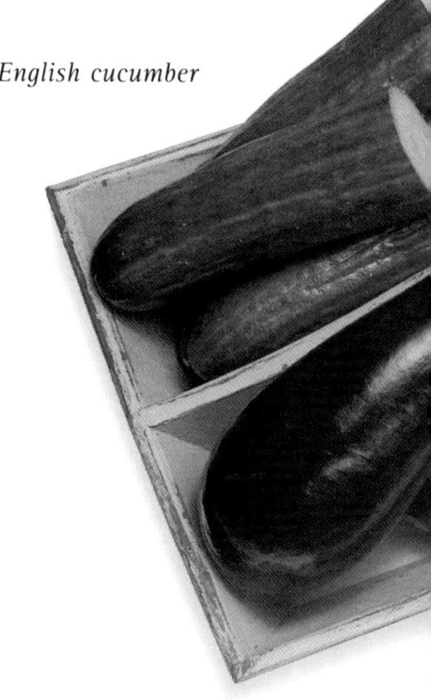
English cucumber

provide beta-carotene, folic acid and vitamin C.

Zucchini are green, with flecks of yellow. The golden variety is yellow with green at the stem end.

Pattypan squash are flattened, ball-shaped vegetables. Usually yellow, they may be mottled or streaked with green. They are generally steamed, sautéd, or pan-fried.

EGGPLANTS (aubergines)

Purple, White

Eggplants (aubergines) come in a range of shapes and sizes. Eggplants are used in numerous dishes. They are wonderful grilled, braised, boiled or stewed, but when fried can absorb large amounts of fat. (A 4oz-/100g-serving contains around 300 calories.) Ratatouille, a famous French vegetable stew, makes liberal use of eggplants.

The common purple variety may have a rounded or elongated pear shape with a deep glossy purple-black skin.

White eggplants may be long or egg-shaped.

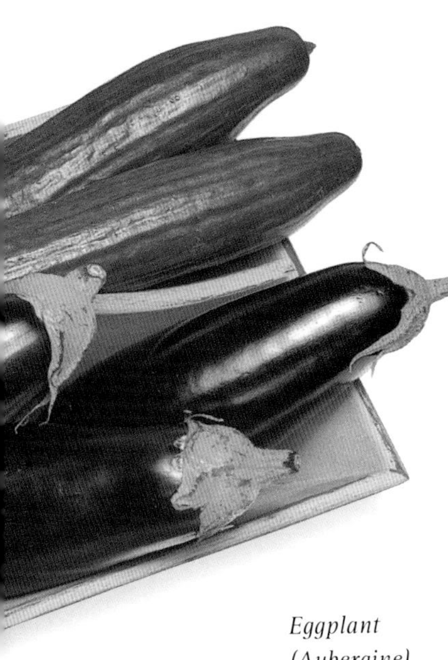

Eggplant (Aubergine)

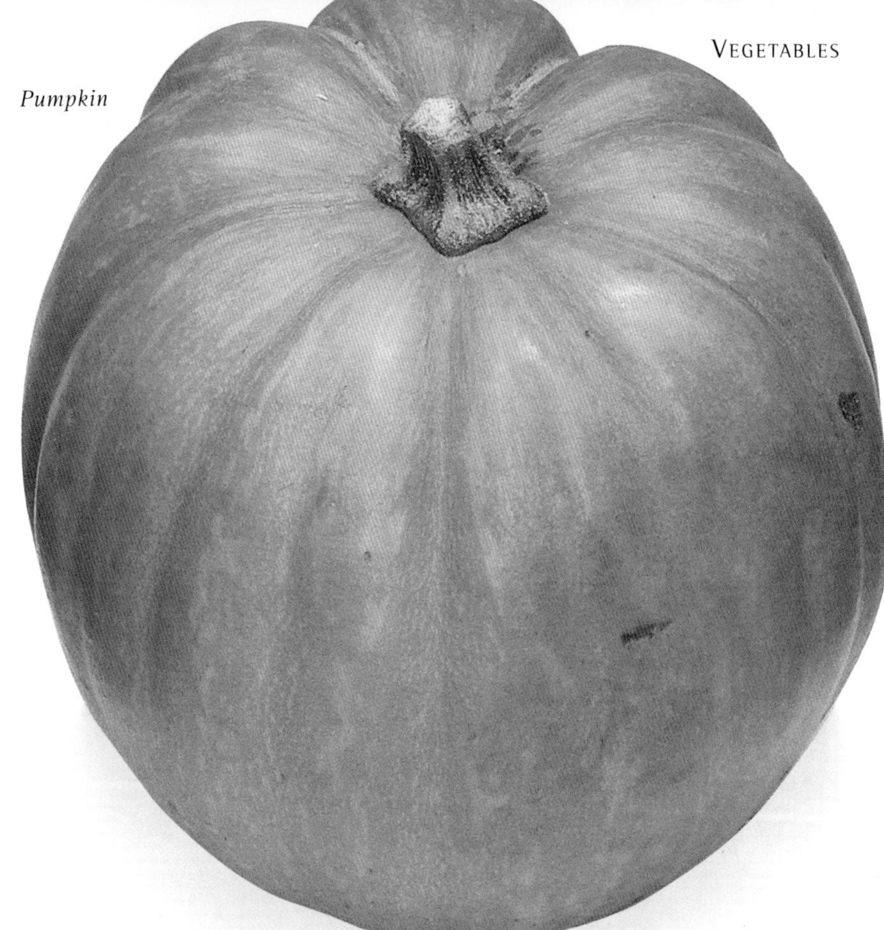

Pumpkin

WINTER SQUASH

Pumpkin, Marrow, Acorn, Spaghetti, Butternut

Winter squash lend themselves to sweet and savory recipes. All varieties are good sources of complex carbohydrates, vitamins and minerals. Those with orange flesh are a source of beta-carotene.

Pumpkin is orange with a rough, deeply ridged skin.

Butternut squash can be sliced, stewed, boiled or baked in a pie.

Marrows are a popular winter vegetable, particularly in the U.K. They grow very large and can be stuffed, baked or boiled. They are low in calories and provide some beta-carotene.

Acorn squash is dark green (some varieties may have an orange blush or be almost completely orange) with deep ridges and an acorn shape.

Spaghetti squash is yellow and has a "zeppelin" shape.

PEPPERS AND GOURDS

	NSP(g)	Vit A(mcg)	Vit C(mg)
Peppers, bell (sweet), red, raw *3 calories (portion 10g)*	0.16	64.00	14.00
Peppers, bell (sweet) and chili, green, raw *2 calories (portion 10g)*	–	2.92	12.00
Eggplant (aubergine), raw *20 calories (portion 130g)*	2.60	15.17	5.20
Cucumber, raw *2 calories (portion 23g)*	0.15	2.21	0.45
Squash, butternut, baked *21 calories (portion 65g)*	0.91	354.25	9.75

Onion Family

Onions and their relations belong to the allium, or lily, family. All varieties, including shallots, scallions (spring onions) and garlic, share a pungent flavor and aroma. Onions are used in so many dishes and in so many guises that they are quite rightly considered indispensable.

Garlic contains sulfur components, which are useful in maintaining healthy blood cholesterol levels and strengthening the immune system. Onions are a significant source of flavonoids in the diet—they are also valuable in cutting the risk of heart disease.

ONIONS

Boiling onions, Cippolini, Red onions, Scallions (spring onions), Shallots, Spanish

Boiling and pickling onions are small and round with white skin.

Cippolini onions are small, round, flattened onions with yellow papery skin; they may be baked, grilled, or used in casseroles.

Red onions are small, round flattened onions with red papery skin. They may be eaten raw in salads, grilled, fried or used in compotes and marmalades.

Scallions (spring onions) are long and slender, with white bulbs and green tops. The entire plant is used. They are picked when young and tender, before the bulb forms and are available from mid-winter to mid-summer. Used fresh in salads, scallions are much higher in vitamin C than other onions.

Shallots, which have light brown papery skins, have a more delicate flavor than large onions. Their flesh is white-purple, and they are used primarily as a flavoring ingredient.

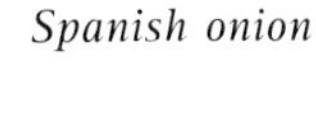

Spanish onion

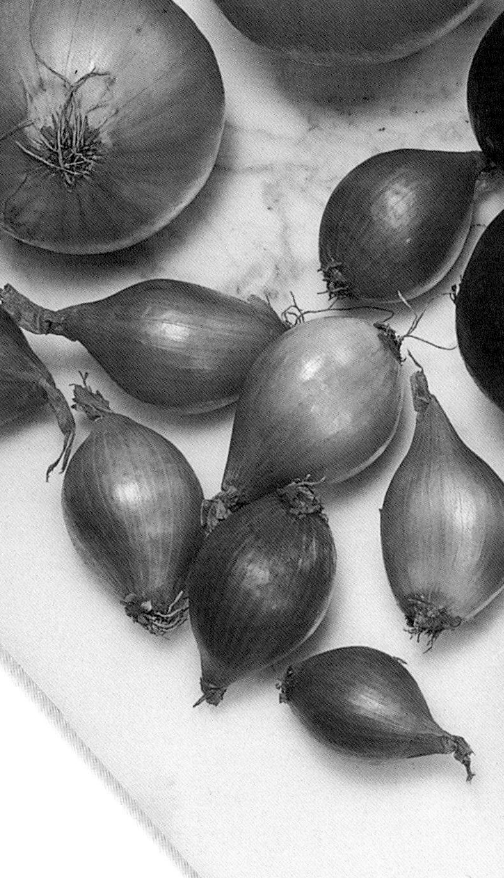

Shallots

Red onions

ONION FAMILY	NSP(g)	Vit C(mg)	FOLAT(mcg)	B_1(mg)
Onions, raw *22 calories (portion 60g)*	0.84	3.00	10.20	0.08
Scallions (spring onions), bulbs and tops, raw *2 calories (portion 10g)*	0.15	2.60	5.40	0.00
Garlic, raw *3 calories (portion 3g)*	0.12	0.51	0.15	0.00
Leeks, raw *18 calories (portion 80g)*	1.76	13.60	44.80	0.23

Spanish onions are large with yellow to yellow-brown skin; they may be used as an aromatic or as an ingredient in soups, stews, sauces or braises. They are the basic component of *mirepoix*.

LEEKS

More delicately flavored than onions, leeks have a white bulb and dark green tops. They may be grilled, steamed, boiled or served "à la grecque." They are used extensively in soups, stews and sauces.

Ramps are wild leeks with small white stem ends and flat green tops; they may be either stewed or sautéed

GARLIC

Standard garlic has a bulb; white or red-streaked papery skin encases individual cloves, which are also covered with papery skin. Garlic is a flavoring ingredient and may be roasted into purée.

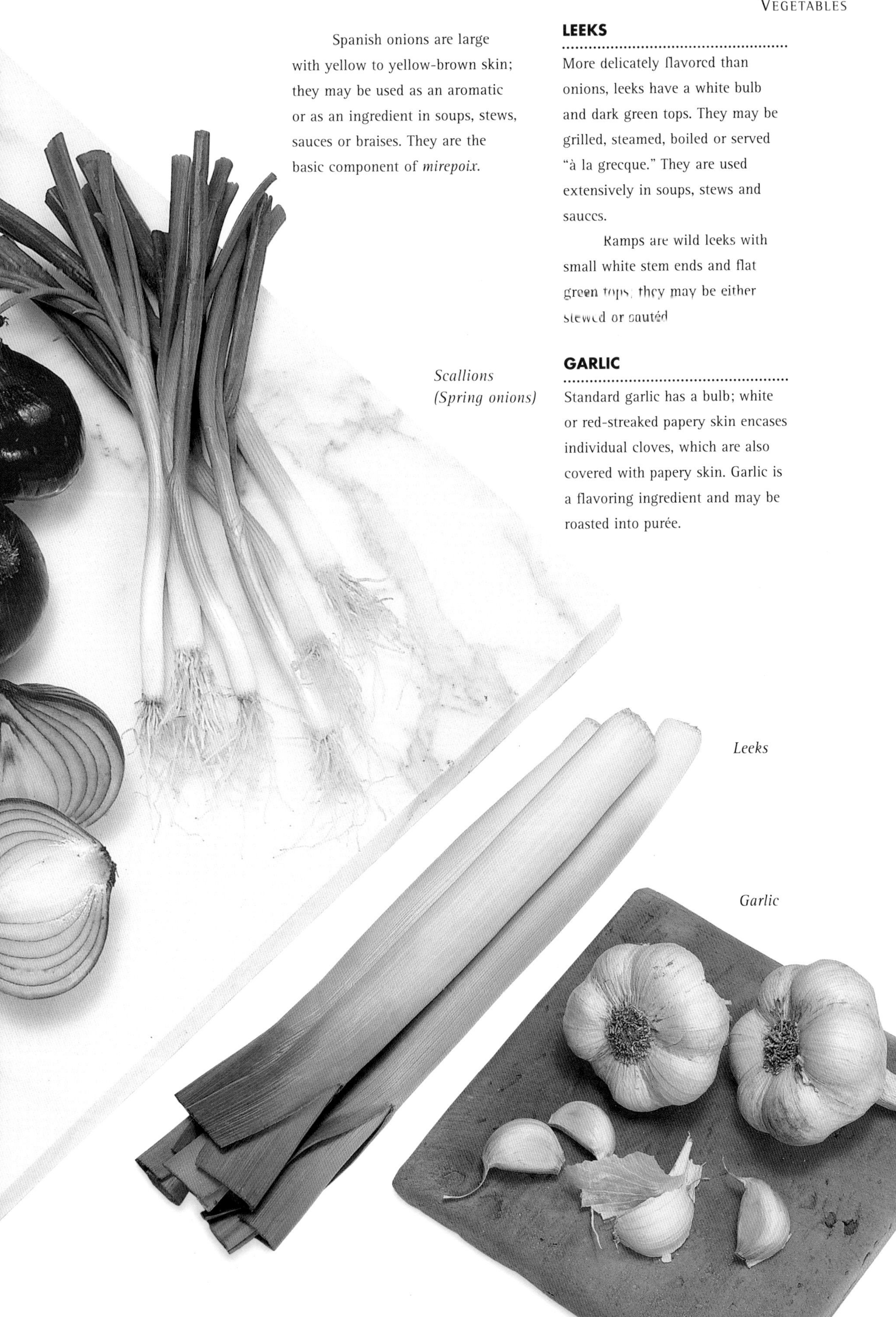

Scallions (Spring onions)

Leeks

Garlic

Roots and Tubers

Roots and tubers serve as nutrient reservoirs for their plants. Consequently, they are rich in sugars, starches, vitamins and minerals. Popular root vegetables include beets (beetroot), carrots, potatoes, parsnips, radishes, rutabagas (swedes) and turnips.

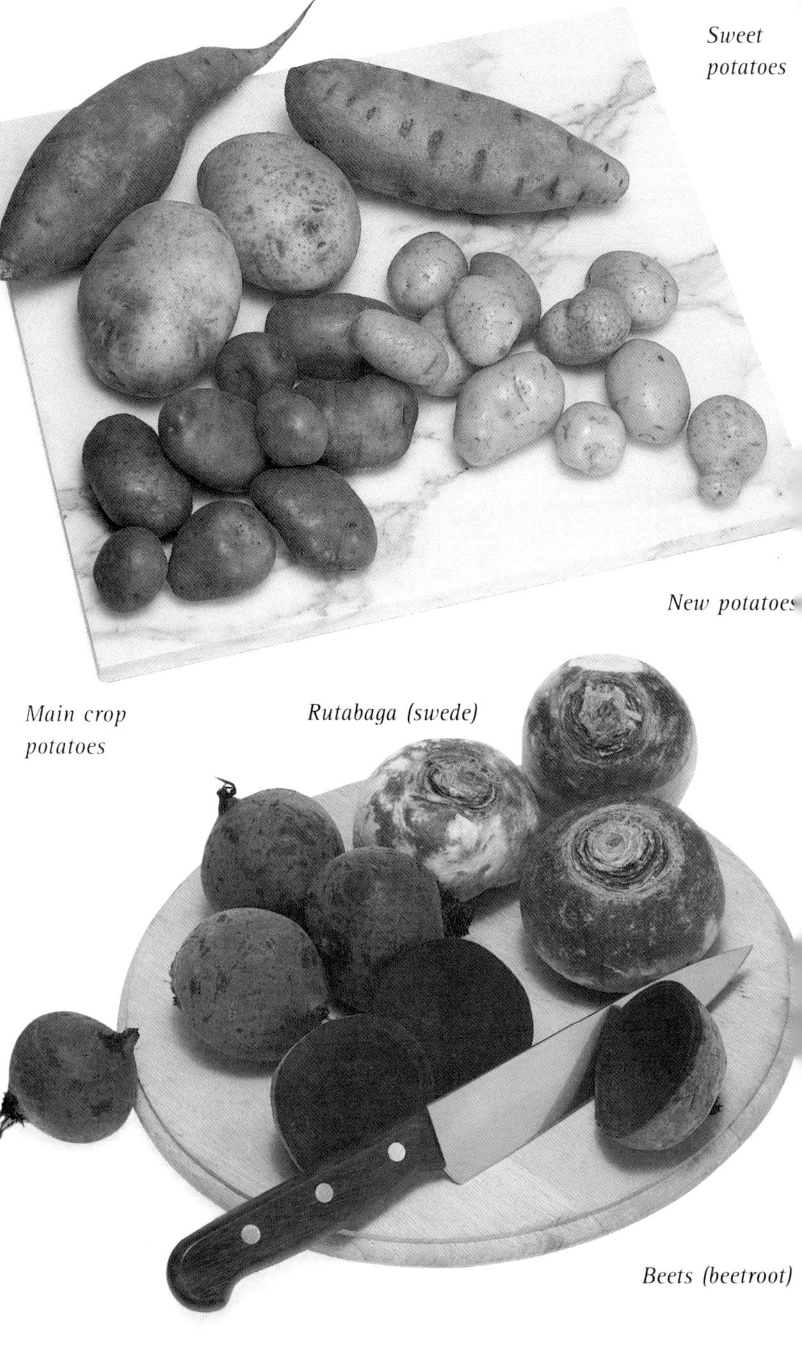

Sweet potatoes

New potatoes

Main crop potatoes

Rutabaga (swede)

Beets (beetroot)

POTATOES

New, Main crop (old), Sweet, Yam (U.S.)

Potatoes are an excellent source of energy; they are starchy carbohydrates and supply around 20 percent of our thiamin (vitamin B_2) intake. They are second only to green vegetables as a source of folic acid in the average diet; they also provide vitamin C. Potatoes should be kept dry, away from excess heat or sunlight, and in a well-ventilated area. Avoid green or sprouting potatoes because they contain the toxin solanin.

New potatoes are the small, firm tubers of early potato varieties, harvested around four months after planting. They may be boiled or oven roasted with herbs.

Main crop (old) potatoes are varieties that are left in the ground longer; they are usually harvested in September for consumption through the winter. New and old potatoes vary in their vitamin C content, with freshly dug new potatoes being richer, and wintered old potatoes being poorer. There are many varieties of potato; for example, Desirée is an all-purpose potato. King Edward is a traditional variety for roasting and mashing, and Marfona is excellent for baking.

Sweet potatoes have a reddish skin with deep orange, moist flesh. They are an excellent source of the

ROOTS AND TUBERS	NSP(g)	Vit A(mcg)	Vit C(mg)	FOLAT(mcg)
New potatoes, boiled in unsalted water *131 calories (portion 175g)*	1.93	–	15.75	33.25
Sweet potatoes, boiled in salted water *109 calories (portion 130g)*	2.99	858.00	22.10	10.40
Yams, boiled in unsalted water *173 calories (portion 130g)*	1.82	–	5.20	7.80
Rutabagas (swedes), boiled in unsalted water *7 calories (portion 60g)*	0.42	16.50	9.00	10.80
Carrots, young, boiled in unsalted water *13 calories (portion 60g)*	1.38	442.50	1.20	10.20
Beets (beetroot), boiled in salted water *18 calories (portion 40g)*	0.76	1.80	2.00	44.00

antioxidant and vitamin A precursor beta-carotene and may be baked, roasted, boiled, puréed or used in casseroles and soups.

Yams (white sweet potatoes) have tan to light brown russeted skin with pale to deep yellow flesh. They are drier and less sweet than red sweet potatoes. (*Note:* Yams in the U.K. are a different vegetable than U.S. yams. British yams are large tubers with a coarse outer bark and white to pale yellow flesh.) All varieties may be peeled and cooked like potatoes.

BEETS (beetroot)

Baby beets are small, red and ball-shaped. Available throughout summer and into fall, they may be served hot or cold.

Larger beets are available throughout summer and into fall. They are usually served hot but may also be pickled or used in soup (borscht). Beets are the richest vegetable source of natural sugars.

TURNIPS

Similar in shape to beets, turnips are available from fall into early winter. They are cooked whole when young and puréed or used in soups when older.

RUTABAGAS (swedes)

These large, ball-shaped vegetables are available throughout winter. They have subtly flavored yellow-orange flesh and can be cooked in the same way as parsnips.

RADISHES

Red, Daikon

Red radishes are small, ball-shaped root vegetables. They may be cherry red, striped, white or special colors (purple or orange, for example). Generally available in spring and summer, they have a spicy flavor and are used in salads and crudités.

Daikon or Japanese radishes are large, carrot-shaped white radishes with a mild flavor.

PARSNIPS

Parsnips are a sweet root vegetable and are at their best in winter. Parsnips can be braised, boiled, roasted or puréed. They are as good a source of folic acid as many green vegetables.

CARROTS

Carrots are the richest natural source of beta-carotene, but cooked ones provide a better absorbed source than raw ones.

Carrots are sometimes sold with their tops still attached; look for unwilted greenery and remove it promptly to prevent softening.

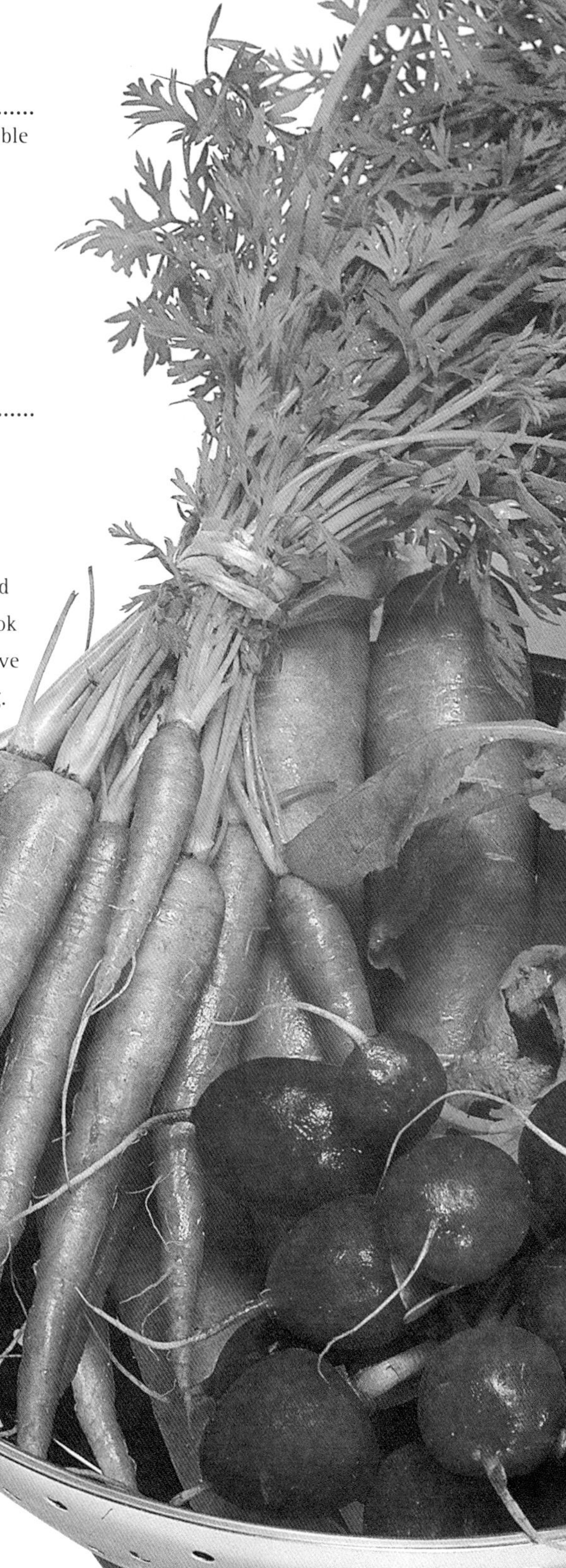

Carrots

Red radishes

Pears

Pears, like apples, are grown in many varieties. Their flesh is extremely fragile. Because they are usually picked for shipping before they have ripened, it is difficult to find perfectly ripe pears in the market. They will become softer after picking but will not actually ripen. For this reason, pears are often poached whole or used in sorbets to compensate for their underdeveloped flavor.

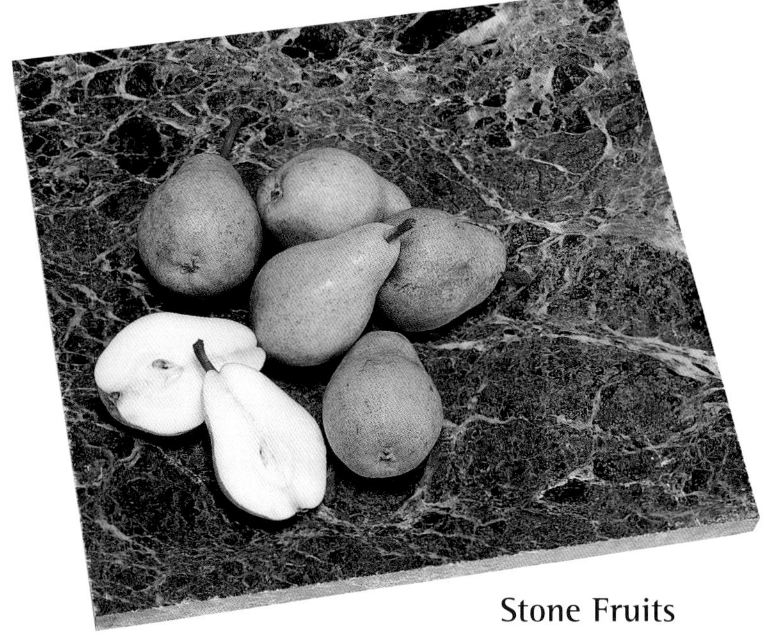

William pears

PEARS

Bartlett, Bosc, D'Anjou, William, Comice, Conference

Bartlett pears have green skin that turns yellow as the fruit ripens; there are also some red varieties.

Bosc pears have a long neck and russeted skin that becomes brown when ripe.

D'Anjou pears have green skin that becomes yellow as it ripens and may have brown scarring.

William pears are slightly bulbous with yellow skin and a strong fragrance. They are eaten fresh and used for preserves and to make the cordial Poire William.

Comice and conference pears become available late in the year and are eaten fresh.

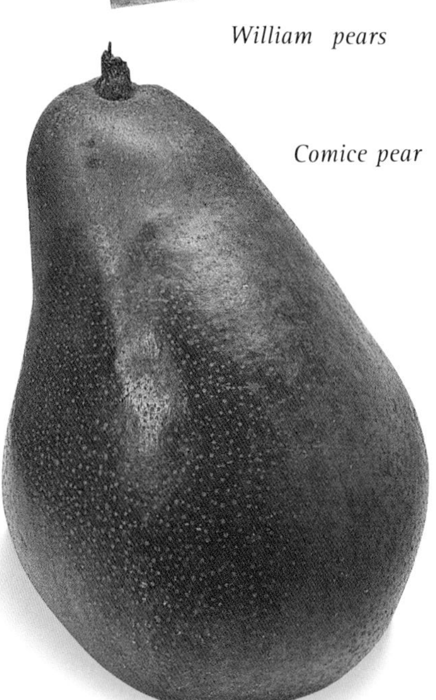

Comice pear

PEARS AND STONE FRUITS

	SUGAR(g)	NSP(g)	Vit A(mcg)	Vit C(mg)
Pears, William, raw *51 calories (portion 150g)*	12.45	3.30	6.00	9.00
Plums, average, raw (weighed with stones) *20 calories (portion 58g)*	4.81	0.87	26.68	2.32
Peaches, raw *36 calories (portion 110g)*	8.36	1.65	11.00	34.10
Nectarines, raw *60 calories (portion 150g)*	13.50	1.80	15.00	55.50
Apricots, raw *12 calories (portion 40g)*	2.88	0.68	26.80	2.40
Cherries, raw *19 calories (portion 40g)*	4.60	0.40	1.60	4.00

Stone Fruits

The stone in stone fruits is simply a large seed. Some fruits cling to the stone, while others separate freely.

CHERRIES

Cherries are grown in numerous varieties and come in many shades of red, from the light crimson Queen Anne to the almost-black Bing. They vary in texture from hard and crisp to soft and juicy, and flavors run the gamut from sweet to sour. They are rich in vitamin C and may be found fresh throughout their growing season (summer). They are also sold canned or dried.

PEACHES, APRICOTS AND NECTARINES

Peaches are sweet and juicy, have distinctively fuzzy skin and come in many varieties. All peaches fall into one of two categories: clingstone, in which the flesh clings to the pit, and freestone, in which the flesh separates easily. Peach flesh comes in a range of colors from white to creamy yellow and yellow-orange to red.

Apricots resemble peaches in

some ways. They have slightly fuzzy skin but are smaller with somewhat drier flesh. Their orange flesh is a good source of beta-carotene.

Nectarines are similar in shape, color and flavor to peaches, but they have a smooth skin.

All three of these fruits are popular eaten fresh, but they are also firm favorites in shortcakes, pies, cobblers and other desserts. They are frequently canned, bottled or frozen. Dried versions of these fruits are also available and make an excellent addition to compotes.

PLUMS

Black friar, Damson, Greengage, Santa Rosa

Plums can vary in size from as small as an apricot to as large as a peach. The possible colors include green, red, purple and various shades between. When ripe, they are sweet and juicy, although some have sour skins. Cooking plums are generally drier and more acidic than dessert plums, but both types can be eaten raw. Greengages are a popular dessert variety, while damsons are probably the best-known cooking plums.

A popular variety in the U.S. is the Black friar—a dark purple plum with a silvery bloom and deep red to purple flesh.

Damsons are small with red to light purple skin and green flesh. They may be eaten fresh but are generally preferred in preserves and pies.

Greengages have green skin, with yellow-green flesh.

Santa Rosa plums are red with light yellow flesh. A popular British variety is the Victoria plum.

Plums are a reasonable source of beta-carotene but are not rich in vitamin C, containing about the same amount as apples.

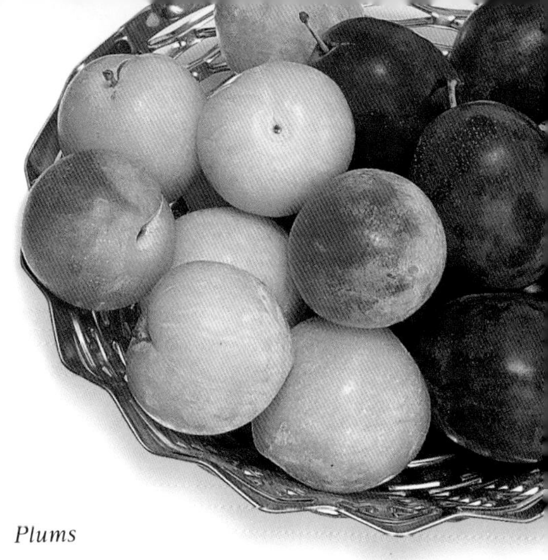

Plums

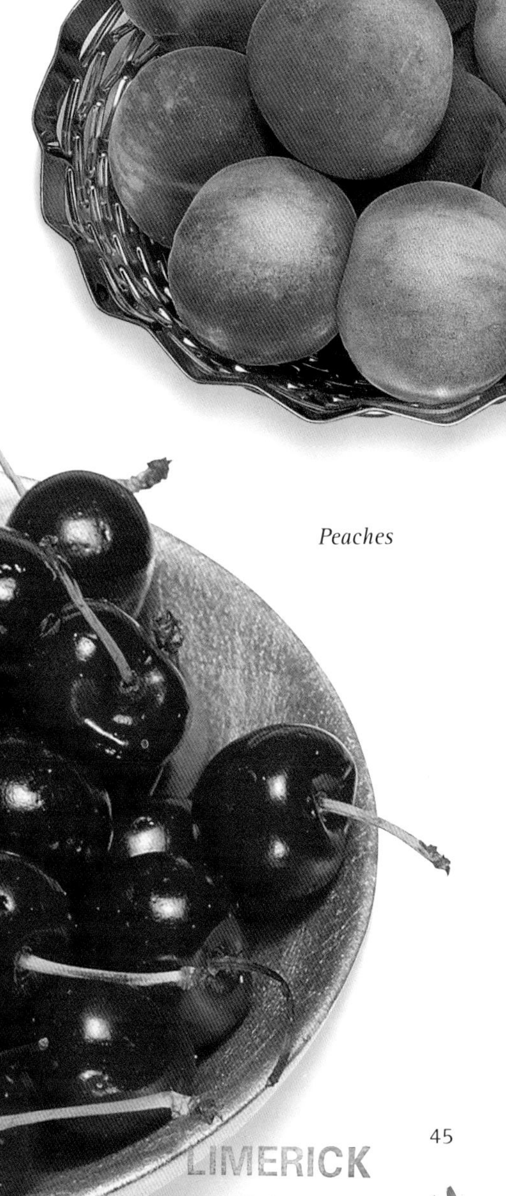

Cherries

Peaches

Berries

The arrival of berries in all their varieties is a sign that spring has arrived or that summer is at its height. Berries are very low in calories and a great source of vitamin C.

They tend to be highly perishable (with the exception of cranberries) and are susceptible to bruising, mold and over-ripening in fairly short order. Inspect all berries and their packaging carefully before you buy them.

When berries are out of season, unsweetened frozen berries are often a perfectly good substitute. Dried berries can be used to great advantage in winter fruit compotes, stuffings, breads or other sweet and savory dishes.

STRAWBERRIES

Strawberries are red, shiny, heart-shaped berries with tiny seeds on the exterior. They are available from late spring into early summer and are delicious eaten fresh or used in shortcakes, baked goods, purées, jams and jellies.

BLUEBERRIES

Blueberries are blue-purple with a dusty, silver-blue "bloom" and are available in late summer.

CRANBERRIES

Cranberries are shiny red berries, some have a white blush. They are dry and sour and are available in fall.

RASPBERRIES

Raspberries are actually clusters of tiny fruits (drupes), each containing a seed; they may have "hairs" on the surface and may be red, black or white (a dewberry is a type of raspberry). They have two seasons: early summer and late summer. Raspberries are eaten fresh and used in baked items, purées, sauces, cordials, syrups and to flavor vinegars.

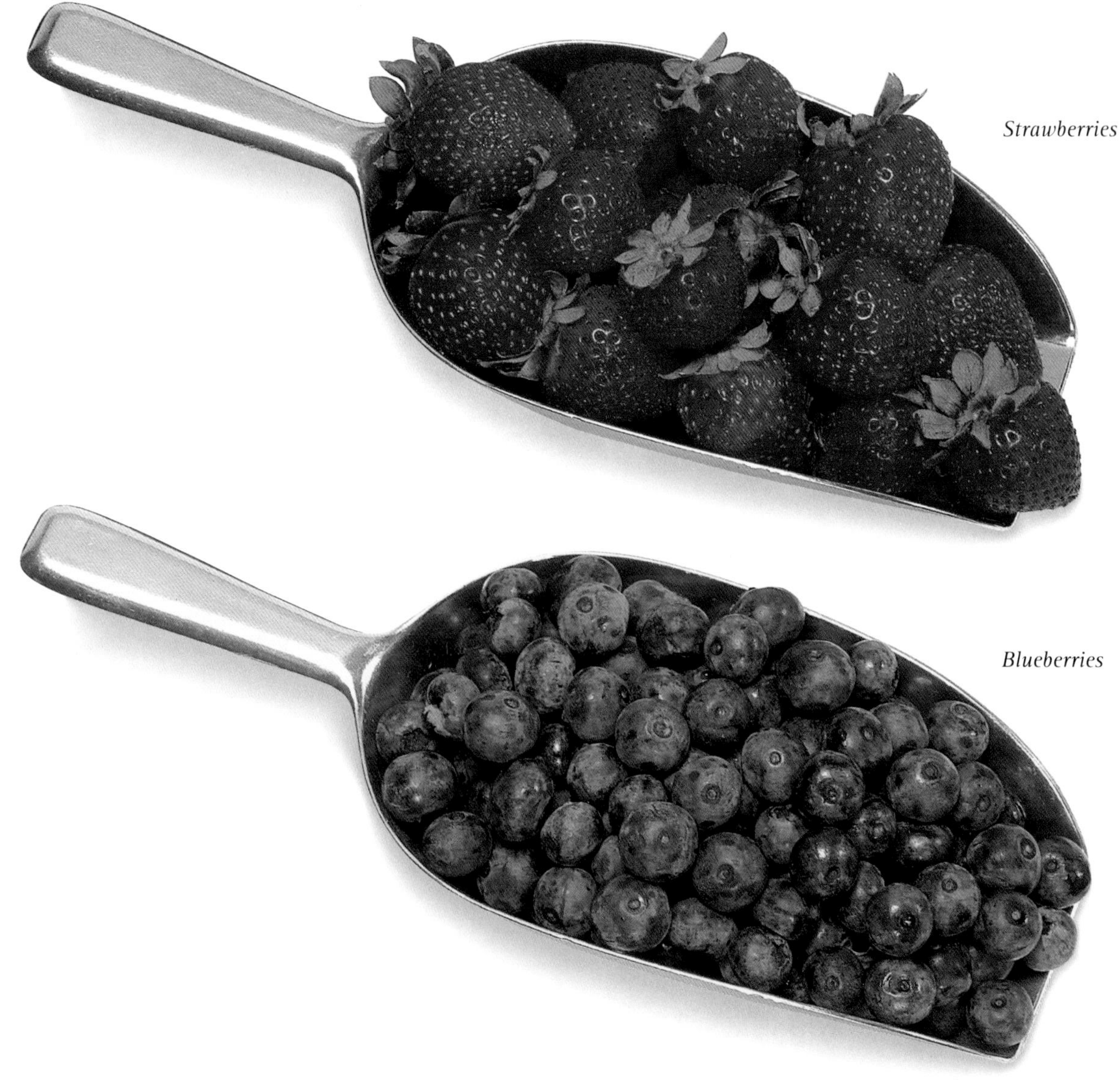

Strawberries

Blueberries

CURRANTS

Currants may be red, black or white; red is generally the sweetest. Black currants are the richest commonly available fruit source of vitamin C, supplying around 200 mg per 4 oz (100 g). Available in mid summer, they are generally cooked for use in relishes, jams, jellies, wines, cordials or syrups.

GOOSEBERRIES

Gooseberries have smooth skin (some with a papery husk still attached). They may be green, golden, red, purple or white; some have fuzzy skins. They are often used crushed in creamy desserts or in compotes, relishes, jams and jellies.

BERRIES *all values per 100g*	*SUGAR(g)*	*NSP(g)*	*K(mg)*	*Vit C(mg)*
Strawberries, raw *27 calories*	6.00	1.10	160.00	77.00
Raspberries, raw *25 calories*	4.60	2.50	170.00	32.00
Cranberries *15 calories*	3.40	3.00	95.00	13.00
Blueberries *30 calories*	6.90	1.80	88.00	17.00
Gooseberries, dessert, raw *40 calories*	9.20	2.40	170.00	26.00
Black currants, raw *28 calories*	6.60	3.60	370.00	200.00

MULBERRIES

Mulberries resemble, but are unrelated to, raspberries. They are juicy with a slightly musty aroma and are available in mid summer.

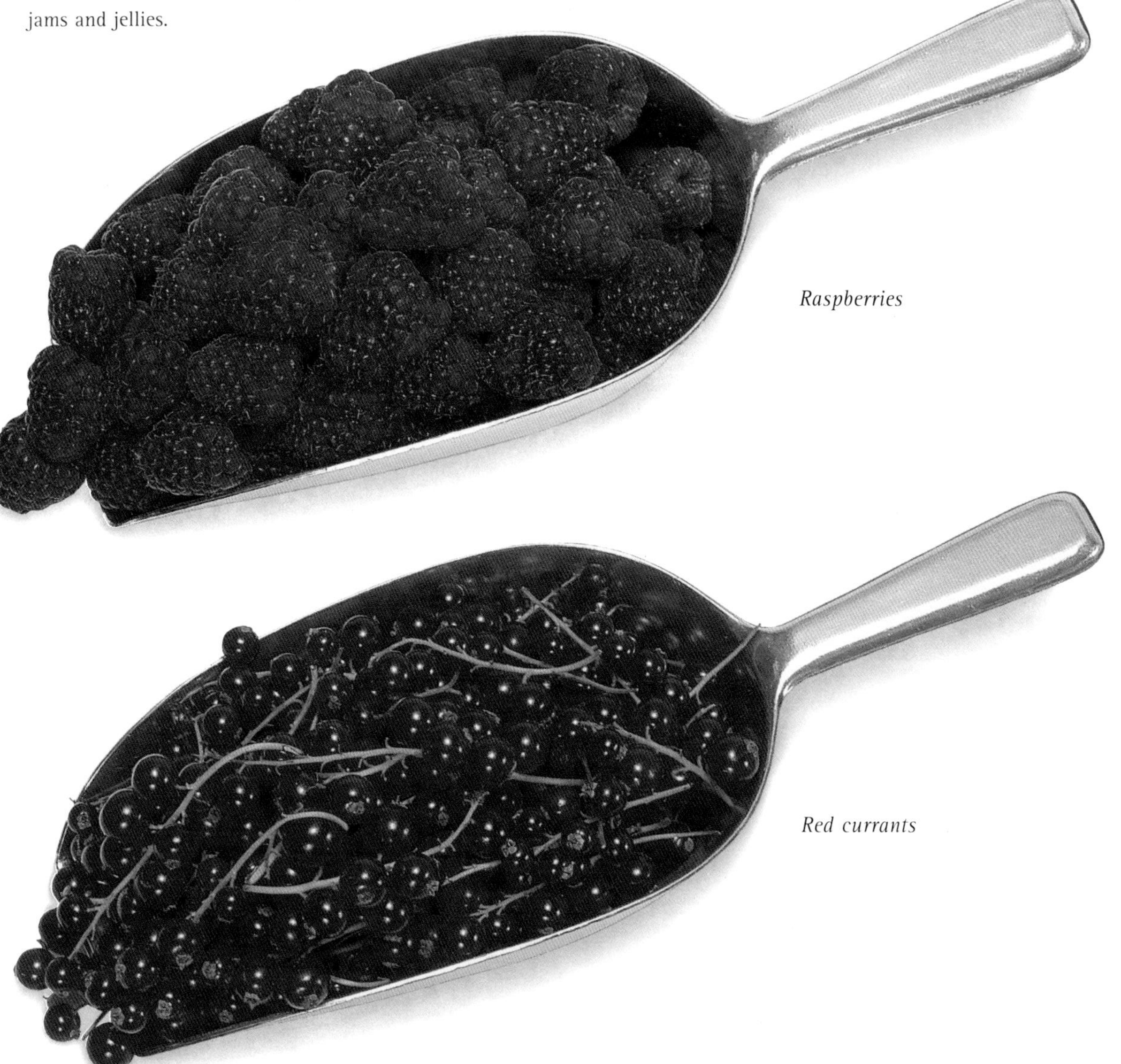

Raspberries

Red currants

GRAPES

Grapes are juicy red (black) or white fruits, most with seeds, some without, that grow in clusters on vines. Technically, they are berries, but because they include so many varieties and have so many different uses, they are grouped into those for eating and those for wine making. Grapes are also dried to form raisins, which are available throughout the year.

Red (black) grapes are an excellent source of antioxidants, so they might help protect the body against heart disease and cancer. These antioxidants are thought to be more active in red wine than they are in fresh grapes.

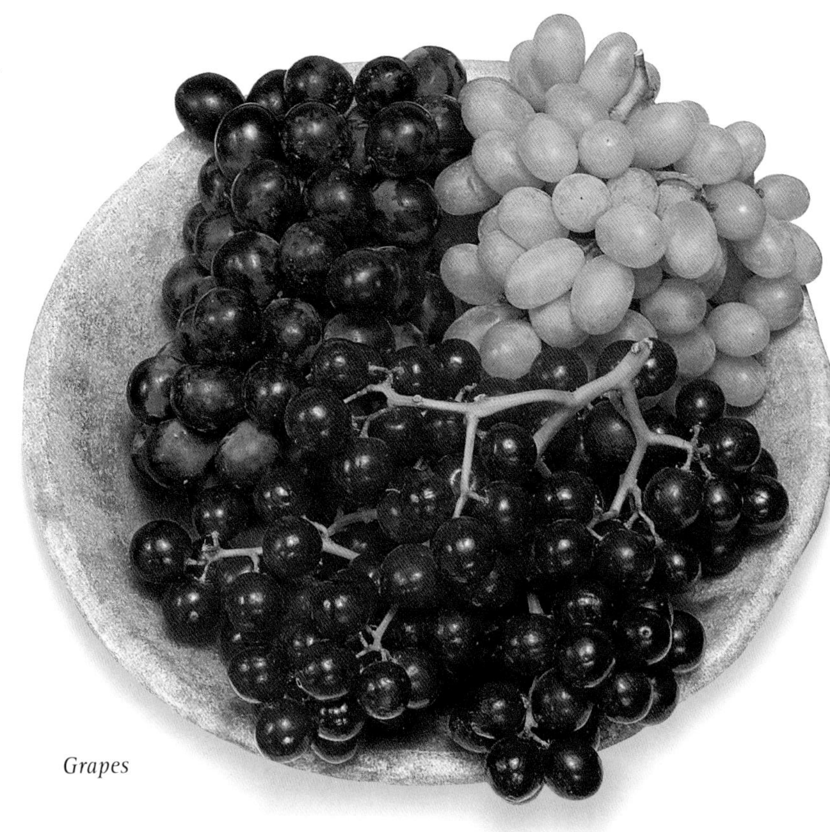

Grapes

Citrus Fruits

Characterized by thick skins that contain aromatic oils, citrus fruits have segmented flesh, which is extremely juicy. The flavors range from the sweetness of oranges to the tartness of lemons.

Citrus fruits are traditionally extolled for their vitamin C content. One orange provides around 90 mg, but kiwis and black currants are better sources. Don't discard the white pithy part of oranges; it is rich in antioxidants called flavonoids.

ORANGES

Blood, Navel, Seville, Tangerines, Satsumas, Clementines

Oranges come in three basic varieties: thin-skinned, thick-skinned and bitter. Thin-skinned oranges are ideal for juicing, while thick-skinned varieties make the best eating oranges. Bitter oranges such as Seville are used almost exclusively for making marmalade.

Blood oranges have orange skin with a blush of red and pockets of dark red (maroon) pigmented flesh. They are eaten fresh or used for juicing, in sauces or as a flavoring ingredient.

Navel oranges have a relatively smooth skin and are seedless. They are suitable for eating fresh or for juicing and may be candied.

GRAPES AND CITRUS FRUITS	*SUGAR(g)*	*NSP(g)*	*NAeq(mg)*	*Vit C(mg)*
Grapes, average *60 calories (portion 100g)*	15.40	0.70	0.20	3.00
Grapefruit, raw *24 calories (portion 80g)*	5.44	1.04	0.32	28.80
Oranges *59 calories (portion 160g)*	13.60	2.72	0.80	86.40
Lemons, whole *4 calories (portion 20g)*	0.64	–	0.06	11.60
Clementines *22 calories (portion 60g)*	5.22	0.72	0.24	32.40
Satsumas *25 calories (portion 70g)*	5.95	0.91	0.28	18.90

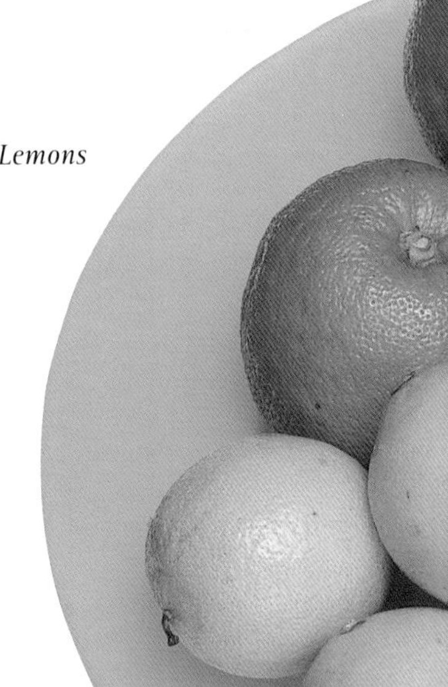

Lemons

Seville oranges have a sour flavor; they are used for marmalade.

Tangerines, satsumas and clementines have orange, lightly pebbled skin that is loosely attached to the fruit. Some varieties have many seeds. These fruits may be eaten fresh or used for juicing.

LEMONS AND LIMES

Lemons, Persian limes, Key limes

Lemons have a yellow-green to deep yellow skin, extremely tart flesh and numerous seeds. They are used for juicing and flavoring and the zest may be candied.

Popular in the U.S., and becoming more available in Europe are Persian and Key limes. Persian limes have dark green, smooth skin and tart, seedless flesh. They are used for juicing and flavoring and the zest may be candied. Key limes are light green and are used for juicing or flavoring.

GRAPEFRUITS

Pink, White, Ugli fruits

Grapefruit are juicy and tart-sweet with either yellow or pink flesh. Pink grapefruit is generally slightly sweeter than other varieties.

Pink grapefruit has yellow skin, possibly with a red blush. It has deep pink flesh, provides some of the carotenoid family of antioxidants and has a mellow, sweet-tart flavor.

White grapefruit has yellow skin and flesh, sometimes with a green tinge. Seedless varieties are available. It is eaten fresh and used for juicing and flavoring and the zest may be candied.

Ugli fruit is a cross between a grapefruit and a tangerine. It has wrinkled yellow-green skin and pink-yellow flesh and is seedless.

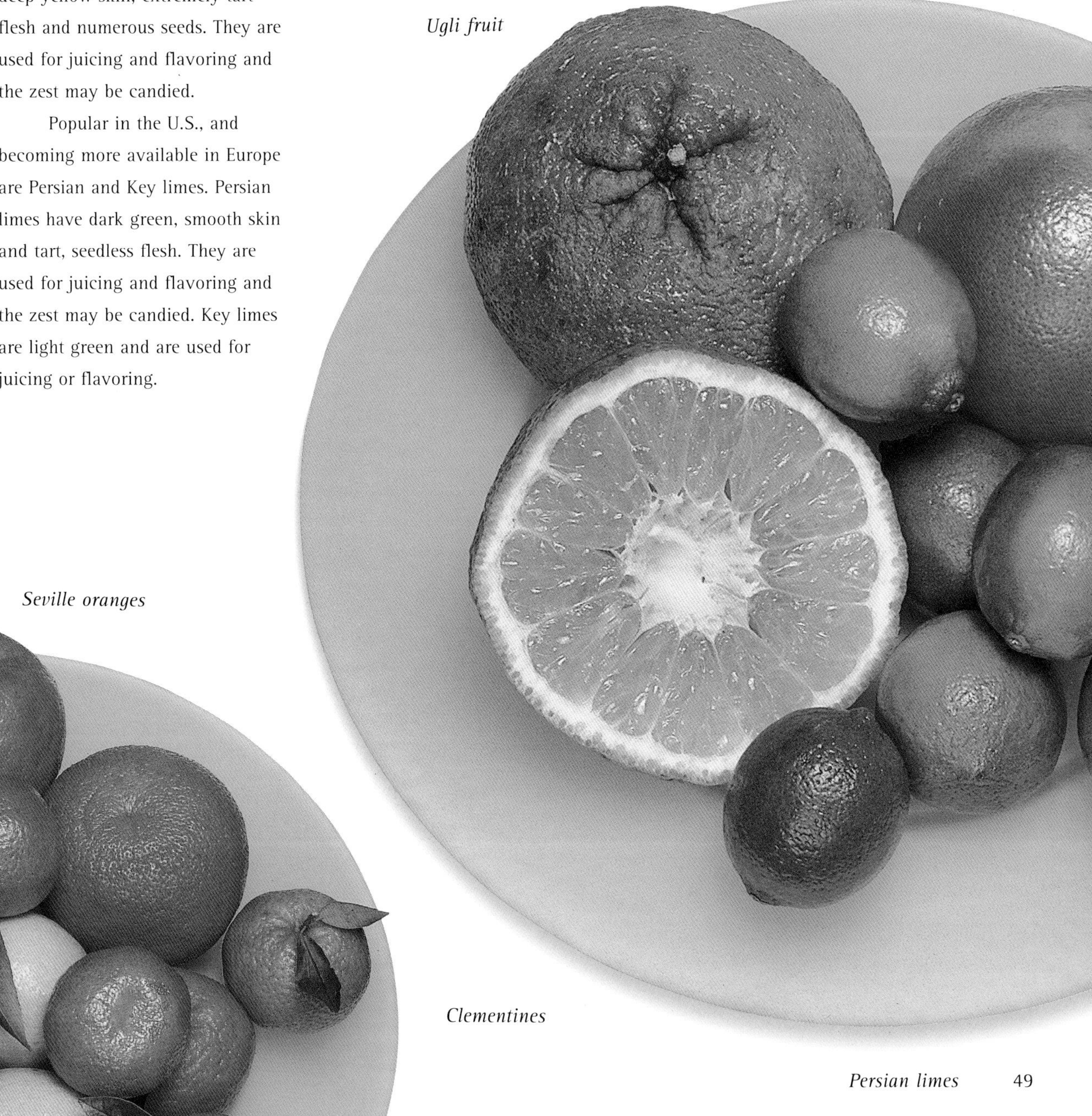

Pink grapefruit

Ugli fruit

Seville oranges

Clementines

Persian limes

Tropical and Exotic Fruits

A wide variety of fruits fall into this category, which is named for the general climatic conditions in which the fruits are grown. Bananas are the most common tropical fruits, but the choices are constantly expanding. Dates, figs, kiwis, mangoes, papayas, plantains, pomegranates and passion fruit also belong to this category.

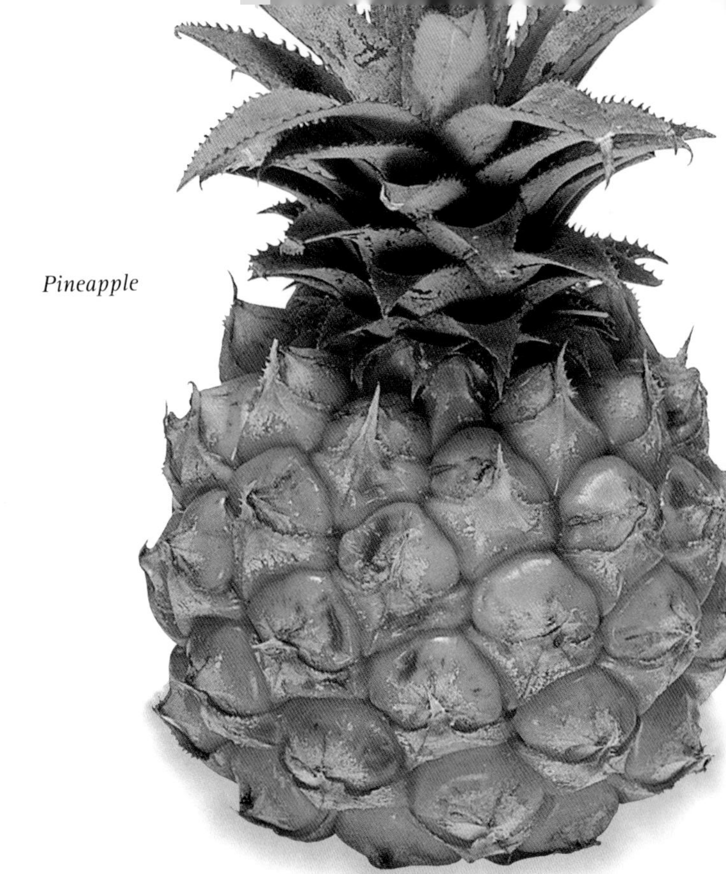

Pineapple

TROPICAL AND EXOTIC FRUITS

Bananas, Kiwis, Mangoes, Pineapples, Pomegranates, Star fruits

Bananas are picked green and allowed to ripen in transit. Sold in bunches, they are eaten fresh or used in cooking. Ripe bananas are rich in carbohydrates and, therefore, a good source of energy.

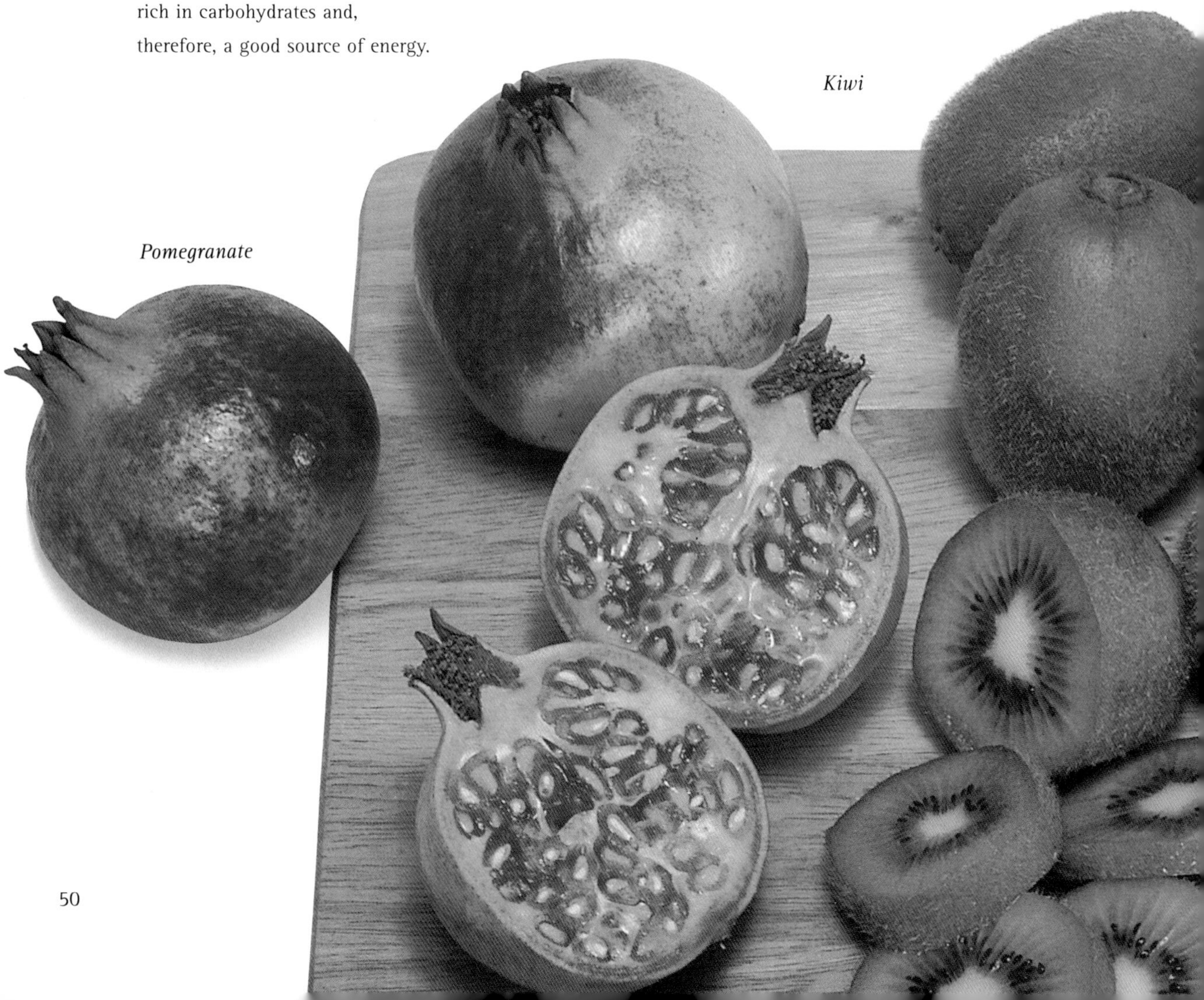

Kiwi

Pomegranate

However, they can be starchy and difficult to digest if under ripe.

Kiwi is a small oval fruit with brown hairy skin; the flesh is deep green and somewhat translucent with tiny, black edible seeds. Kiwi is very rich in vitamin C.

Mango is a carotenoid-rich, bottle-shaped fruit with skin that turns yellow as it ripens. It is used as a vegetable when green and as a fruit when ripe.

Pineapples should be picked fully mature. They are eaten fresh or grilled and are also available in canned forms, packed in syrup or natural juice. Pineapple contains natural digestive enzymes.

Pomegranate is a rounded brownish-pink fruit with a thick rind. The edible portion is the fleshy seeds found inside.

Star fruit, or carombola, is a deeply ridged fruit that ripens to yellow tipped with brown.

TROPICAL AND EXOTIC FRUITS	*SUGAR(g)*	*K(mg)*	*Vit C(mg)*	*Vit A(mcg)*
Mangoes, ripe, raw *86 calories (portion 150g)*	20.70	270.00	55.50	450.00
Kiwis *29 calories (portion 60g)*	6.18	174.00	35.40	3.60
Bananas *95 calories (portion 100g)*	20.90	400.00	11.00	3.00
Pomegranate *79 calories (portion 154g)*	18.17	369.60	20.02	7.70

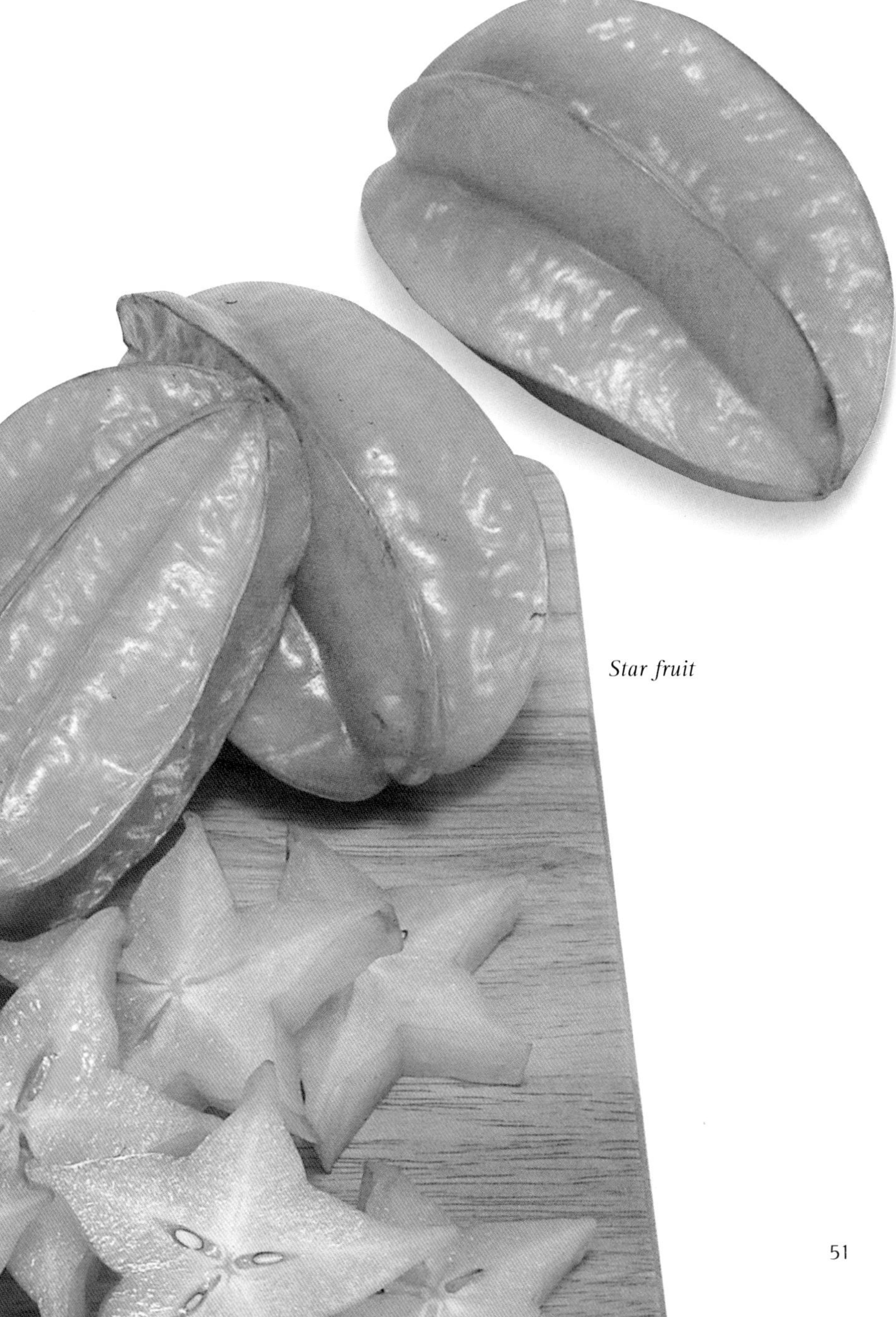

Star fruit

Melons

Fragrant and succulent, melons are available in many varieties. The main types include cantaloupes, watermelons, honeydew charentais and gallia.

Determining when a melon is ripe depends upon the type. Cantaloupe should have a "full slip," meaning that it grew away from the stem, leaving no rough edge. Other melons may become slightly soft at the stem end. Aroma is one of the best keys to determining ripeness; the biochemical changes in the fruit as it ripens strengthen the aroma.

All melons have a good supply of beta-carotene, which has been linked with lower rates of lung and other cancers.

HONEYDEW

Honeydew melon has green, juicy flesh and a velvety, even slightly sticky skin that is yellow with no greenish cast.

MELONS	*SUGAR(g)*	*K(mg)*	*Vit A(mcg)*	*WATER(g)*
Cantaloupe *29 calories (portion 150g)*	6.30	315.00	247.50	138.15
Gallia *36 calories (portion 150g)*	8.40	225.00	–	137.55
Honeydew *56 calories (portion 200g)*	13.20	420.00	16.00	184.40
Watermelon *62 calories (portion 200g)*	14.20	200.00	76.00	184.60

CANTALOUPE AND GALLIA

Cantaloupe and gallia melons have coarse netting, or veining, over the surface of their skins. Cantaloupes have smooth, orange, juicy, fragrant flesh. The gallia has green flesh. The smooth-skinned charentais also has orange flesh which is rich in beta-carotene.

WATERMELON

Watermelon is a large, often oblong-shaped melon with red or yellow flesh. There are some seedless varieties. It is available in mid- to late summer. Watermelons provide lycopene, the same anticancer factor found in tomatoes.

Honeydew melon

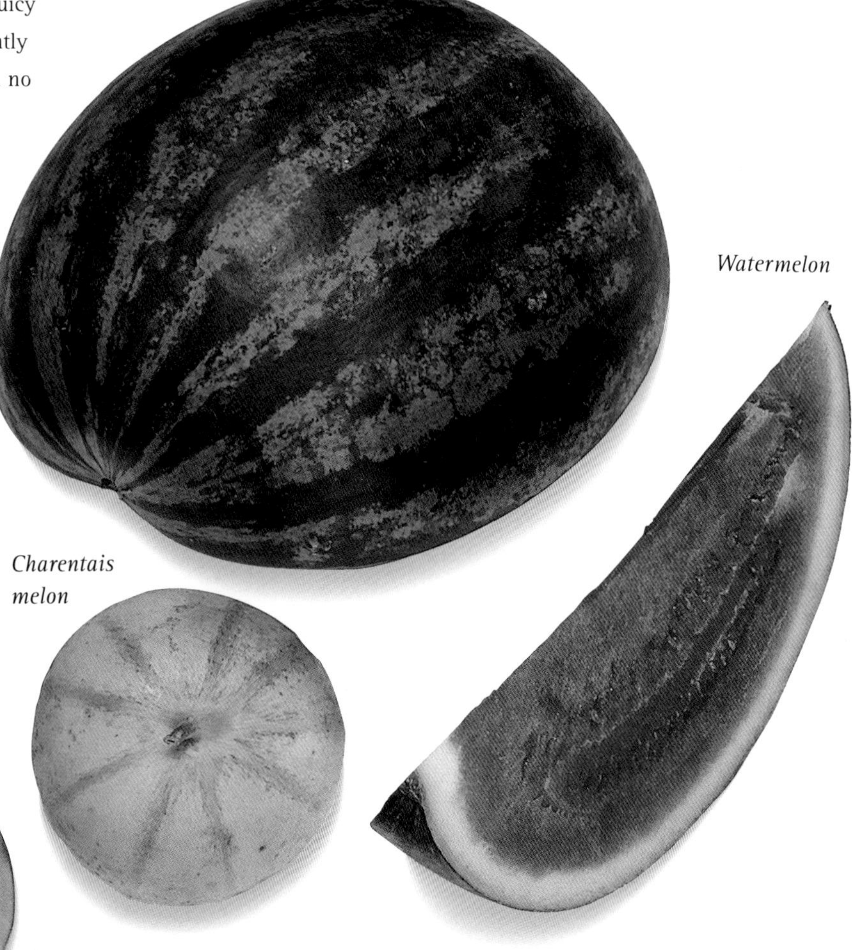

Watermelon

Charentais melon

Dried Fruits

Fruit that is grown to be dried is allowed to mature fully before it is harvested. Premium dried fruits (dried to a high level of moisture) may need refrigeration and have short shelf-lives. Traditionally, dried fruits are not as perishable as fresh ones, but they should be carefully stored in a cool, dry area. There is great variation in price and quality.

Dried fruits are a concentrated source of sugar. They are also good sources of iron—which helps prevent anemia—and magnesium, which is needed for energy release and a healthy nervous system.

A wide range of dried fruits is readily available, including the following: apples, apricots, bananas, blueberries, cherries, cranberries, currants, dates, figs, peaches, prunes, raisins, strawberries, golden raisins (sultanas).

DRIED FRUITS	*SUGAR(g)*	*NSP(g)*	*Ca(mg)*	*Fe(mg)*
Figs *45 calories (portion 20g)*	10.58	1.50	50.00	0.84
Apricots *15 calories (portion 8g)*	3.47	0.62	7.36	0.33
Golden raisins (sultanas) *66 calories (portion 24g)*	16.66	0.48	15.36	0.53
Raisins *82 calories (portion 30g)*	20.79	0.60	13.80	1.14
Dates *41 calories (portion 15g)*	10.20	0.60	6.75	0.19
Prunes *16 calories (portion 10g)*	3.84	0.65	3.80	0.29

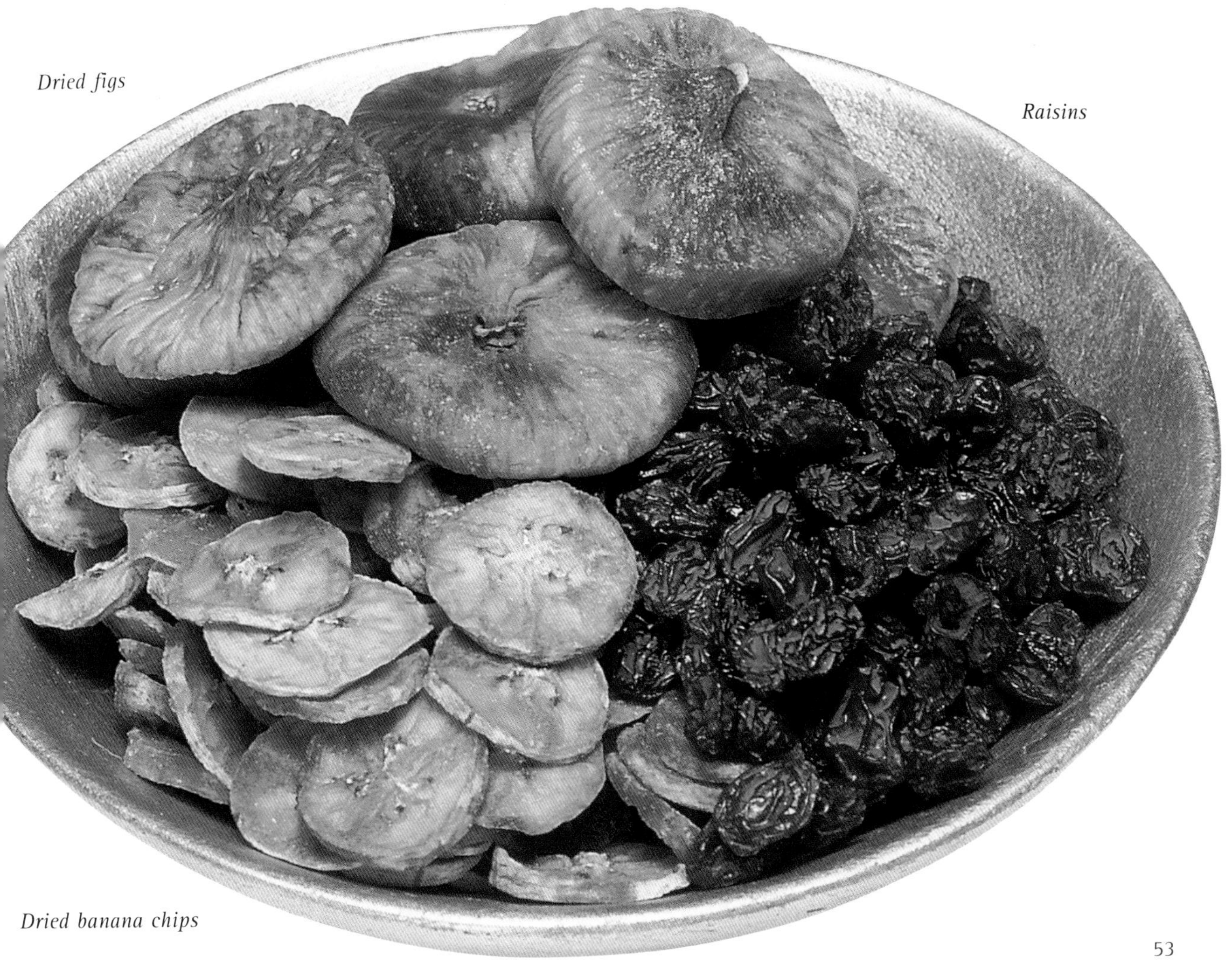

Dried figs

Raisins

Dried banana chips

Herbs

Herbs are the leaves of aromatic plants and are used primarily to add flavor to foods. They may be quite rich in nutrients, but in the small amounts usually used in cooking they are unlikely to make a significant contribution to the diet. Most herbs are available both fresh and dried, although some dry more successfully than others.

Aroma is a good indicator of quality in both fresh and dried herbs. The scent of herbs can be best tested by crumbling a few leaves and then smelling them. A weak or stale aroma indicates old, less potent herbs. Fresh herbs may also be judged by appearance. They should have good color (usually green), fresh-looking leaves and stems, and no wilting, brown spots, sunburn or pest damage.

Fresh herbs should be minced, chopped or cut into fine shreds just before they are needed. They are usually added to a dish toward the end of the cooking time to prevent their flavor from being lost. Dried herbs are usually added early in the process. For uncooked preparations, fresh herbs should be added well before serving to give them a chance to blend with the other elements.

Herbs should be stored wrapped loosely in damp paper or cloth. If desired, the wrapped herbs may be placed in plastic bags and refrigerated to help retain freshness.

The following section presents a selection of the hundreds of herbs and spices available.

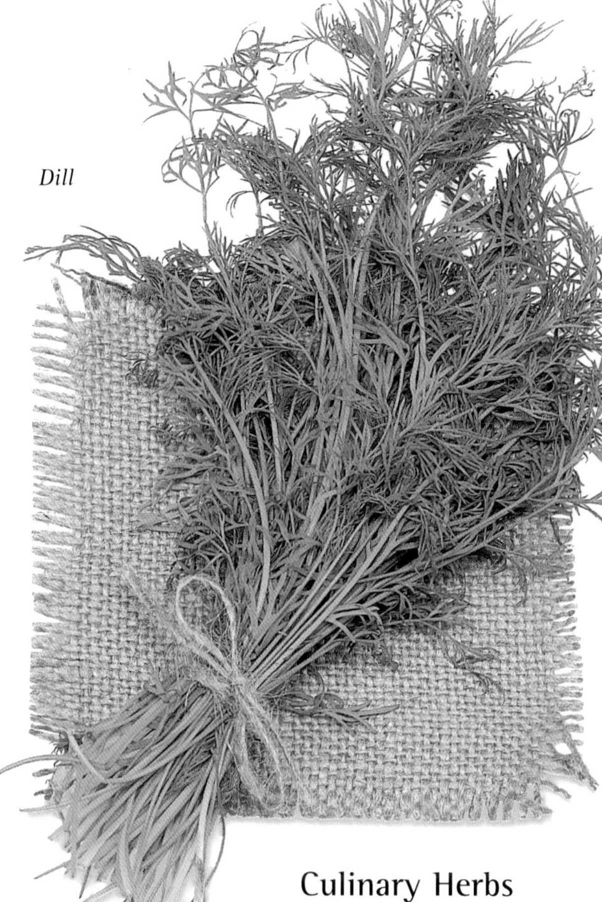

Dill

Thyme

Culinary Herbs

Herbs are the perfect way to add flavor to food. They can give subtle or strong accents to soups, sauces, stews and casseroles. Culinary herbs also make a good, healthy alternative to salt, which contains sodium and may raise blood pressure.

CILANTRO (coriander)

Cilantro (coriander) looks similar to parsley but has larger leaves and a pronounced, unique flavor.

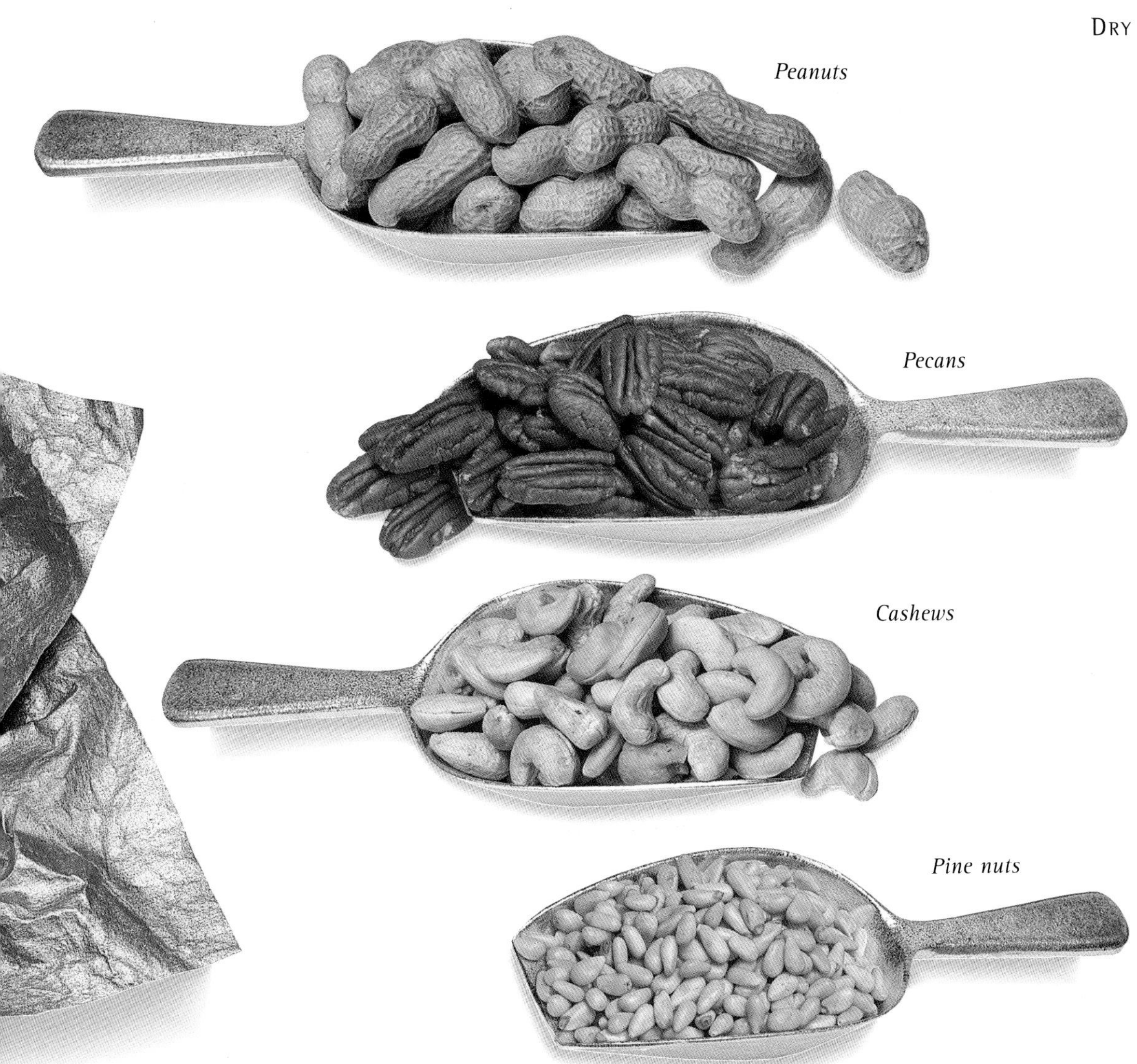

available whole or as pastes and should be stored in the same way as nuts. Sunflower seeds are a particularly rich source of the anti-oxidant vitamin E, which may help prevent heart disease and cancer.

NUTS

Peanuts, Pecans, Cashews, Pine, Brazil, Chestnuts

Nuts have a number of culinary uses, adding a distinctive flavor and texture to dishes. They are relatively expensive and should be stored carefully to prevent them from becoming rancid. Nuts that have not been roasted or shelled will keep longer. Shelled nuts may be stored in the freezer or in a cooler (crisper) drawer, if space allows. In any case, they should be stored in a cool, dry, well-ventilated area and checked periodically to be sure they are still fresh.

Brazil nuts are very high in selenium, an antioxidant that has been associated with a lowered risk of cancer. Chestnuts are the only nuts that are not high in fat.

NUTS AND SEEDS *all values per 100g, average portion = 13g*	*PROT(g)*	*FAT(g)*	*CHO(g)*	*NSP(g)*
Almonds *612 calories*	21.10	55.80	6.90	7.40
Brazil nuts *682 calories*	14.10	68.20	3.10	4.30
Cashew nuts *573 calories*	17.70	48.20	18.10	3.20
Peanuts, plain *564 calories*	25.60	46.10	12.50	6.20
Coconut, desiccated *604 calories*	5.60	62.00	6.40	13.70
Sesame seeds *598 calories*	18.20	58.00	0.90	7.90

Red kidney beans

Flageolet beans

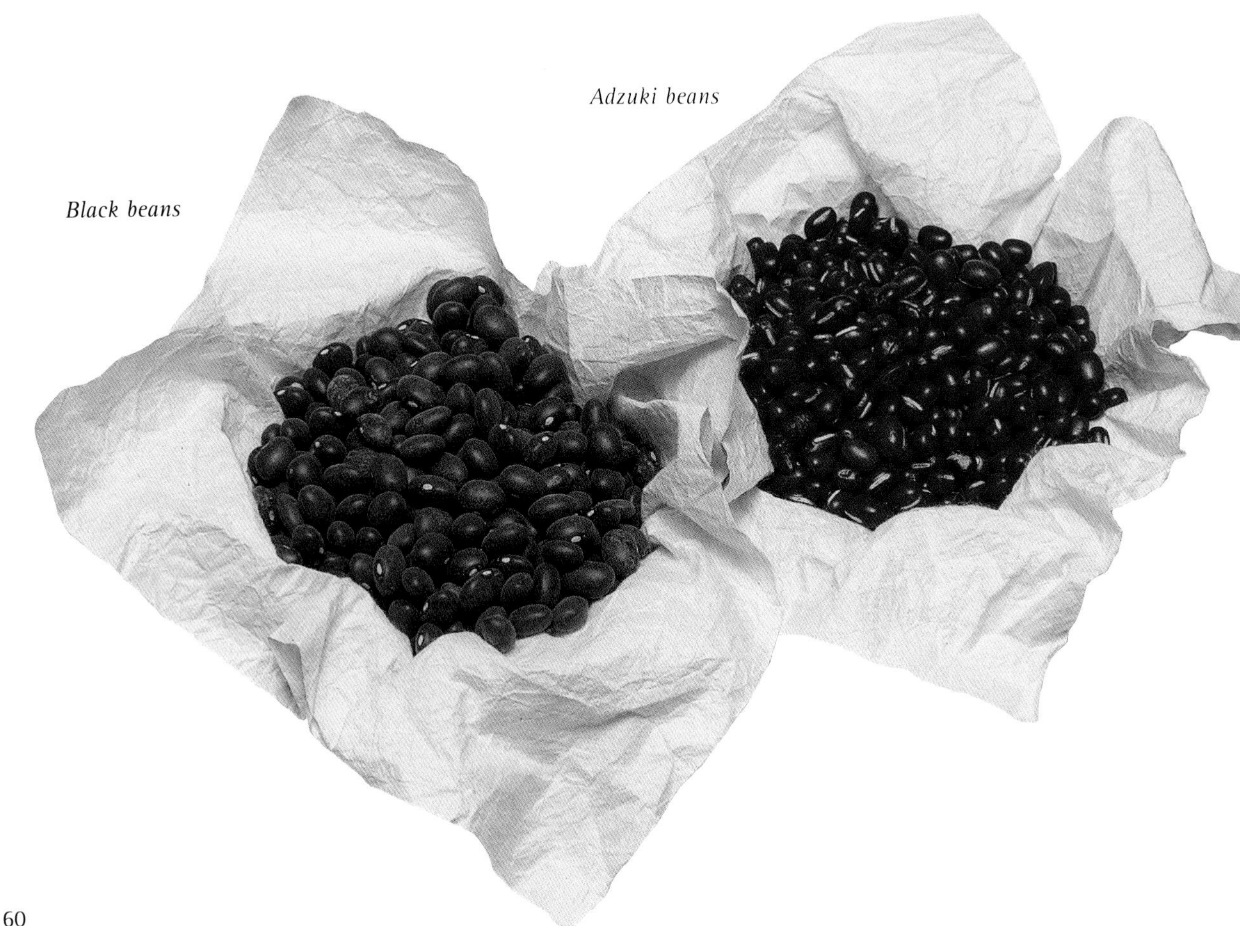

Adzuki beans

Black beans

BEANS AND BEAN PRODUCTS *all values per 100g*	*CHO(g)*	*PROT(g)*	*FAT(g)*	*NSP(g)*
Adzuki beans, dried, boiled in unsalted water *123 calories*	22.50	9.30	0.20	5.50
Black-eyed peas, dried, boiled in unsalted water *116 calories*	19.90	8.80	0.70	3.50
Mung beans, dried, boiled in unsalted water *91 calories*	15.30	7.60	0.40	3.00
Soybeans, dried, boiled in unsalted water *142 calories*	5.10	14.00	7.30	6.10
Tofu, soybean product, steamed *73 calories*	0.70	8.10	4.20	–

Dried Legumes

Legumes or pulses (beans, peas and lentils) are the seeds from pod-producing plants and are a nutritious meat alternative as they are a good source of protein. They are rich in fiber, including soluble fiber, which helps maintain healthy cholesterol levels.

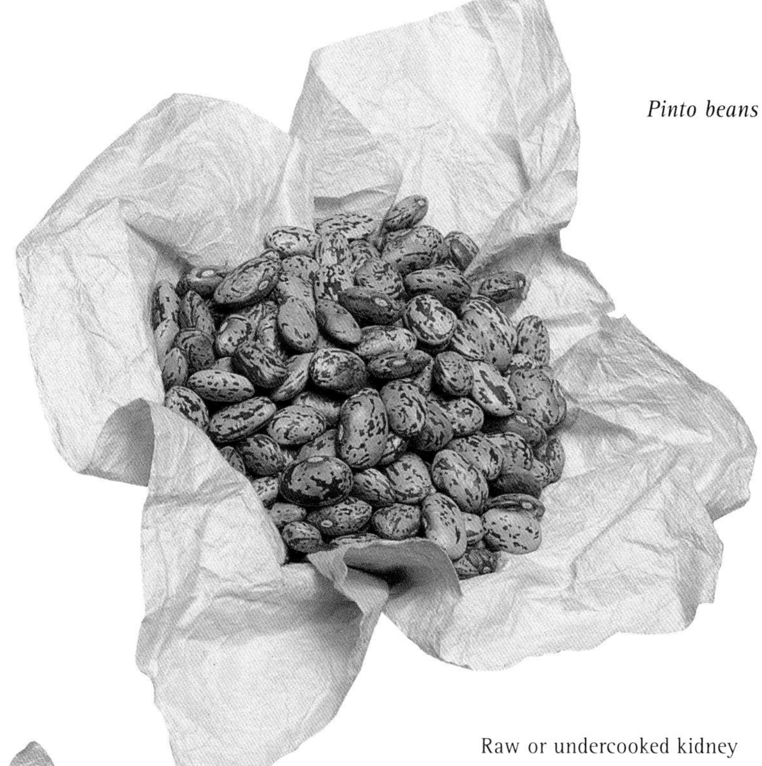

Pinto beans

BEANS

Kidney beans, Soybeans, Flageolet beans, Pinto beans, Haricot beans, Adzuki beans, Black beans

Store dried beans in a cool, dry, well-ventilated area. Before using, discard any that appear moldy, damp or wrinkled. Note that old beans take longer to cook.

Haricot beans

Raw or undercooked kidney beans may cause severe food poisoning. Be sure to boil kidney beans rapidly for 15 minutes to make them safe.

Soybeans are exceptional in that they have an almost perfect amino acid profile, which is similar to that of animal protein. They also contain traces of phytoestrogens, which may be important in preventing breast cancer.

All other beans (haricot, black, flageolet, pinto and adzuki) are also good sources of protein and provide B vitamins essential for a healthy nervous system.

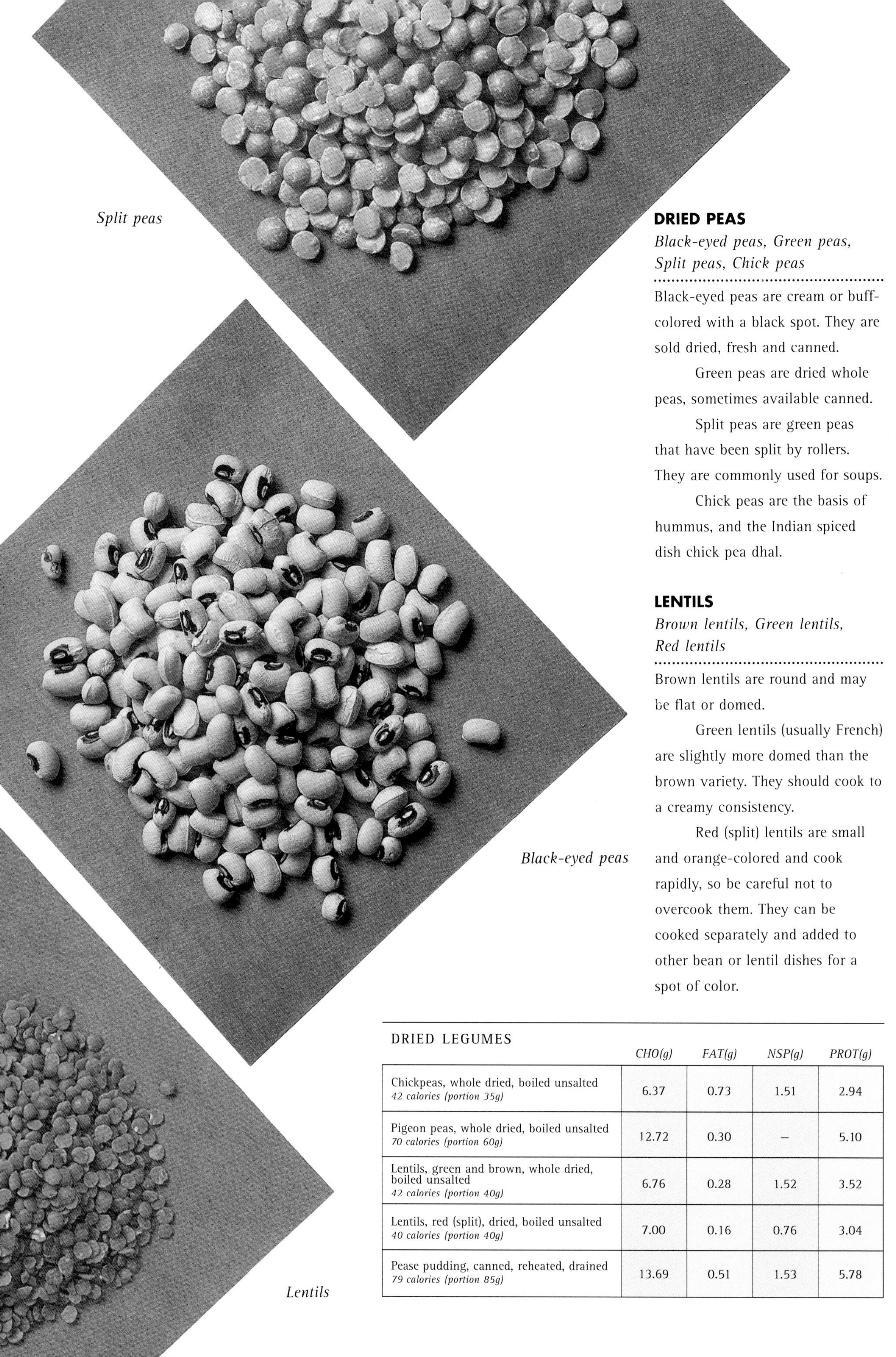

Split peas

Black-eyed peas

Lentils

DRIED PEAS

Black-eyed peas, Green peas, Split peas, Chick peas

Black-eyed peas are cream or buff-colored with a black spot. They are sold dried, fresh and canned.

Green peas are dried whole peas, sometimes available canned.

Split peas are green peas that have been split by rollers. They are commonly used for soups.

Chick peas are the basis of hummus, and the Indian spiced dish chick pea dhal.

LENTILS

Brown lentils, Green lentils, Red lentils

Brown lentils are round and may be flat or domed.

Green lentils (usually French) are slightly more domed than the brown variety. They should cook to a creamy consistency.

Red (split) lentils are small and orange-colored and cook rapidly, so be careful not to overcook them. They can be cooked separately and added to other bean or lentil dishes for a spot of color.

DRIED LEGUMES	CHO(g)	FAT(g)	NSP(g)	PROT(g)
Chickpeas, whole dried, boiled unsalted *42 calories (portion 35g)*	6.37	0.73	1.51	2.94
Pigeon peas, whole dried, boiled unsalted *70 calories (portion 60g)*	12.72	0.30	–	5.10
Lentils, green and brown, whole dried, boiled unsalted *42 calories (portion 40g)*	6.76	0.28	1.52	3.52
Lentils, red (split), dried, boiled unsalted *40 calories (portion 40g)*	7.00	0.16	0.76	3.04
Pease pudding, canned, reheated, drained *79 calories (portion 85g)*	13.69	0.51	1.53	5.78

Grains

Grains are of great significance in many cuisines. Wheat and corn are particularly important in Western countries, while rice, barley or oats may be favored in other parts of the world.

Many Western societies have so severely restricted the quantities of whole, unrefined grains included in a "typical" diet that traditional methods of preparing and serving grains have been virtually lost to a whole generation of cooks. It is worth relearning these methods because the health benefits of a diet based on grains, cereals, bread and pasta are being reaffirmed wherever we look. In fact, nutritionists now advise that all meals should be based on starches and carbohydrates.

Whole grains tend to have a shorter lifespan than milled grains, so they should be purchased in amounts that can be used over a period of two to three weeks.

The less refined the grain, the higher the nutritional value, although in both the U.S. and U.K. certain nutrients such as iron and thiamin (vitamin B_1) are added back to white flour. In addition to complex carbohydrates, whole grains provide B vitamins for energy release, the antioxidant vitamin E, protein and fiber.

RICE

Rice is available in many different varieties. Short-grain varietiess tend to be stickier than long-grain. Brown rice retains some of the bran and the germ. White rice has usually been polished and in the process loses a high proportion of its B vitamins. Special rices, such as basmati, wehani, arborio or sticky rice, may be suggested by specific recipes. Wild rice is a grass rather than a grain.

WHOLE GRAINS

Wheat grains, Oats, Corn, Quinoa, Millet, Flaked wheats, Wheat germ, Pearl barley

Whole wheat grains take a long time to cook, and are often soaked before simmering or boiling. They may be sprouted and added to breads, salads or sandwiches. Cracked wheat, or bulgur, can be prepared in the same way as rice and served as a hot side dish, a stuffing or a cold salad. Flaked wheat is the basis of many breakfast cereals.

Oats are similar to wheat grains in appearance and handling requirements. A regular daily consumption of oats can help lower cholesterol levels. The effect is due to a large amount of soluble fiber in oats, which binds cholesterol and prevents it from being absorbed by the intestines.

Quinoa is an old South American grain that has recently been rediscovered. It is prepared in the same way as rice.

Whole dried corn is known as hominy; when treated with lye, it may be referred to as pozole. Hominy is available dried or canned.

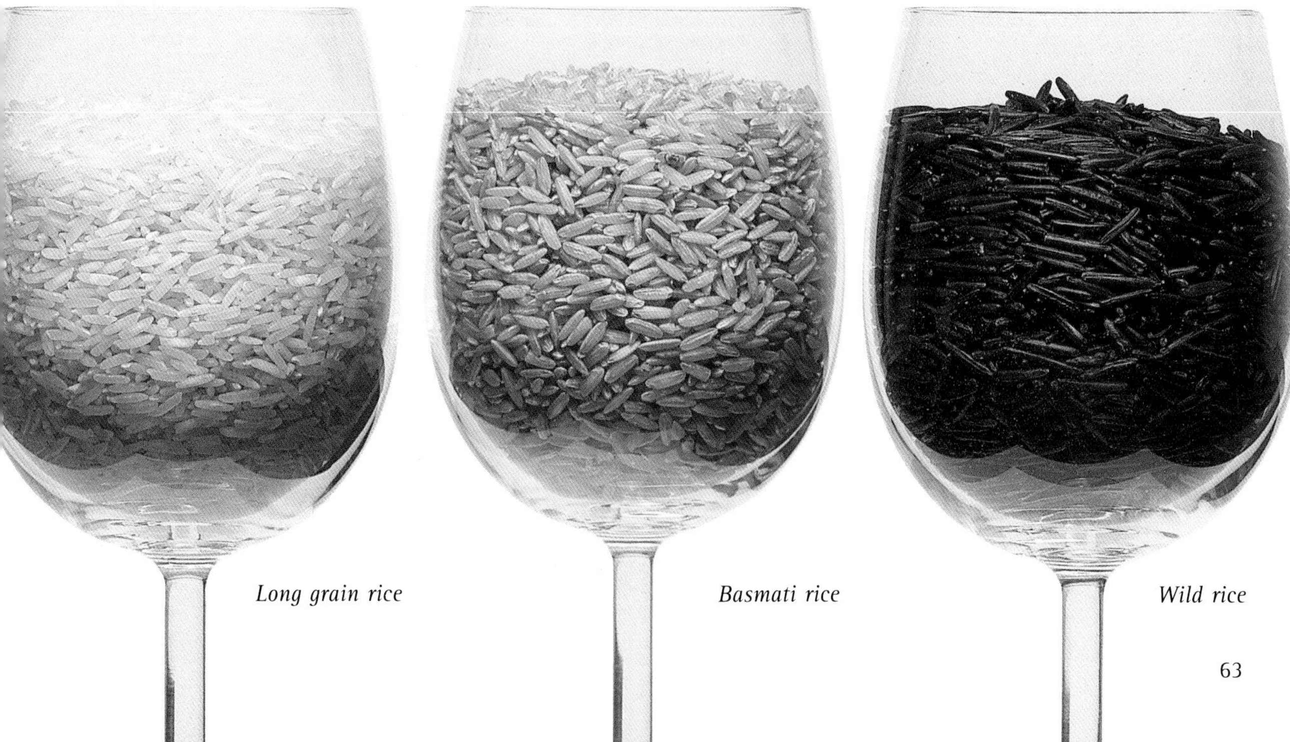

Long grain rice *Basmati rice* *Wild rice*

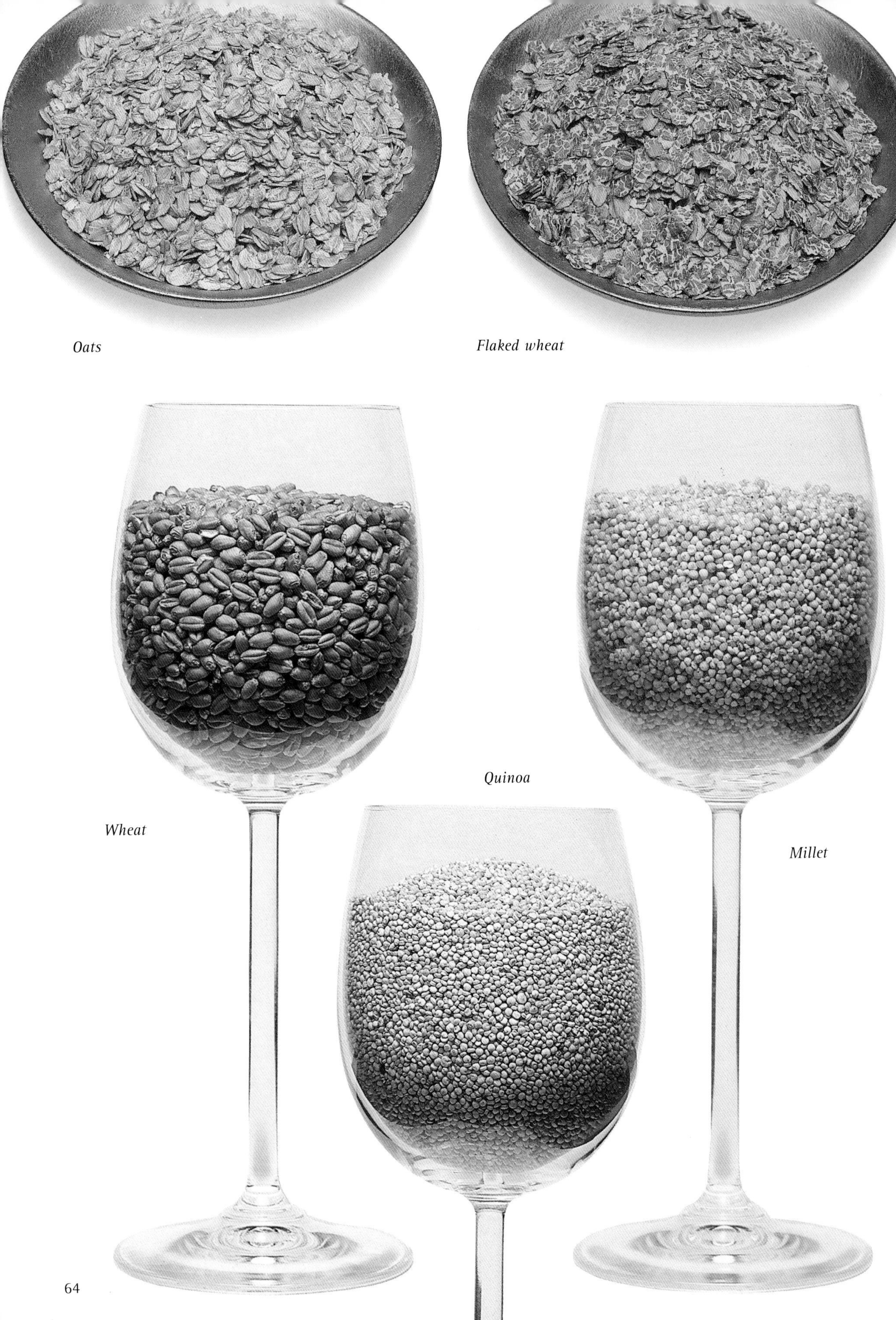

Oats

Flaked wheat

Wheat

Quinoa

Millet

Wheat germ is the "embryo" of the wheat grain and is rich in many nutrients including vitamin E.

Pearly barley—dehulled and polished barley grains—makes a wholesome addition to soups and is also used to make beverages.

Millet is not widely popular but holds a special place in African cuisines. It is a round grain with a deep yellow color and subtle flavor.

Rye and buckwheat are associated with the cuisines of northern and eastern Europe. These brown grains have a distinctive aroma and flavor. Both are ground into flour.

GRAINS, CEREALS AND MEALS *all values per 100g*	*CHO(g)*	*NSP(mg)*	*B_1(mg)*	*NAeq(mg)*
Bulgur wheat *353 calories*	76.30	–	0.48	6.10
Rice, brown, boiled *141 calories*	32.10	0.80	0.14	1.90
Oatmeal, quick cooked, raw *375 calories*	66.00	7.10	0.90	3.40
Cornmeal, unsifted *353 calories*	71.50	–	0.30	2.80
Quinoa *309 calories*	55.70	–	0.20	4.80
Millet flour *354 calories*	75.40	–	0.68	2.80

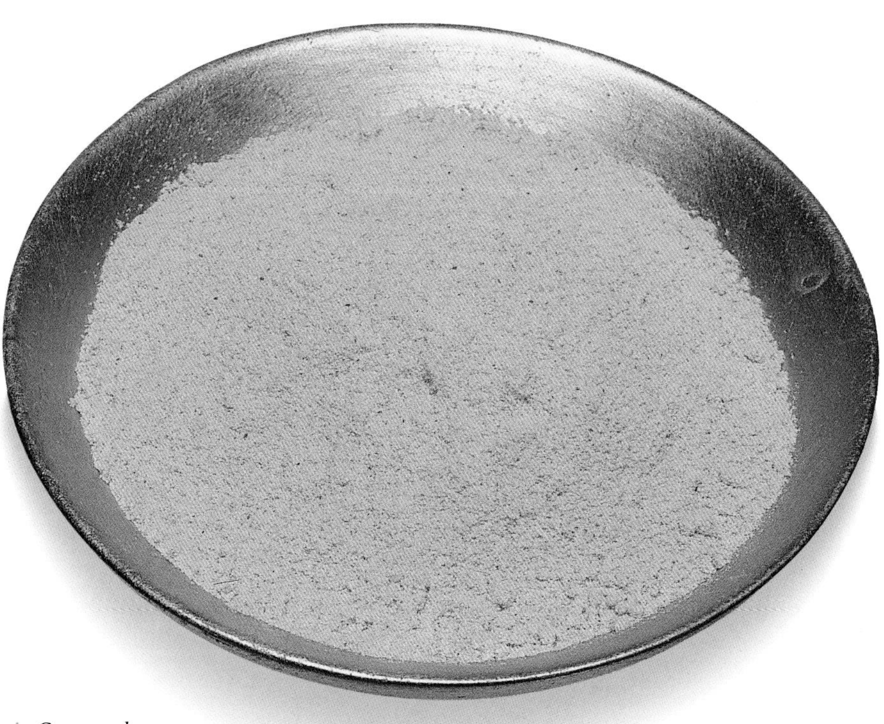

Cornmeal

Cereals and Meals

When whole grains are milled, they are essentially crushed into successively smaller particles. Various methods are used for milling: for example, crushing between metal rollers, grinding between stones or cutting with steel blades in an action similar to that of a food processor. Grains ground between stones are called "stone-ground"; these may be preferred in some cases because they retain more of their nutritive value because of the lower temperature used in processing.

Milled grains that are broken into coarse particles may be referred to as "cracked." If milled again, meals and cereals (cornmeal, farina, cream of rice) are formed. Finally, the grain may be ground into a fine powder, known as flour.

INGREDIENT PRODUCT: BREADS	*CHO(g)*	*NSP(g)*	*Ca(mg)*	*Fe(mg)*
Whole wheat (wholemeal) bread *77 calories (portion 36g)*	14.98	2.09	19.44	0.97
White bread *85 calories (portion 36g)*	17.75	0.54	39.60	0.58
Chapatis, made without fat *111 calories (portion 55g)*	24.03	–	33.00	1.15
Naan bread *538 calories (portion 160g)*	80.16	3.04	256.00	2.08
Pumpernickel bread *72 calories (portion 33g)*	15.11	2.47	26.40	0.82
Pitta bread, white *199 calories (portion 75g)*	43.43	1.65	68.25	1.28

FLOURS

Wheat flours are available in the following forms: cake/pastry, graham/whole wheat, semolina (whole) and unbleached.

Other flours that can be purchased in specialty shops include: oat, pumpernickel, rice and rye.

The following flours are used as thickeners: arrowroot, cornstarch (corn flour) and tapioca (the pearl form of tapioca is also used to prepare desserts).

FLOUR AND PASTA *all values per 100g*	*CHO(g)*	*NSP(g)*	*B_1(mg)*	*NAeq(mg)*
Wheat flour, whole wheat (wholemeal) *310 calories*	63.90	9.00	0.47	8.20
Corn flour *354 calories*	92.00	0.10	–	0.10
Wheat flour, white, all-purpose (plain) *341 calories*	77.70	3.10	0.31	3.60
Spaghetti, regular, boiled *104 calories*	22.20	1.20	0.01	1.20
Noodles, plain, boiled *62 calories*	13.00	0.70	0.02	0.80
Noodles, egg, boiled *62 calories*	13.00	0.60	0.01	0.70

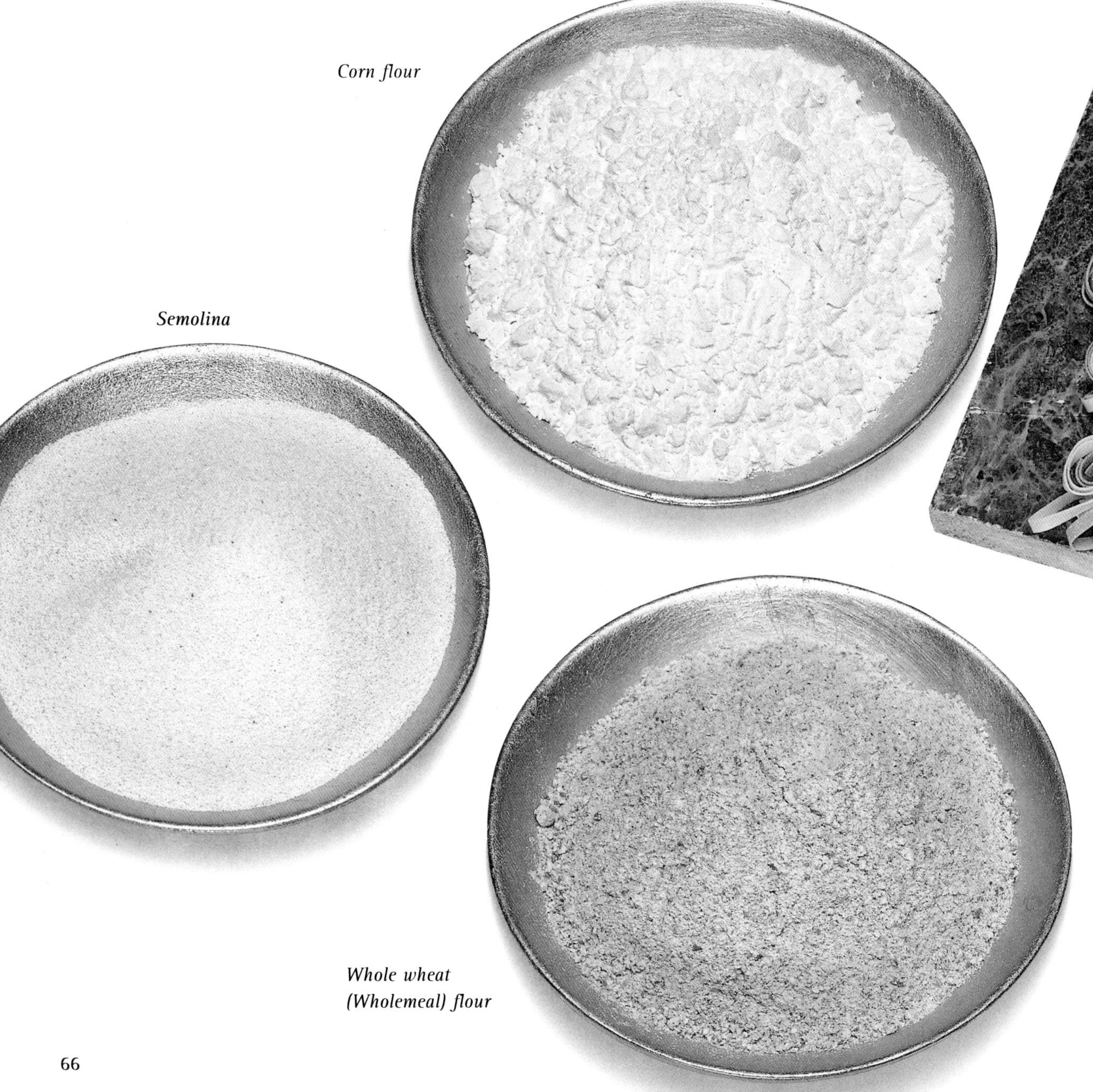

Corn flour

Semolina

Whole wheat (Wholemeal) flour

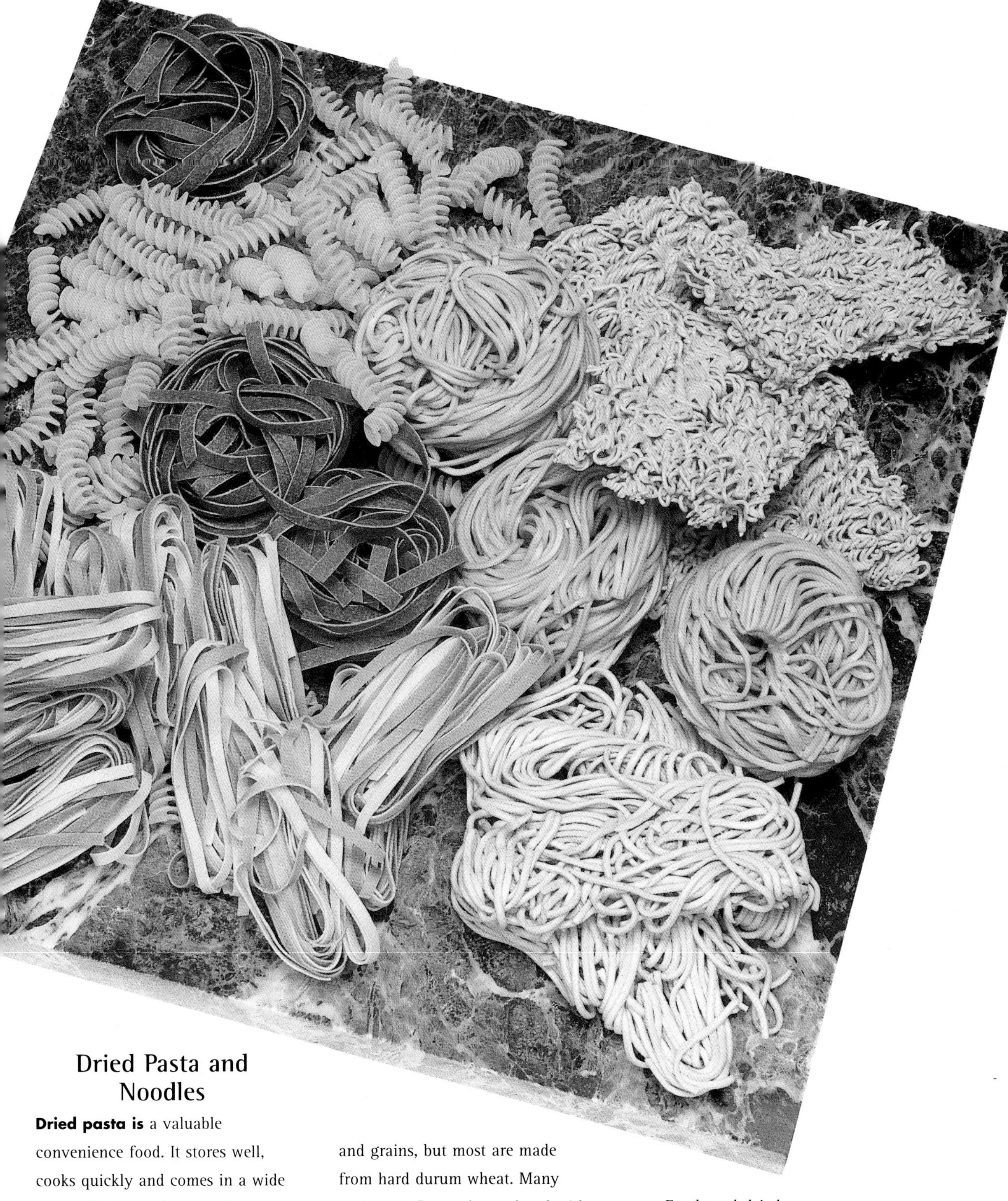

Fresh and dried pasta and noodles

Dried Pasta and Noodles

Dried pasta is a valuable convenience food. It stores well, cooks quickly and comes in a wide array of shapes, sizes and flavors. This range provides a base for a number of preparations, from simple spaghetti dishes to Oriental and Middle Eastern specialties.

Pasta and noodles are made from a number of different flours and grains, but most are made from hard durum wheat. Many pastas are flavored or colored with vegetables such as spinach, peppers and tomatoes. Pasta has a stodgy image, but it is not in itself fattening—it is the rich sauces with which it is often served that pile on the calories.

Savory and Sweet

As well as judicious use of fats and oils, most diets include small amounts of savory and sweet condiments of varying nutritional value. These help to overcome any blandness that may otherwise make a healthy diet unpalatable. Vinegars, mustards and relishes can add flavor with the minimum of calories: Sugars, jams and jellies also add some culinary excitement at the other end of the taste spectrum. However as with shortenings and oils, too much sugar in the diet is undesirable.

Think of all those savory and sweet culinary items that turn your food from acceptable to exciting. Many of them have little nutritional value and should only be used in moderation. But what pantry would be complete without items such as oil, vinegar, relishes and jellies? The secret is to buy wisely and use such items with restraint and care.

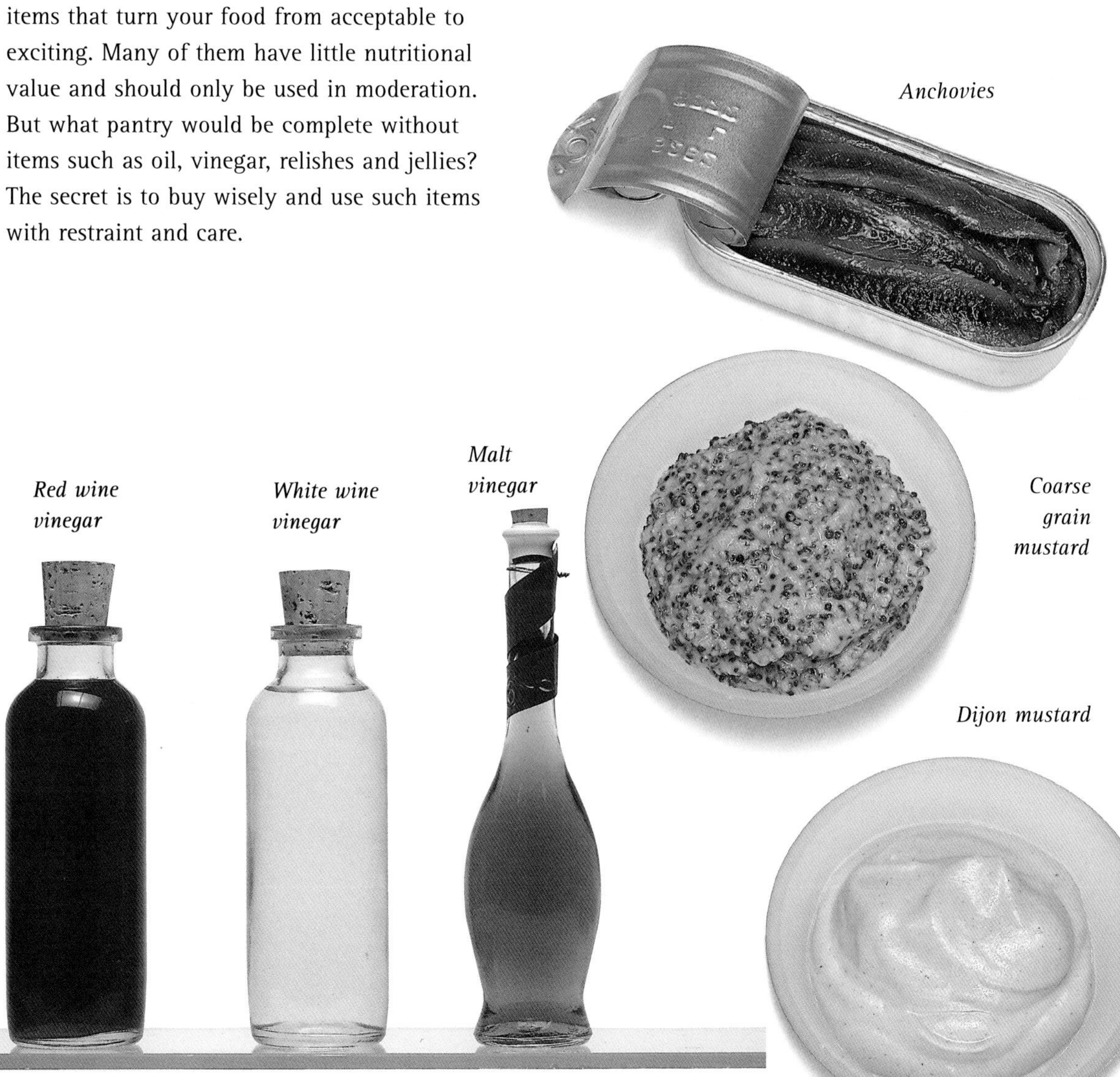

Anchovies

Coarse grain mustard

Dijon mustard

Red wine vinegar

White wine vinegar

Malt vinegar

Savory Condiments

There are a variety of savory condiments that can be used instead of salt and pepper. Some provide moisture, texture and color as well as flavor.

VINEGAR

Vinegar is known chemically as acetic acid. It adds piquancy to oily dishes (such as the traditional British fish and chips) and is a major ingredient of vinaigrette-type dressings, marinades and pickles. Malt vinegar is an all-purpose, quite strongly flavored vinegar; wine vinegar and cider vinegar are more delicately flavored for use in more subtle dishes. One specialist vinegar which can be highly expensive, is balsamic vinegar. Vinegar has no nutritional value and is virtually calorie free.

ANCHOVIES

Anchovies are tiny, very fatty fishes that are cured in a way that removes most of the fat through pressure and fermentation. They are then usually filleted, brined and sold in jars or cans. Anchovies have a strong flavor and are used in canapes, pizzas, anchovy butter and salad Nicoise.

RELISHES

Relishes are usually added to "spice" up burgers and other meat dishes. Some can be filled with additives and flavors and high in fat. However, tomato ketchup is a rich source of a carotenoid called lycopene and is fat-free.

SALSAS

Salsas are normally tomato or chili-based dips. They are generally healthier than many relishes and cheese-based dips. They are traditionally eaten with tortillas or crudites.

MUSTARD

(Dijon, English, American)

Mustard is a condiment produced from the seeds of three different plants of the Cruciferae family. Although most mustards are thought of as hot, English mustard is one of only a few that are really fiery. Dijon mustard is a popular French mustard ideal for flavoring beef, and American mustard is mild and an excellent accompaniment to hot dogs.

OLIVES

(Green, black)

Olives are rich in monounsaturated fatty acids that can help lower cholesterol levels. Black olives are simply green olives ripened. Some olives are stoned, stuffed and eaten as canapes or with pasta dishes.

VINEGARS AND SAVORY CONDIMENTS

	FAT(g)	SFA(g)	Na(mg)	CHOL(mg)
Vinegar *1 calories (portion 5g)*	0.00	0.00	0.25	0.00
Tomato ketchup *23 calories (portion 20g)*	0.02	–	326.00	0.00
Mustard, coarse (wholegrain) *20 calories (portion 14g)*	1.43	0.08	226.80	0.00
Chutney, mango, sweet *19 calories (portion 10g)*	0.01	–	130.00	0.00

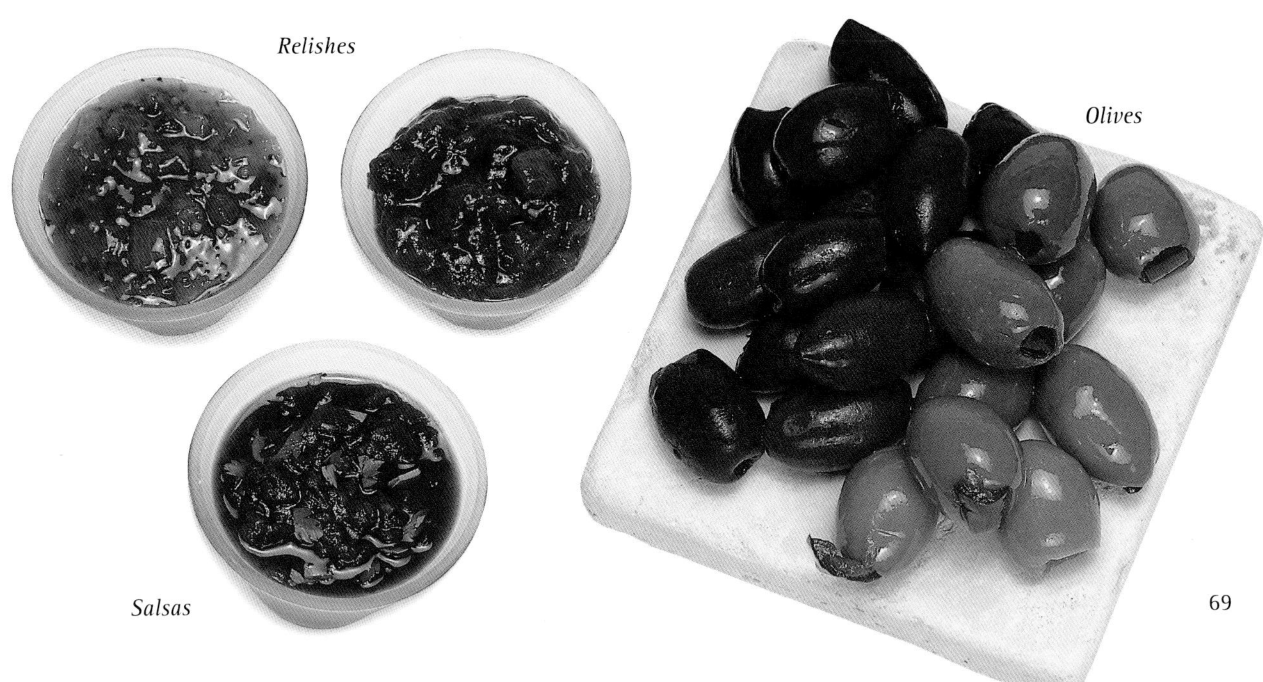

Relishes

Olives

Salsas

Oils and Shortenings (solid fats)

Oils are produced by pressing foods high in fat such as olives, nuts, corn, avocados and soybeans. The oil may then be filtered, clarified or hydrogenated (hardened) in order to produce a fat that has the appropriate characteristics for its intended use.

The hydrogenation process causes the oil to remain solid at room temperature and converts the unsaturated fatty acids of vegetable oils into more harmful saturated fats that can raise blood cholesterol and clog the arteries. Vegetable shortening (solid fat) is made from vegetable oil; those without this label may contain animal fats.

Although several different oils and shortenings (solid fats) are required in every kitchen, we should make an effort to consume less of them because excess fat is known to lead to heart disease, obesity and some cancers. Oils for salads and other cold dishes should be of the best possible quality, with a perfectly fresh flavor. First pressings of olive oil or nut oils are often chosen for these purposes because of their delicate flavors.

Cooking oils should have a neutral flavor; those used for frying should also have a high smoking point. Shortenings (solid fats) used for baking should also be neutral in flavor.

Oils should be stored in a dry place away from extremes of heat and light. Shortenings (solid fats) should be refrigerated.

Mayonnaise

OLIVE OIL

Try to use olive oil in place of other oils because it contains a high level of monounsaturated fats, which help improve the balance of cholesterol in the blood.

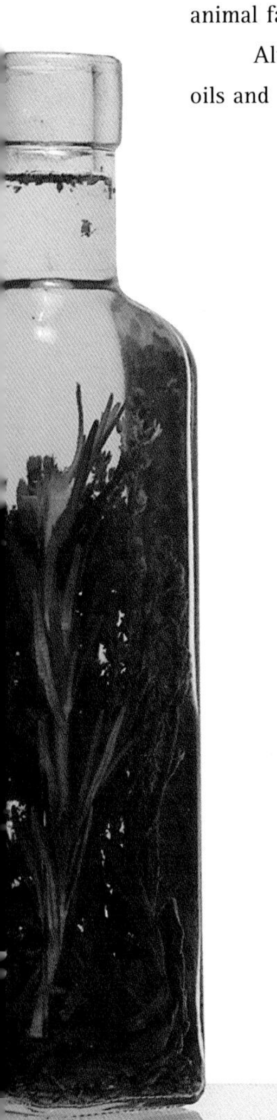

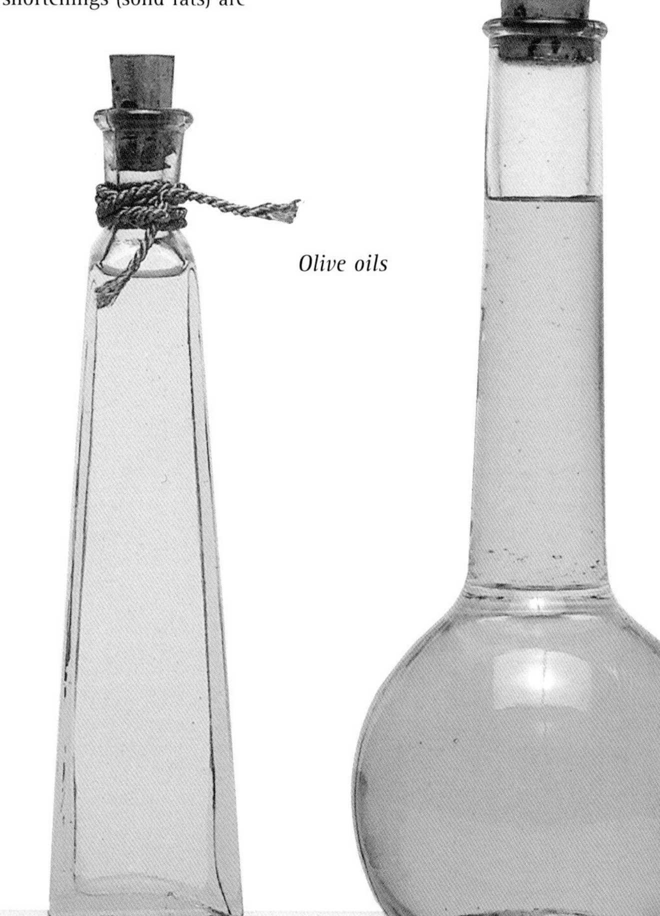

Olive oils

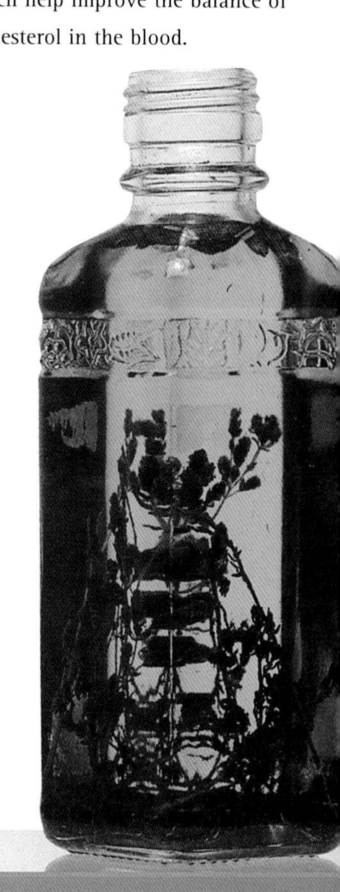

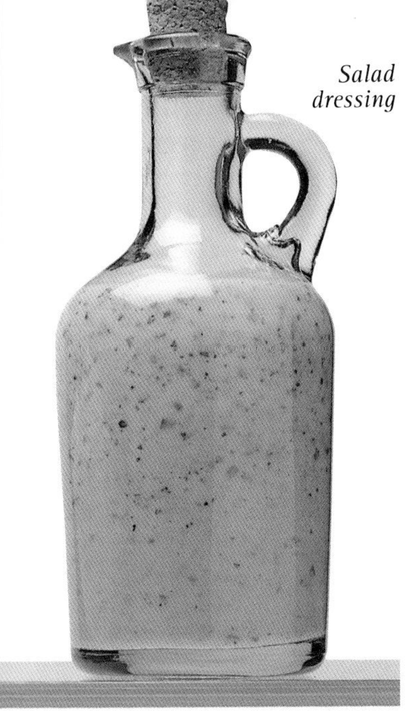
Salad dressing

FATS AND OILS *all values per 100g unless otherwise stated*	FAT(g)	PUFA(g)	MUFA(g)	SFA(g)
Olive oil *899 calories*	99.90	8.20	73.00	14.30
Butter *737 calories*	81.70	2.70	20.00	54.30
Low-fat spread *390 calories*	40.50	9.90	17.60	11.20
Very low-fat spread (20–25% fat, not polyunsaturated) *247 calories*	23.80	4.80	11.90	6.20
Mayonnaise *207 calories (portion 30g)*	22.68	–	–	3.33
Dressing, French *69 calories (portion 15g)*	7.41	–	–	–

VEGETABLE OILS

Oils made from such things as sunflower seeds, corn, peanuts, rapeseed (canola) and sesame seeds are usually high in polyunsaturated fats, so using them can help to keep down cholesterol levels. Avoid coconut oil and palm oil because they are high in saturated fats.

MARGARINE

Margarine has the same fat content as butter, and may be highly saturated if hydrogenated. Using low-fat spreads instead of butter or margarine can significantly reduce the fat content of your diet.

MAYONNAISE AND SALAD DRESSINGS

Both mayonnaise and salad dressings made with oil have very large amounts of fat and need to be consumed sparingly in the diet. Mayonnaise is 73 percent fat, but reduced-fat versions are available and should be used every time mayonnaise is called for.

Salad dressings such as vinaigrette can be much healthier than mayonnaise if they are based on olive oil which is high in "heart friendly" monounsaturated fats. But it is still important to go easy with them because of their high calorie content.

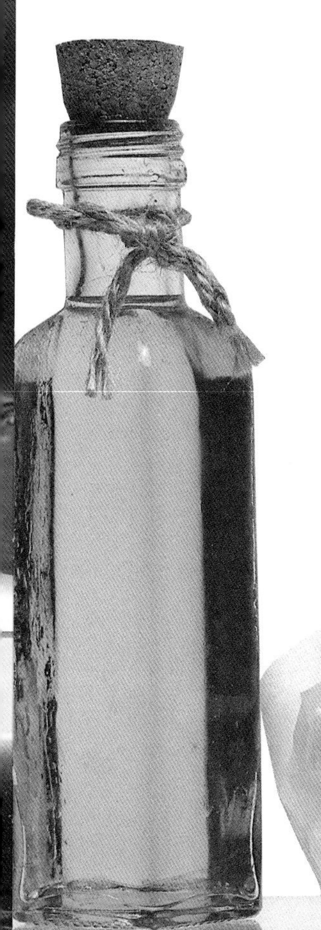

Hard margarine

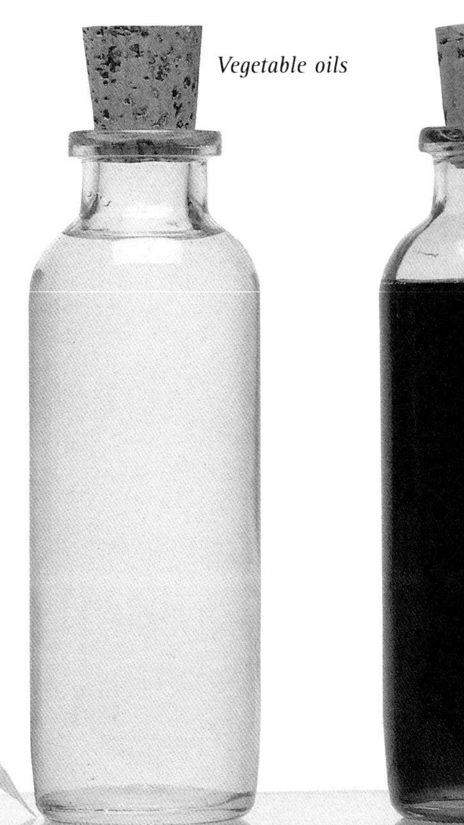
Vegetable oils

Dairy Products and Eggs

A concentrated source of many nutrients—especially protein and calcium—dairy products and eggs hold an important place in most diets. Nutritionists recommend around two servings of dairy products per day. Eggs can be eaten as an alternative to meat or fish up to a few times a week. Milk and milk products are used not only as beverages but also as ingredients in numerous dishes. Cheeses may be served as a separate course with fruit or as part of another dish.

Low-fat or non-fat milk, yogurt and cheese provide a rich source of calcium, which is especially important for women hoping to avoid osteoporosis. A good calcium intake when young and up to the age of 30 is most important in ensuring healthy bones in later life. Yogurt in particular is credited with maintaining a healthy digestive tract and improving the overall functioning of the immune system.

Some cheeses are so high in fat that they can only be considered occasional treats by most of us. These include rind-ripened cheeses, Cheddar and blue-veined cheeses. However, there is no reason to exclude them completely from your diet since they are concentrated sources of protein, vitamins and minerals.

Eggs have been linked to heart disease, so moderation should be the key. If you are sensitive to cholesterol, then the presence of cholesterol in egg yolks might make them off-limits in your diet. Otherwise, three eggs a week is hardly a cause for concern.

Milk

Most milk sold in Western countries has been pasteurized. The process of pasteurization heats the milk to 145°F (63°C) for 30 minutes, or to 161°F (72°C) for 15 seconds, and in order to kill bacteria or other organisms that could cause infection or contamination. Milk may also be fortified with vitamins A and D (low fat or skim milk is almost

DAIRY PRODUCTS

Dairy products are an important dietary source of protein, calcium and B vitamins. To maintain strong bones, it's recommended that we consume at least two servings of dairy products a day. Low-fat versions are healthiest, for example, a cup of skim milk and a bowl of cottage cheese.

Milk, cream and butter should be stored away from foods with strong odors whenever possible. Cheeses should be carefully wrapped in waxed paper or foil, both to maintain moistness and to prevent their odors from permeating other foods and vice-versa.

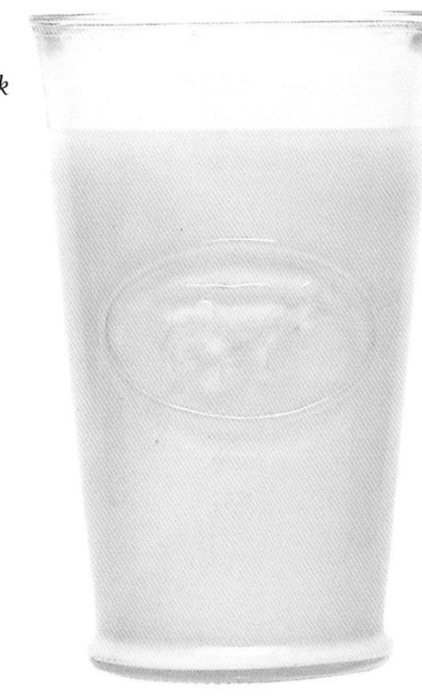

Milk

always fortified because removing the fat also removes fat-soluble vitamins).

Standards for milk are fairly consistent in Western countries. Milk products are carefully inspected before and after production. Farms and animals (cows and goats) are also inspected to ensure that sanitary conditions are upheld.

Avoid combining milk or cream from separate containers because contamination may occur.

When used in hot dishes, milk or cream should be brought to a boil before it is added to other ingredients. If it curdles, it should not be used.

Milk comes in various forms and is classified according to its percentage of fat:

Type	**Fat content %**	
	U.S.	**U.K.**
Whole milk	4	4
Low-fat (semi-skimmed)	2	1.7
Skim (skimmed)	1	0 (approx.)
Non-fat	0	0

MILK AND CREAM *all values per 100g*	*FAT(g)*	*PROT(g)*	*Ca(mg)*	*B_2(mg)*
Skim (skimmed) milk *33 calories*	0.10	3.30	120.00	0.17
Low-fat skim milk, pasteurized *46 calories*	1.60	3.30	120.00	0.18
Whole milk, pasteurized *66 calories*	3.90	3.20	115.00	0.17
Soy milk, plain *32 calories*	1.90	2.90	13.00	0.27
Goats' milk, pasteurized *60 calories*	3.50	3.10	100.00	0.13
Cream, fresh, light (single) *198 calories*	19.10	–	91.00–	–
Cream, fresh, heavy (double) *449 calories*	48.00	–	50.00	–

Cream

Cream, like milk, is usually pasteurized and may also be stabilized (ultra-heat treated) to help extend its shelf life. Two types of cream are used for cooking and baking in most kitchens: heavy (double) cream, which has 48 percent fat, and light (single) cream, which has 19 percent fat.

CLOTTED CREAM

Clotted cream, also known as Devon or Devonshire cream in the U.S., is prepared by gently heating unpasteurized milk until a thick layer of semisolid cream forms on the top. This layer of clotted cream is skimmed away once the milk has been cooled. Clotted cream keeps for only around four days but is considered a great treat when paired with fresh berries. It contains a hefty 63 percent fat.

CLABBERED CREAM

Clabbered cream or milk is a popular dish in southern parts of the U.S. It is produced by souring unpasteurized milk until it thickens to the desired firmness. It is similar to the French sour cream called *crème fraîche.*

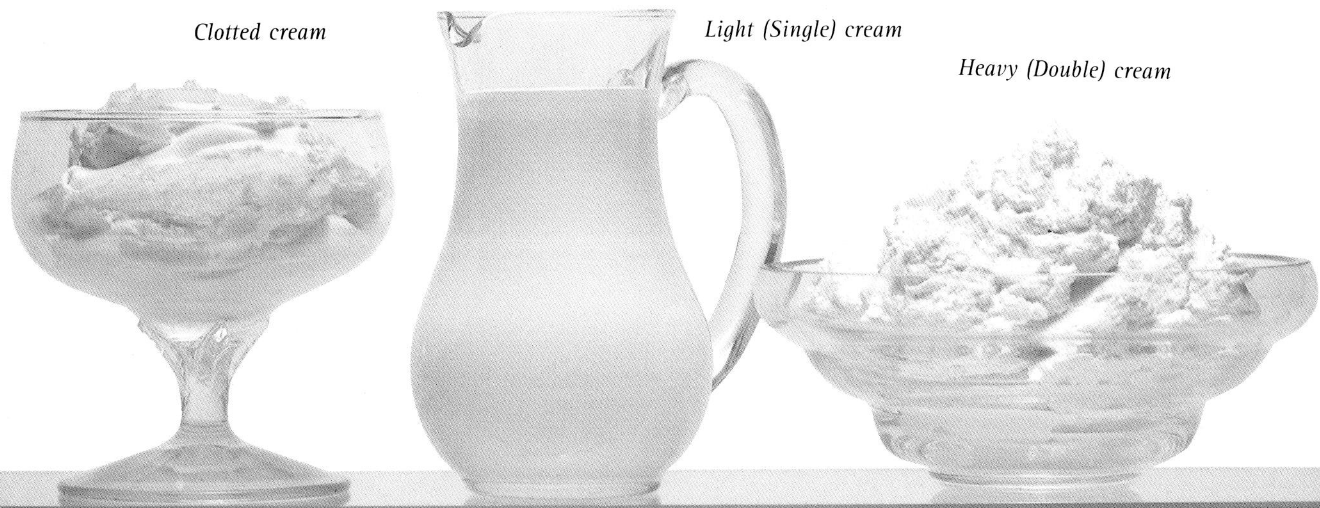

Clotted cream

Light (Single) cream

Heavy (Double) cream

Butter

The best butter has a sweet flavor, similar to very fresh heavy (double) cream. If salt has been added, it should be barely detectable. The color of butter will vary depending upon the breed of cow and time of year, but it is usually a pale yellow. The cow's diet differs from season to season, which affects both the color and flavor of the butter.

Salted butter may contain no more than a maximum of 2 percent salt. This added salt will aid in extending butter's shelf-life. The best-quality butter is made from sweet cream, which imparts a superior flavor, color, aroma and texture.

Unfortunately, all butter is extremely high in saturated fats, which can lead to heart disease. Use it only occasionally, and spread it thinly.

Cultured Milk Products

Cultured milk products are all produced by inoculating milk or cream with a bacterial strain that causes fermentation. This process thickens the milk and gives it a pleasantly sour flavor.

BUTTERMILK

Despite its name, buttermilk contains only a very small amount of butterfat. Most buttermilk sold today is actually skim milk to which a bacterial strain has been added.

CRÈME FRAÎCHE

Crème fraîche is a French sour cream that has a slightly more rounded flavor than regular sour cream. It is often preferred in cooking since it curdles less easily in hot dishes.

Butter

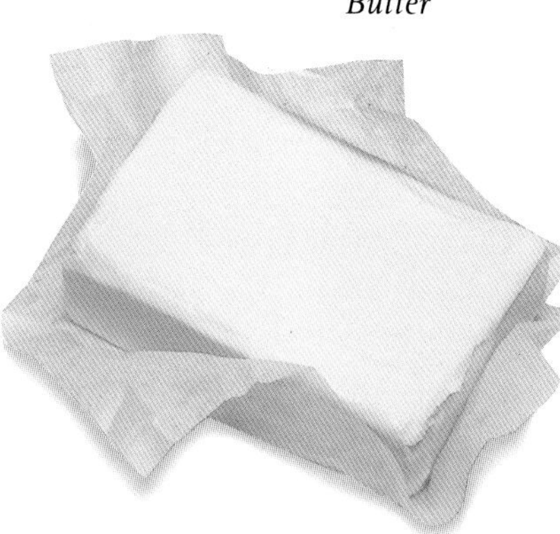

Buttermilk

Creme fraiche

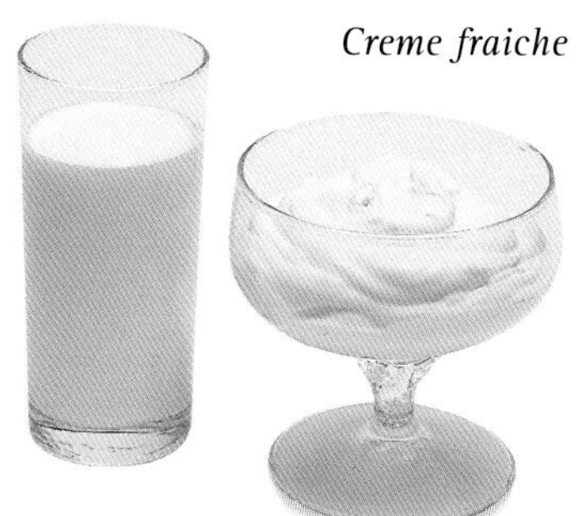

YOGURT AND SOUR CREAM

Yogurt is made by introducing the appropriate culture into milk (whole, low-fat [semi-skimmed], or skim may be used). Yogurts can contain varying levels of fat, so check the labels carefully. "Bio" or "acidophilus" yogurts are claimed to be especially beneficial for the digestive tract; they may reduce the risk of food poisoning and thrush.

Sour cream is a cultured sweet cream that contains between 16 and 22 percent fat. Low-, reduced- and non-fat versions of sour cream are also available.

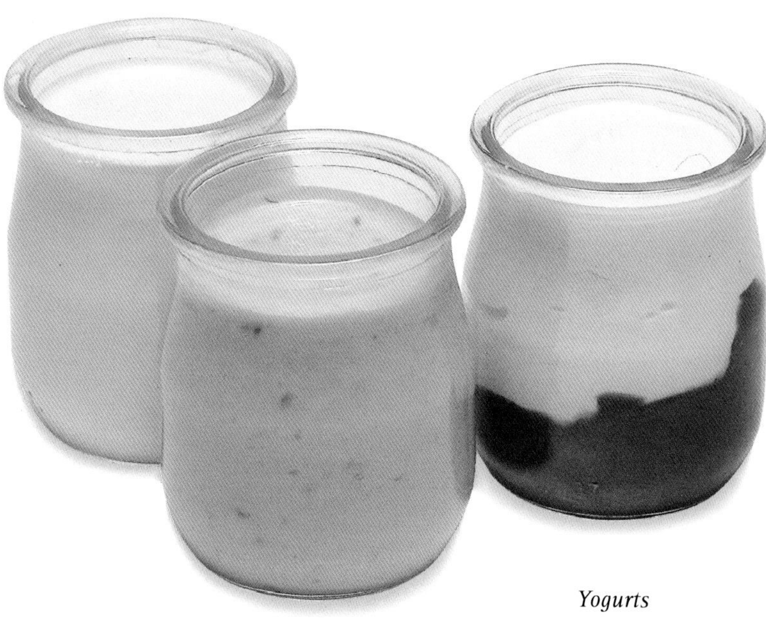

Yogurts

YOGURTS AND FROMAGE FRAIS *all values per 100g*	FAT(g)	SFA(g)	Ca(mg)	P(mg)
Low-fat yogurt, plain *56 calories*	0.80	0.50	190.00	160.00
Strained (Greek) yogurt, cows' milk *115 calories*	9.10	5.20	150.00	130.00
Fromage frais, plain *113 calories*	7.10	4.40	89.00	110.00
Cream, fresh, sour (crème fraîche) *205 calories*	19.90	12.50	93.00	81.00

FRESH CHEESES	FAT(g)	SFA(g)	Ca(mg)	Mg(mg)
Cream cheese *75 calories (portion 17g)*	8.06	5.05	16.66	1.70
Cottage cheese, plain *110 calories (portion 112g)*	4.37	2.69	81.76	10.08
Quark (German curd cheese) *41 calories (portion 55g)*	–	–	66.00	6.05
Goats' milk soft cheese *109 calories (portion 55g)*	8.69	5.72	104.50	7.70
Mozzarella *159 calories (portion 55g)*	11.55	7.21	324.50	14.85

Cheese

A huge variety of cheese is produced around the world, ranging from bland cottage cheese to powerful Gorgonzola. Hard cheeses such as Cheddar are usually excellent for both cooking and eating fresh.

Cheese is made from a variety of different milks–cows', goats', ewes', and even buffaloes'. The type of milk used will help to determine the cheese's ultimate flavor and texture. Natural cheeses are produced by inoculating milk with a bacterium or mold and allowing the milk to ferment. They are allowed to age to maturity (ripen) and then spoil (overripen). However, processed or pasteurized cheeses do not ripen and age.

Cheeses may be grouped according to the type of milk from which they are made, their texture, their age or the ripening process. The terms used are: fresh cheese; soft, or rind-ripened, cheese; semisoft cheese; hard cheese; grating cheese; and blue-veined cheese.

FRESH CHEESES

Cottage, Goat, Mozzarella, Fromage blanc, Ricotta, Quark

Among the best-known fresh cheeses are cottage cheese, goat's cheese, mozzarella, fromage blanc, ricotta, cream cheese and quark. These cheeses are moist and very soft. Although their flavor is generally described as mild, those made from goat's or sheep's milk may seem strong to some tastes.

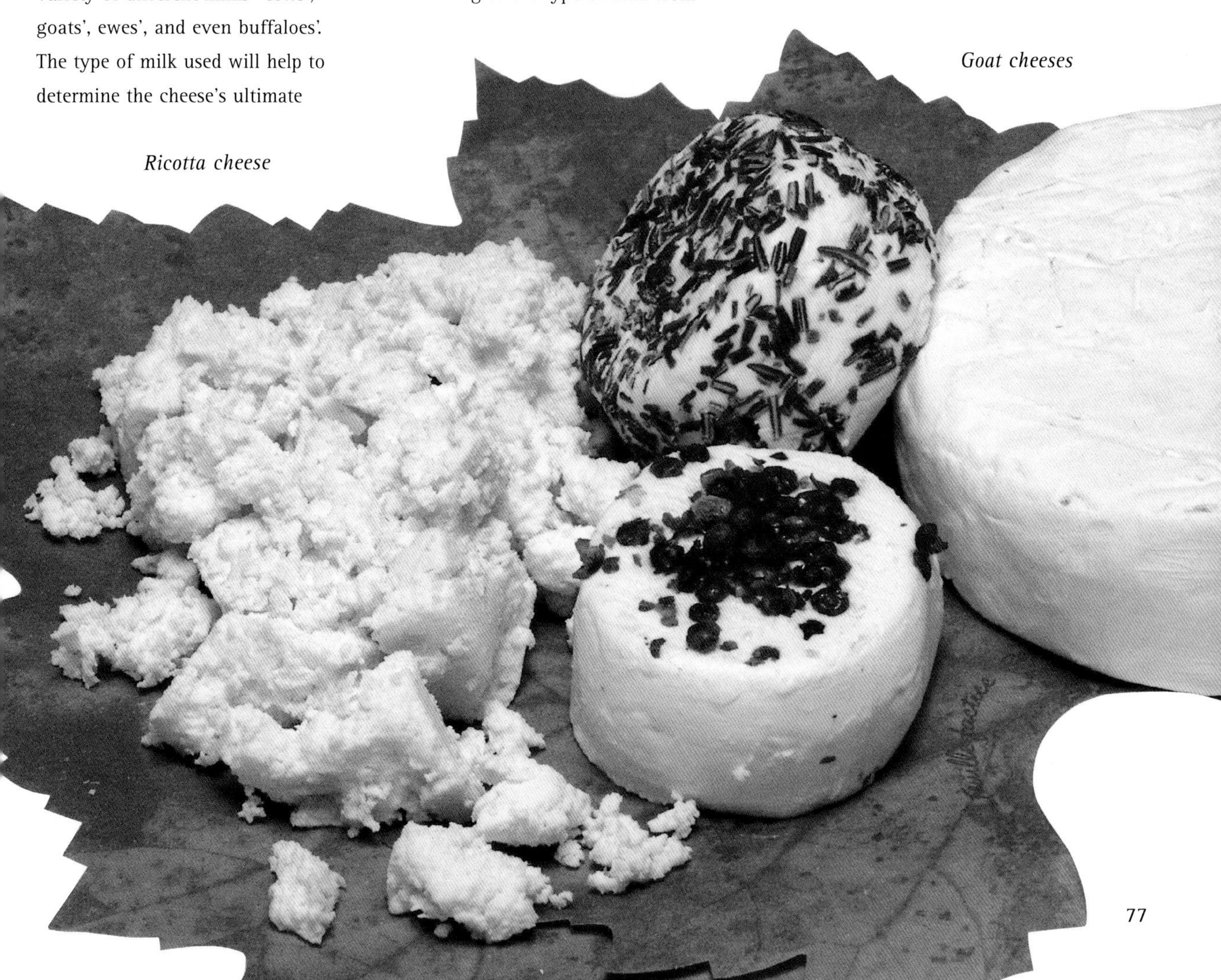

Ricotta cheese

Goat cheeses

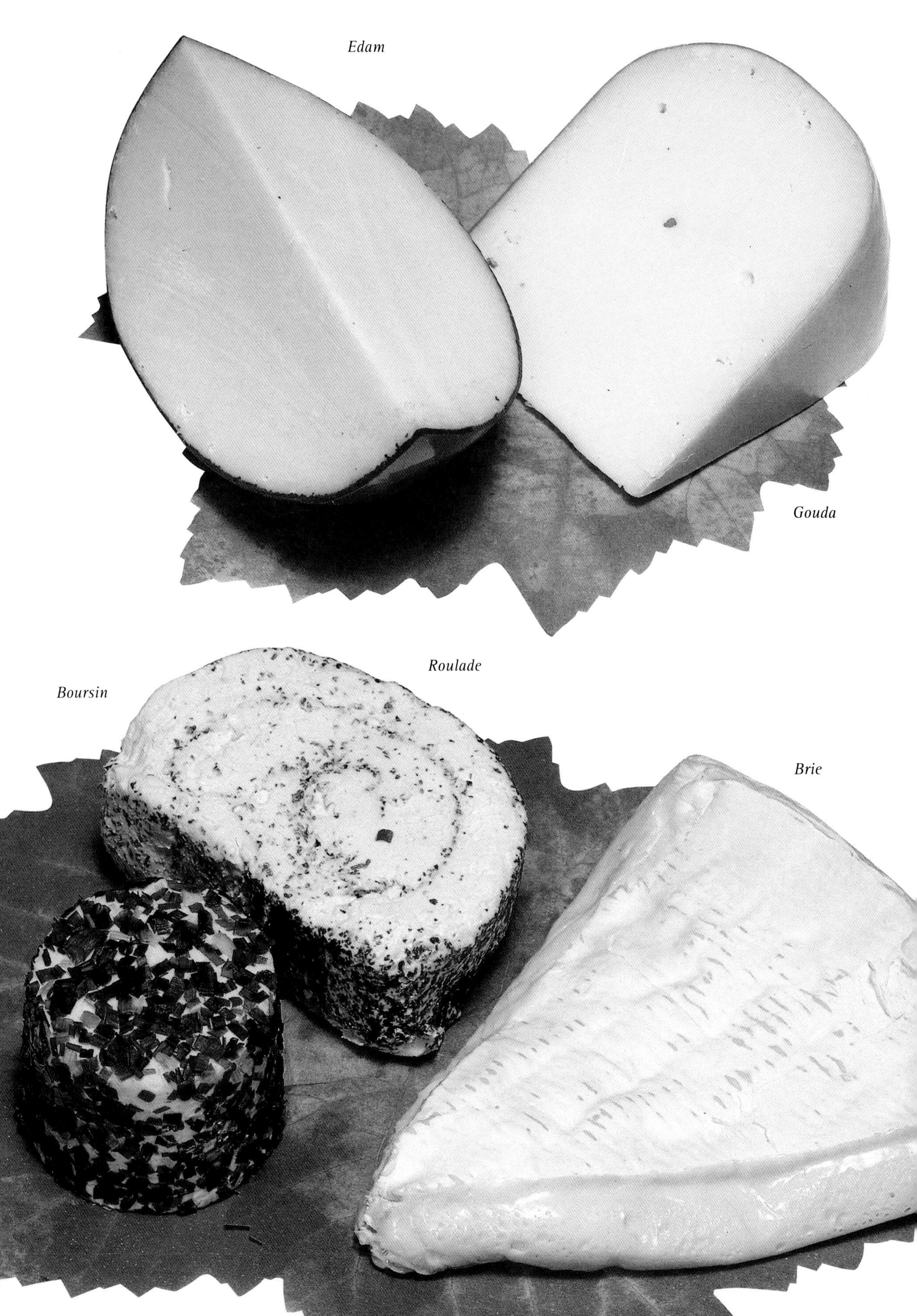
Edam
Gouda
Roulade
Boursin
Brie

SOFT, OR RIND-RIPENED, CHEESES

Brie, Camembert, Boursin, Roulade, Feta

Soft cheeses, such as Brie, Camembert, Boursin or roulade have a surface mold. Others such as the popular Greek feta do not. This soft, velvety skin is often edible, though some people find it too strong to enjoy. Soft, ripened cheeses should not be eaten by pregnant women because they carry a small risk of containing listeria bacteria which may cause miscarriage.

SEMISOFT CHEESES

Gouda, Edam, Munster, Port Salut, Manchego

Gouda, Edam, Munster and Port Salut are among the better known semisoft cheeses. Some are covered with an inedible wax rind in order to preserve moisture and extend its shelf-life. These cheeses are allowed to age for specified periods of time, though not for quite as long as hard or grating cheeses. They can be sliced but do not grate easily.

Manchego cheese, one of Spain's most famous cheeses, is a rich golden cheese that melts evenly in baked dishes. It was originally made from the milk of sheep that grazed the famous plains of La Mancha.

SEMISOFT CHEESES	*FAT(g)*	*MUFA(g)*	*SFA(g)*	*PROT(g)*
Brie *128 calories (portion 40g)*	10.76	3.12	6.72	7.72
Camembert *119 calories (portion 40g)*	9.48	2.76	5.92	8.36
Edam *133 calories (portion 40g)*	10.16	2.96	6.36	10.40
Gouda *150 calories (portion 40g)*	12.40	3.60	7.76	9.60
Soy cheese *96 calories (portion 30g)*	8.19	–	–	5.49

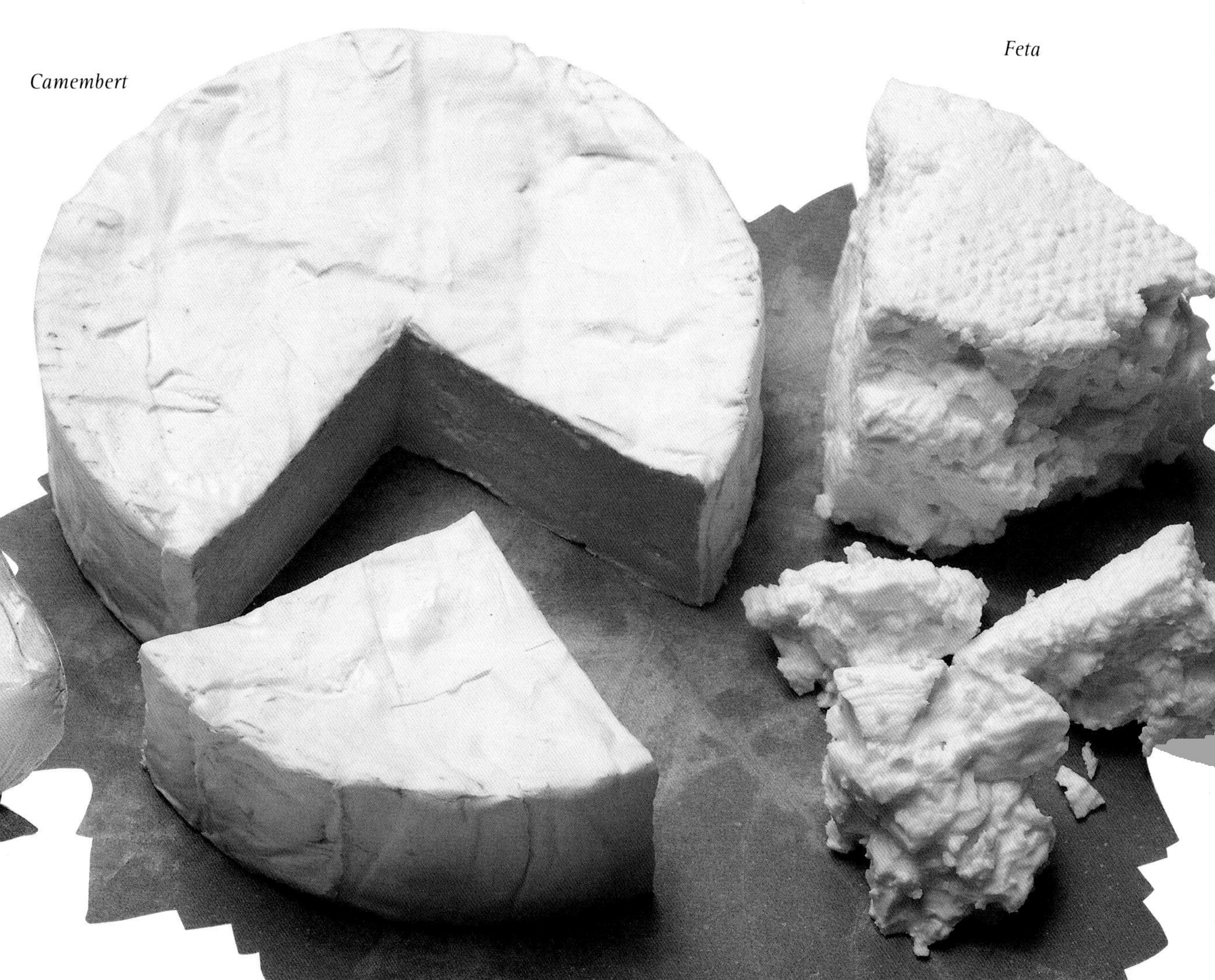

Camembert

Feta

HARD, OR CHEDDAR-TYPE, CHEESES

Gruyère, Provolone, Cheddar, Cheshire, Emmenthal

Hard cheeses, such as Gruyère, provolone and Cheddar, have a firm consistency and a drier texture than semisoft cheeses. They slice and grate easily.

Emmenthal is a famous Swiss cows' milk cheese with a sweet, nutty flavor.

Crumbly Cheshire cheese is a good snack cheese with a slightly salty, tangy taste.

GRATING CHEESES

Parmesan, Pecorino, Sapsago, Sbrinz

Parmesan, pecorino and sapsago cheeses are typically grated or shaved rather than sliced because of their crumbly texture. The best-quality Parmesan is imported from the Reggiano region of Italy. It is used as a table or cooking cheese. An aged version of Monterey Jack cheese, known as Dry Jack, is produced in the U.S. and used in ways similar to Parmesan and pecorino.

Sapsago is a hard Swiss cheese; it is pale green in color because clover is added to the curd. It is a good, all-purpose cooking cheese.

Sbrinz is a Swiss cheese made from cows' milk. It takes over two years to make and mature.

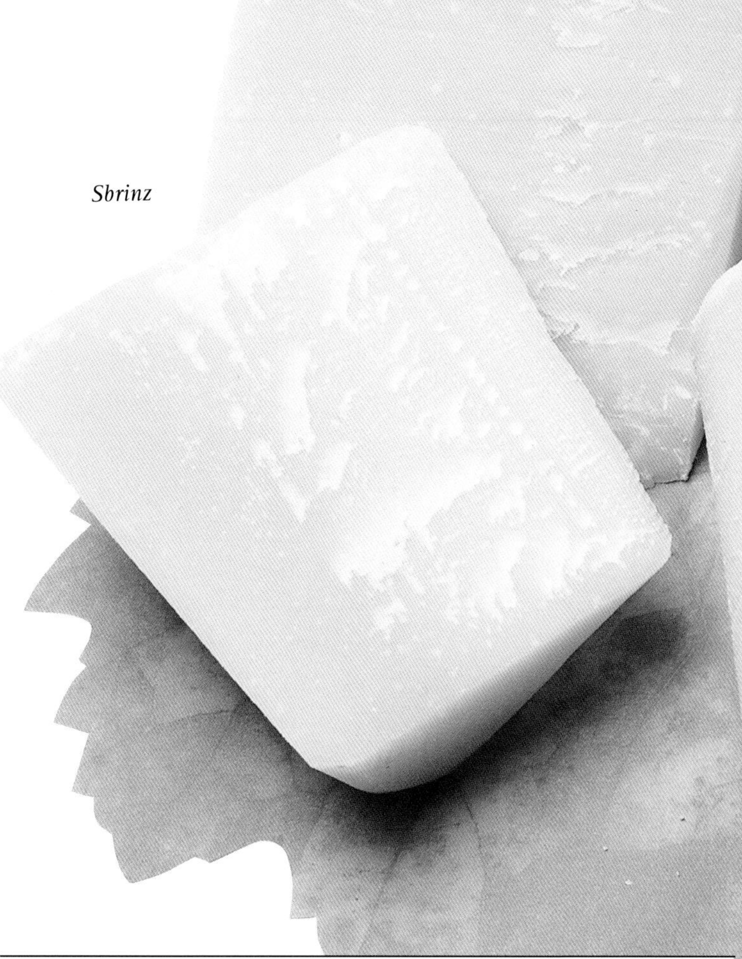

Sbrinz

HARD CHEESES	*FAT(g)*	*SFA(g)*	*MUFA(g)*	*Zn(mg)*
Cheddar, average *165 calories (portion 40g)*	13.76	8.68	3.76	0.92
Cheddar-type, reduced fat *104 calories (portion 40g)*	6.00	3.76	1.76	1.12
Parmesan *45 calories (portion 10g)*	3.27	2.05	0.95	0.53
Emmenthal *153 calories (portion 40g)*	11.88	7.44	3.44	1.76

Cheese is a reasonable source of zinc. Other sources include beef (6–12.0 mg per 5 oz [140 g] serving), bran breakfast cereals (2.7 mg per 1.5 oz [40 g] bowl) and canned mackerel (5.4 mg per 7 oz [200 g] serving).

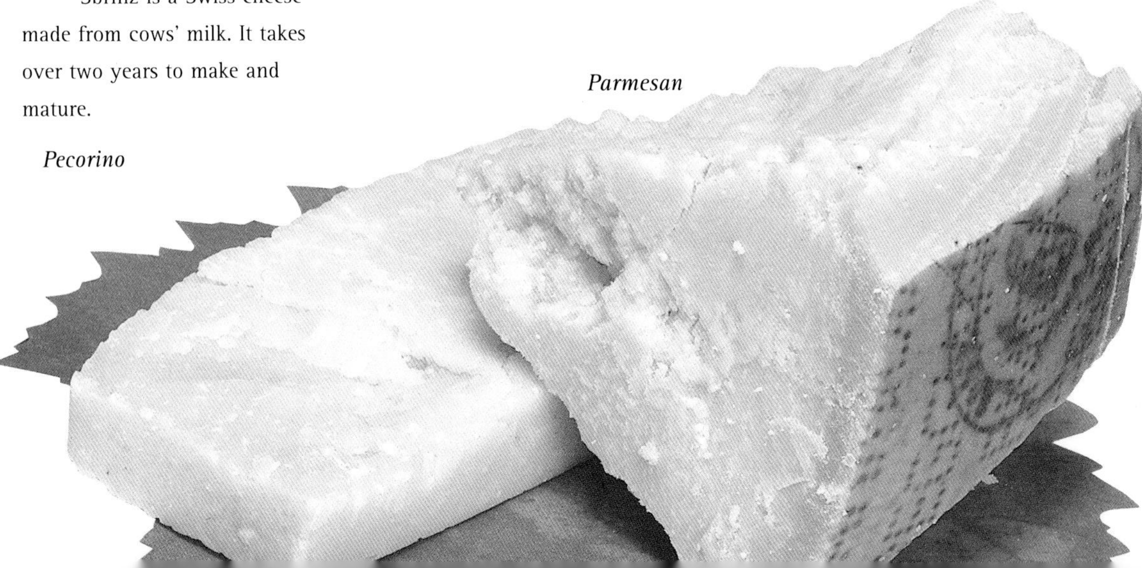

Parmesan

Pecorino

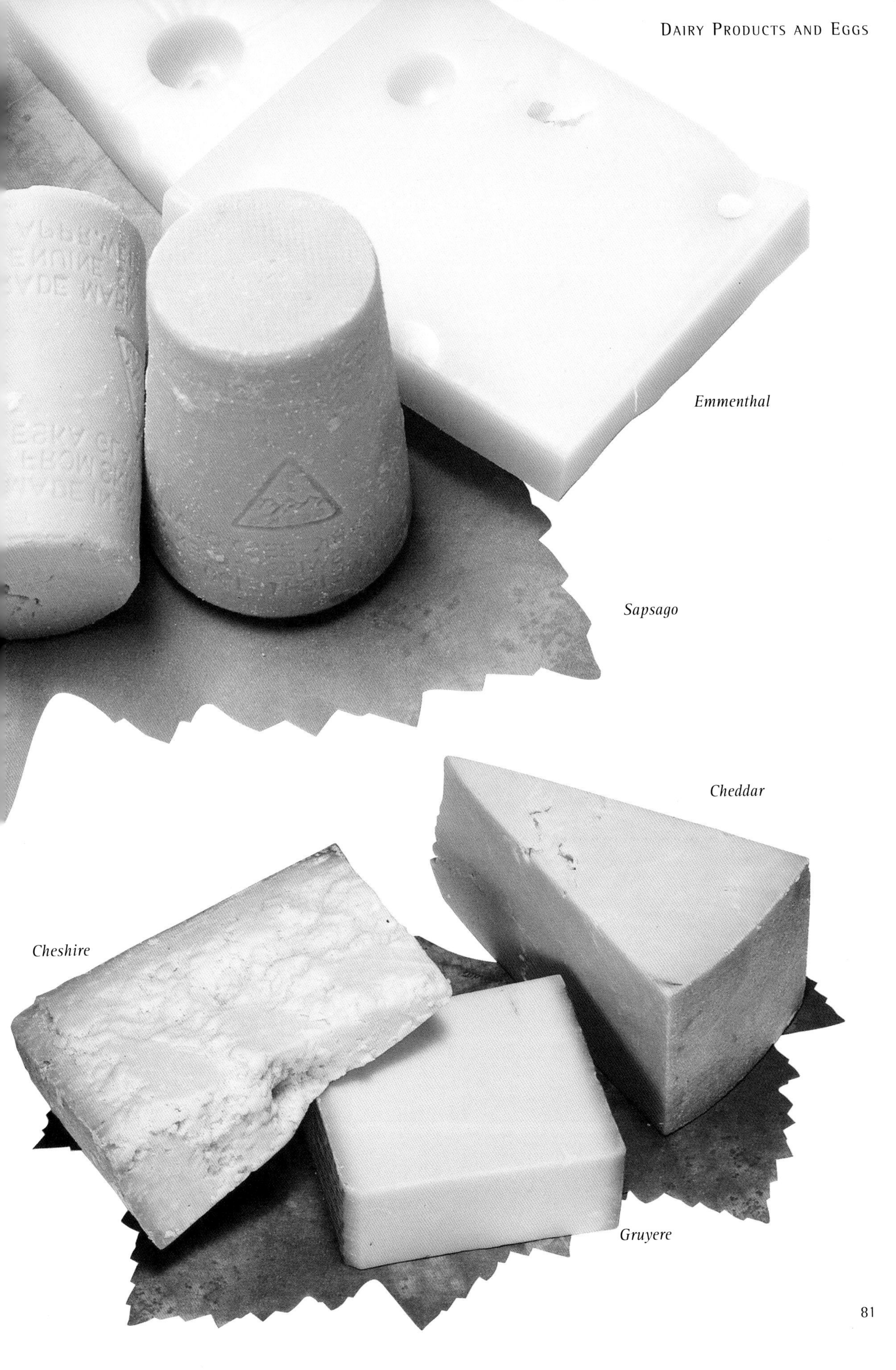

Emmenthal

Sapsago

Cheddar

Cheshire

Gruyere

BLUE-VEINED CHEESES	FAT(g)	SFA(g)	Zn(mg)	I(mcg)
Stilton, blue *144 calories (portion 35g)*	12.43	7.77	0.88	16.10
Danish blue *104 calories (portion 30g)*	8.88	5.55	0.60	2.70
Roquefort *131 calories (portion 35g)*	11.52	7.25	0.56	–

Cheese provides the next richest source of iodine (I) after fish or milk.

BLUE-VEINED CHEESES

Roquefort, Stilton, Gorgonzola

Blue-veined cheeses have consistencies that range from smooth and creamy to dry and crumbly. Their blue veining is the result of a special mold being injected into the cheese before it ripens. Some believe that the mold may have health benefits as a natural antibiotic, but any such benefit would have to be weighed against the amount of fat, cholesterol and sodium you would take in as part of an average serving. Blue cheeses should not be eaten by pregnant women.

Roquefort, from France, is produced from ewes' milk. Being one of the world's oldest and most famous cheeses, it is sometimes referred to as the "king of cheese."

Stilton is an equally famous blue cheese produced in England. It received its name from the town of Stilton in Cambridgeshire, where it was first sold. This cheese is allowed to age for four to six months.

Gorgonzola is a soft, creamy and intensely flavored blue cheese made in Italy.

Other blue-veined cheeses include: Maytag, a blue cheese produced in the US, and Danish Blue, particularly popular in Europe.

Eggs

Eggs are one of the most important foodstuffs in the kitchen. From mayonnaise to meringues, soups to sauces, appetizers to desserts, they are prominent on any menu. Today's consumer is well aware of the potential for food-borne illness through eggs. Below, therefore, are a few basic rules about safe handling.

- All eggs in the shell should be free from cracks, leakage, or obvious holes.
- Eggs should be stored in a refrigerator and the "best before" date observed.
- Eggs should be cooked to a minimum of 165°F (74°C) to kill any salmonella bacteria. Pregnant women, the elderly and the very young should avoid soft-boiled eggs.
- If any foods containing eggs are to be reheated, cool them quickly to refrigerator temperature, and warm them thoroughly within 24 to 48 hours.

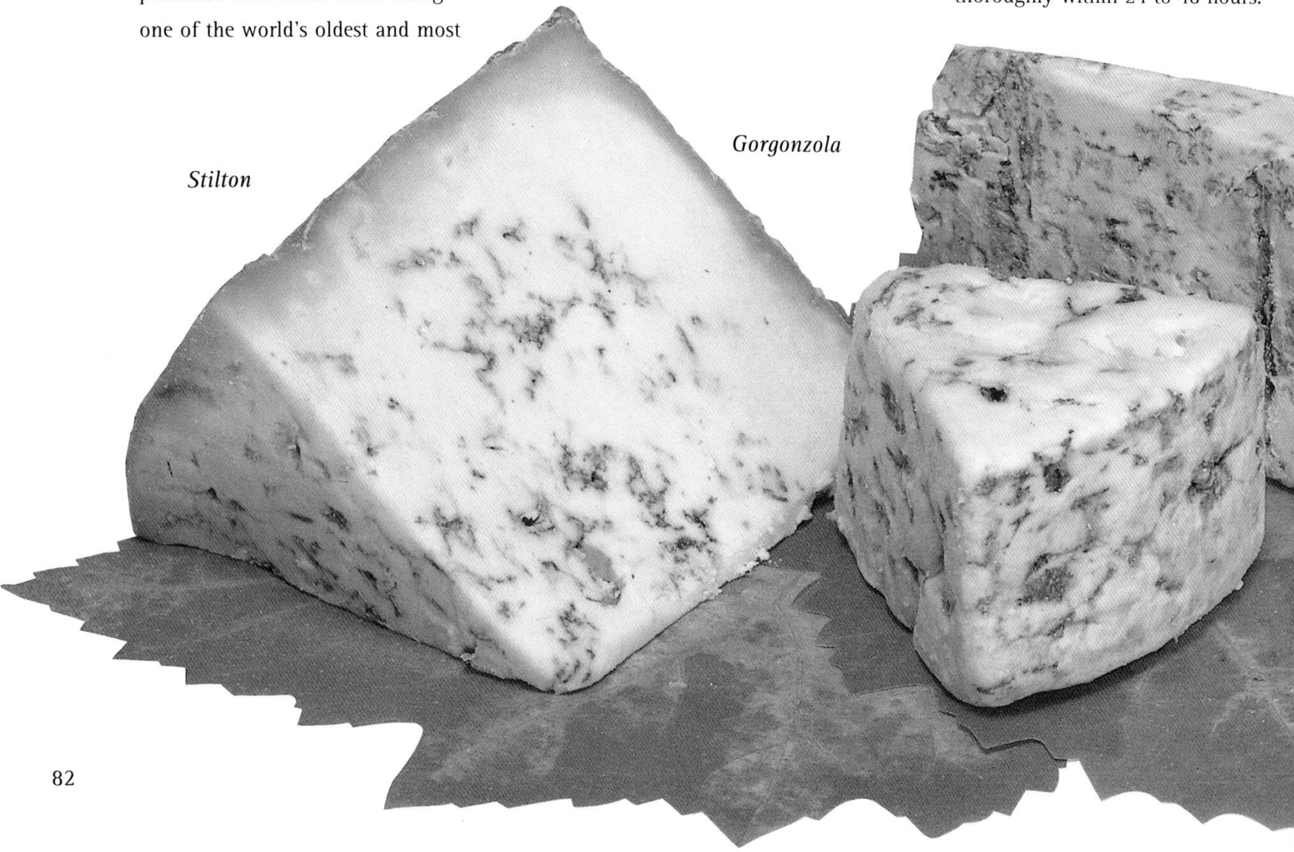

Stilton

Gorgonzola

Eggs in cooking

The white of an egg consists almost exclusively of protein and water. The protein, known as albumen, is highly nutritious, providing all eight essential amino acids in the ratio required by the body's tissues. Its ability to form a relatively stable foam is crucial to the development of proper structure in many items such as soufflés and meringues. It is also a key ingredient in clarifying stocks and broths to produce consommés.

Egg yolks are essential in the preparation of items such as mayonnaise and hollandaise. The yolk contains many vitamins, including B_{12} and D; protein; significant amounts of fat and cholesterol; and a natural emulsifier called lecithin.

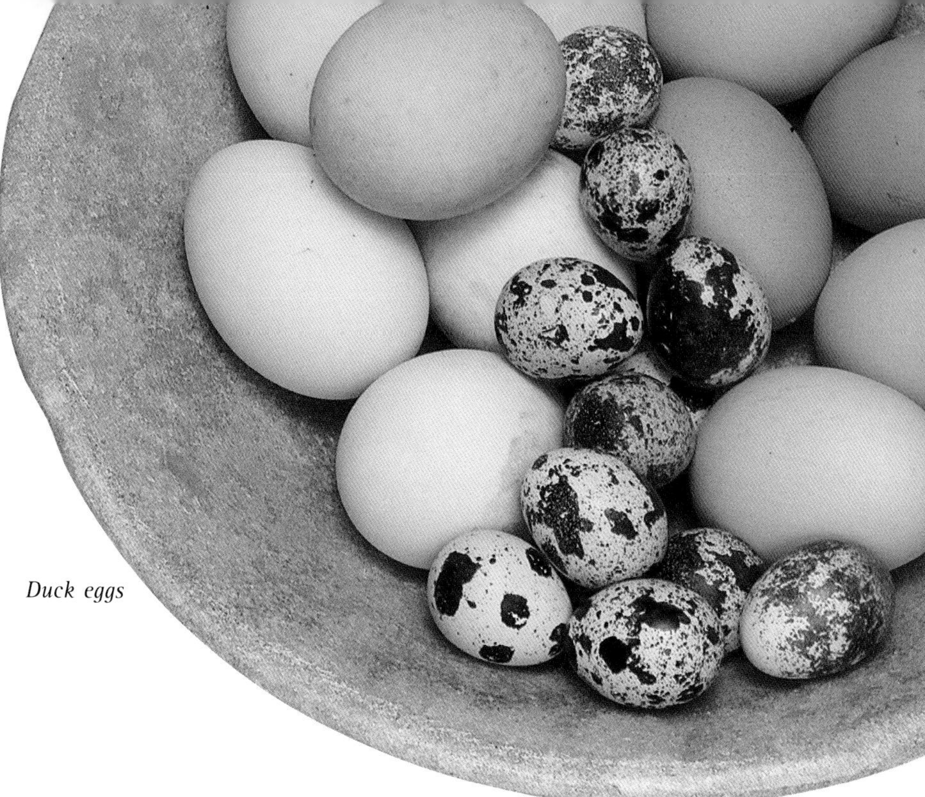

Duck eggs

Quails' eggs

Hens' eggs

TYPES OF EGG

Hens', Ducks', Quails', Dried, Powdered, Egg substitute

Hens' eggs are available in a number of sizes. Medium eggs (size 3 in the U.K.) are generally used for cooking and baking where the liquid content is critical. Ducks' and quails' eggs are tasty alternatives.

Dried or powdered eggs can be useful for certain baked goods, or in specific circumstances such as long sea voyages, when it may not be possible to store fresh eggs properly.

Egg substitutes may be entirely egg-free or may be produced from egg whites, with dairy or vegetable products substituted for the yolks. These substitutes are important for people who require a reduced-cholesterol diet.

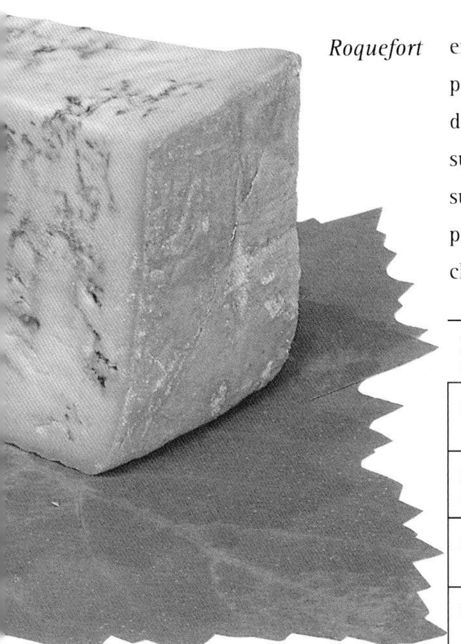

Roquefort

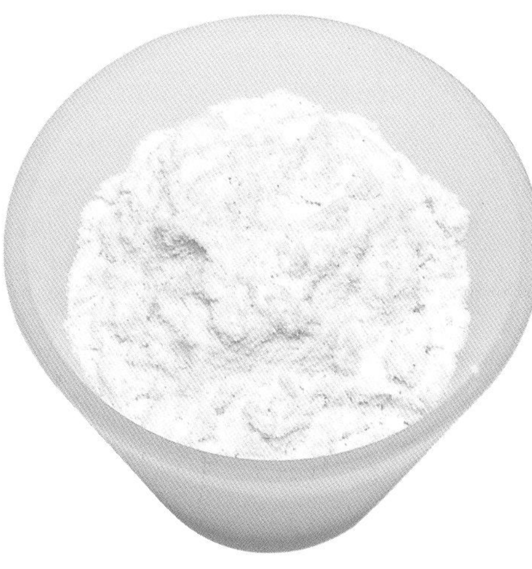

Powdered eggs

EGGS *all values per 100g*	*PROT(g)*	*FAT(g)*	*Fe(mg)*	*Vit A(mcg)*
Eggs, hen's, poached *147 calories*	12.50	10.80	1.90	190.00
Eggs, hen's, scrambled, with milk *247 calories*	10.70	22.60	1.60	307.00
Eggs, duck, boiled and salted *198 calories*	14.60	15.50	3.20	–
Eggs, quail, whole, raw *151 calories*	12.90	11.10	3.70	–

The majority of vitamin A in eggs is present as retinol, though some is also present as carotenes. The iron found in eggs is not fully available as it is bound by albumin.

Meat

The various food guides on pages 9–10 show clearly that meat, while an excellent source of many nutrients, should be included with discretion in most diets. It is not necessary for you to become a vegetarian in order to eat healthily and feel your best, but diets that are high in animal protcin arc also oftcn high in calorics, fat and cholcsterol. Organic meats may taste better, but they are no better for you nutritionally.

Shifting away from large, daily servings of meat toward a menu plan that includes more fish and smaller portions of meat (especially red meat) has many benefits. Too much protein in the diet tends to leach calcium from the bones and, thus, increases the risk of osteoporosis.

When you do select meat for a meal, take the time to pick a cut that is lean and well-suited to the recipe you intend to prepare. Cuts from various parts of animals respond differently to different cooking methods. In general, dry-heat techniques (broiling/grilling, roasting and sautéing) are best done with cuts from the loin or rib. Moist-heat methods (poaching or boiling) are good for cheaper cuts from the shank, leg or shoulder. The combination methods known as braising and stewing are equally good for these flavorful but tougher cuts. Stir-fries, stews and soups are a good way to serve smaller portions of meat without the meal looking skimpy.

KOSHER MEATS

Kosher meats are specially slaughtered, bled and processed in order to comply with religious dietary laws. Generally, only beef and veal forequarters, poultry and some game are used for kosher preparations. Kosher meats come from animals that have been slaughtered by a scholet, or specially trained rabbi. The animal must be killed with a single stroke of a knife and then fully bled. All the veins and arteries must be removed from the meat. This process would essentially mutilate the flesh of loins and legs of beef and veal; therefore, they are generally not sold as kosher meat.

CUTS OF MEAT

After slaughtering, inspection and grading, the animal carcass is cut into manageable pieces. These divisions break the animal into what are referred to as sides, quarters and saddles, depending upon your region or country. Sides are prepared by making a cut down the length of the backbone. Quarters are made by cutting sides into two pieces, dividing them between specifically determined vertebrae. Saddles are made by cutting the animal across the belly, again at a specified point or vertebrae. The exact standards for individual animal types govern where the carcass is to be divided.

The next step is cutting the animal into what are referred to as primal cuts in some countries. Again, the uniform standards and terminology for these cuts will vary from region to region and country to country.

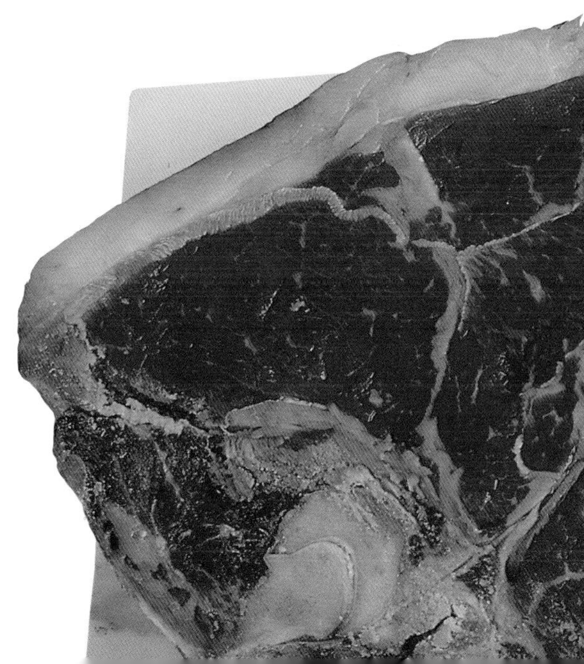

Beef

All beef provides a good source of iron and vitamin B_{12} for healthy blood. Beef is traditionally thought of as being very high in undesirable saturated fats but lean cuts trimmed of all visible fat can actually be 95 percent fat free.

CHUCK OR SHOULDER

This large portion of the animal contains some of its most exercised muscles. This means that, as a general rule, cuts from the shoulder will be best when prepared by one of the moist or combination cooking methods. Long, slow cooking brings out the flavor of these cuts, while lessening any toughness.

In addition to cuts and steaks for braising, stewing meat and ground (minced) beef are often prepared from the chuck.

RIB

The rib contains many of the most prized roasts and steaks. These cuts are tender, and well suited to dry-heat cooking methods. Steaks cut from the rib may be bone-in or boneless.

LOIN

The loin also yields a variety of cuts prized by those who value tenderness in beef. Some terms often used in conjunction with cuts from the tenderloin include Châteaubriand, tournedos, medallions, filet mignon and tenderloin tips.

Roasts from the loin may be referred to in the US as strip loins or New York strips. A variety of other steaks are also available from the loin.

BEEF CUTS

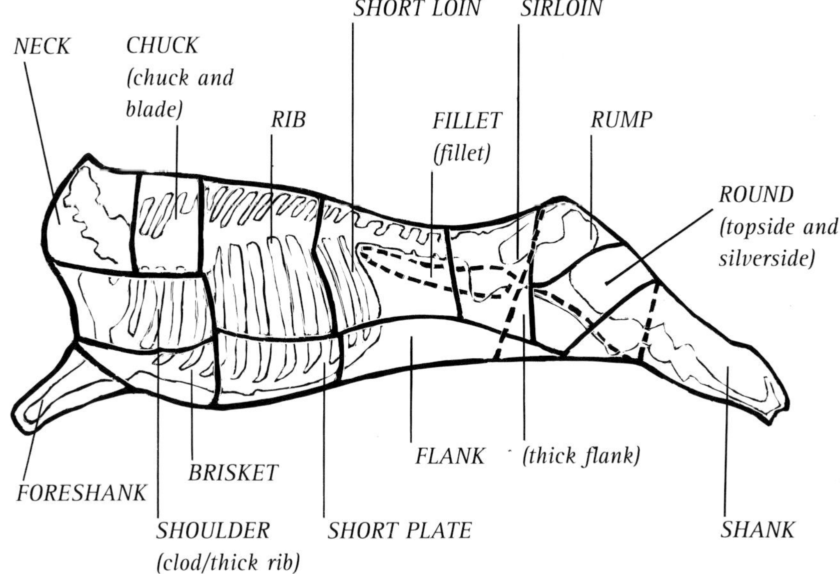

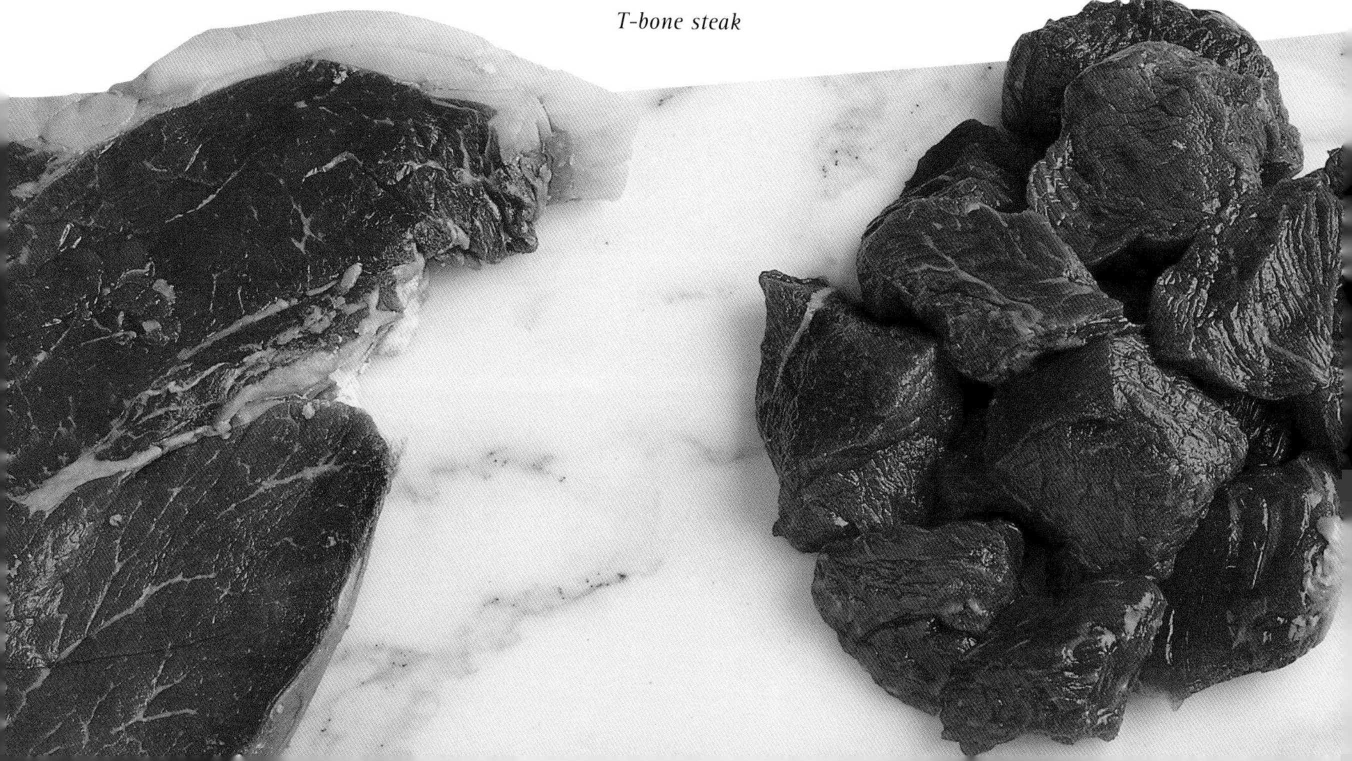

Cubed chuck steak

T-bone steak

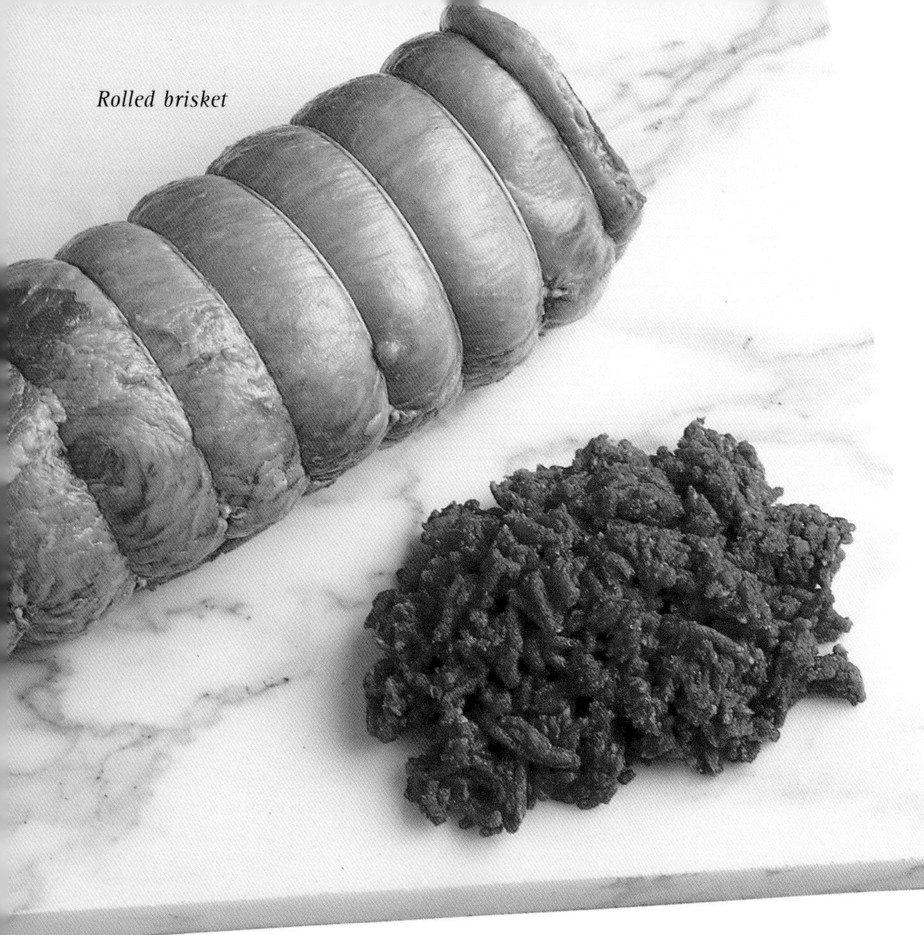

Rolled brisket

Ground (Minced) beef

ROUND (Silverside)

This section of the animal produces a range of meats. Some cuts are best when braised, stewed or simmered, while others, if handled properly, can be roasted with great success.

Good-quality, lean ground (minced) meats are made from the round (silverside) as well.

SHANK (Shin)

The foreshank (shin) is occasionally available and may be used for braising or stews.

FLANK AND SKIRT STEAK

These steaks are found along the very edge of the rib and loin portion of the animal. The fibers, though long and relatively coarse, are even. There is enough intramuscular fat to ensure that the meat stays tender as long as it is not overcooked.

BRISKET

Brisket may be found fresh or corned (salted). Fresh brisket is often favored for pot roasts and other braises. It responds well to slow cooking in a sauce. Corned (salt) beef has been brined and cured with spices. It is traditionally prepared by simmering, with or without root vegetable accompaniments.

MISCELLANEOUS CUTS OF BEEF

Oxtail, Heart, Liver, Tongue

Oxtail is an intensely flavored cut, and is excellent in stews, soups and braises. It may be purchased whole or as cross-cuts.

Fresh heart can be prepared in the same way any other well-exercised part of the animal is handled – by braising or stewing. Though not particularly common nowadays, hearts are highly respected in many ethnic cuisines.

Beef (ox) liver is darker and more deeply flavored than other livers. Like heart, it is not a particularly popular cut.

Tongue is available fresh, smoked or cured. Although it has declined in popularity in Western countries, tongue is highly regarded in Japan and other Asian countries. This cut is best prepared by simmering it in a flavored bouillon or broth and is often served pickled.

Veal

Veal is considered by some to be the finest meat available, but the practices used in raising calves for slaughter have caused many people concern. Like other meats, veal is a good source of protein and B

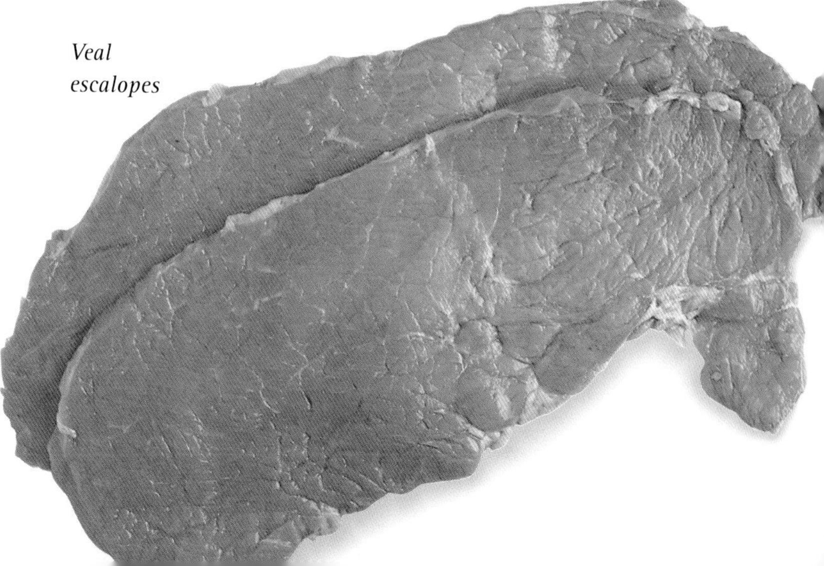

Veal escalopes

vitamins. It is also lower in saturated fat than beef.

SHOULDER (Chuck)

Cuts may be handled in the same way as beef chuck cuts. Stewing meat and ground (minced) meat are commonly taken from cheaper cuts, or may be the trimmings from roasts (joints).

SHANK

The veal foreshank is most commonly available, though it may be possible to procure the hindshank as well. The foreshank is generally meatier and usually braised. Osso bucco is one of the most famous dishes made from the shank. There are many regional variations on this dish.

RACK (Rib)

The rib may be roasted whole (bone-in or as a boneless rolled roast). Portion-sized cuts from the rib are referred to as chops. The rib bones may be left attached and are generally "frenched," which means that the bone has been scraped free of all meat, cartilage and sinew.

LOIN

Veal loin is one of the most expensive cuts. Chops, medallions and roasts are all easily prepared from the loin. Tenderloins of veal may also be prepared from this cut but should be ordered from your butcher well in advance.

LEG

The leg yields numerous cuts, perhaps the most familiar of which is the cutlet. Veal cutlets formed from the top round (best end of neck) have the best texture and cook most evenly. It is possible to make cutlets from other areas of the leg, including the bottom round.

There are many names for cutlets, and they vary from one cuisine to another: Scallops, scaloppine and escalope are some of the more familiar.

BEEF AND VEAL	*FAT(g)*	*SFA(g)*	*B_{12}(mcg)*	*Fe(mg)*
Beef, fillet steak, broiled (grilled), lean *316 calories (portion 168g)*	13.44	6.05	3.36	3.86
Beef, braising steak, slow-cooked, lean *276 calories (portion 140g)*	11.06	4.76	4.20	3.50
Hamburgers (beefburgers), fried *106 calories (portion 40g)*	6.92	3.20	0.80	1.24
Veal, escalope, fried *294 calories (portion 150g)*	10.20	2.70	6.00	1.35
Kidney, ox, stewed *155 calories (portion 112g)*	4.93	1.57	42.56	10.08
Liver, calf, fried *176 calories (portion 100g)*	9.60	–	58.00	12.20
Tripe, dressed, raw *33 calories (portion 100g)*	–	–	–	0.20

VEAL CUTS

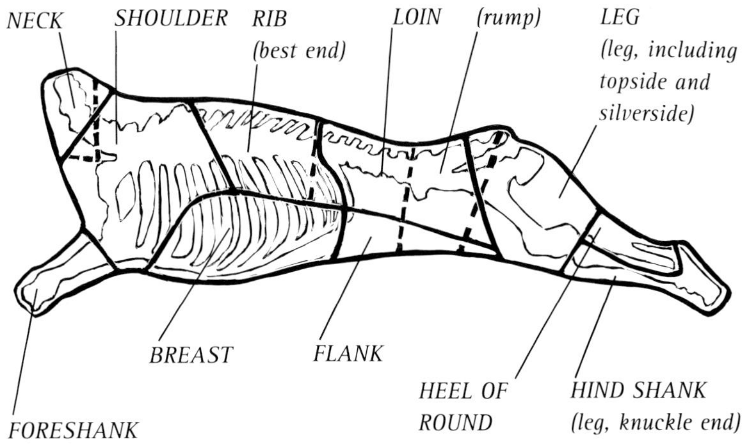

BREAST

Veal breast is often prepared as a bone-in roast, as a rolled and tied boneless roast or simply boned, butterflied, stuffed and rolled. Long cooking methods such as braising are best for this cut.

ORGAN MEATS AND BY-PRODUCTS

Veal or calf's liver, heart, tongue and bones are the most familiar organ meats and by-products used in Western kitchens. Sweetbreads (the thymus gland) and brains may also be found. In the U.K., bovine and sheep sources of these organ meats have been banned due to concern over the diseases bovine spongiform encephalopathy (BSE) and scrapie. There is relatively little call for these specialty items in the U.S., however.

Pork

Pigs have been specially bred over many generations to produce leaner meat, and some cuts now have less fat than chicken. The animals are slaughtered and butchered in facilities that handle no other type of meat to prevent the spread of infections and diseases such as trichinosis.

The pork carcass, once split into two halves along the backbone, is divided somewhat differently than other meats. Instead of a primal rib, the loin is cut long. This is done to maximize the number of cuts possible from the prized loin. However, chops cut from the rib end are generally indicated as rib chops. Those from the leg end may be referred to as sirloin chops.

SHOULDER OR BUTT

Roasts, stewing meat and ground (minced) pork are often made from this cut and the smaller cuts from the shoulder. The ratio of fat to lean is somewhat higher than in other portions of the animal. This makes it better suited for use in sausages and other items such as pâtés and terrines.

PORK CUTS

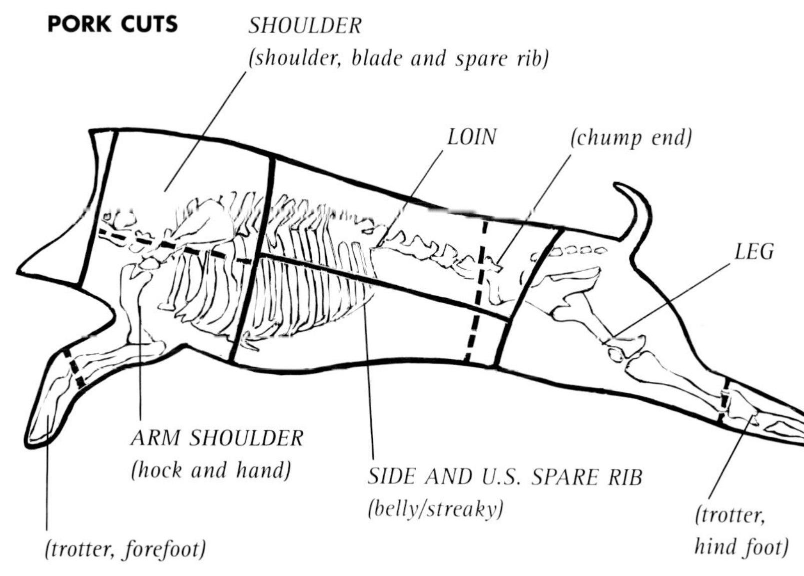

LOIN

This is the largest single primal cut from the pig. It is intentionally cut longer than the loins for beef, veal or lamb. The loin is often roasted, bone-in or boneless. One rather impressive cut produced from the rib portion of the loin is crown roast of pork.

Cuts from the loin include chops of varying thicknesses. The composition of the chop varies greatly from one end of the loin to the other. Boneless cutlets are also prepared from the loin. They are generally sautéd or broiled (grilled). Chops from the shoulder end of the loin may be braised.

The tenderloin, a prized subprimal of the loin, is widely available. Noisettes and medallions are often cut from the tenderloin.

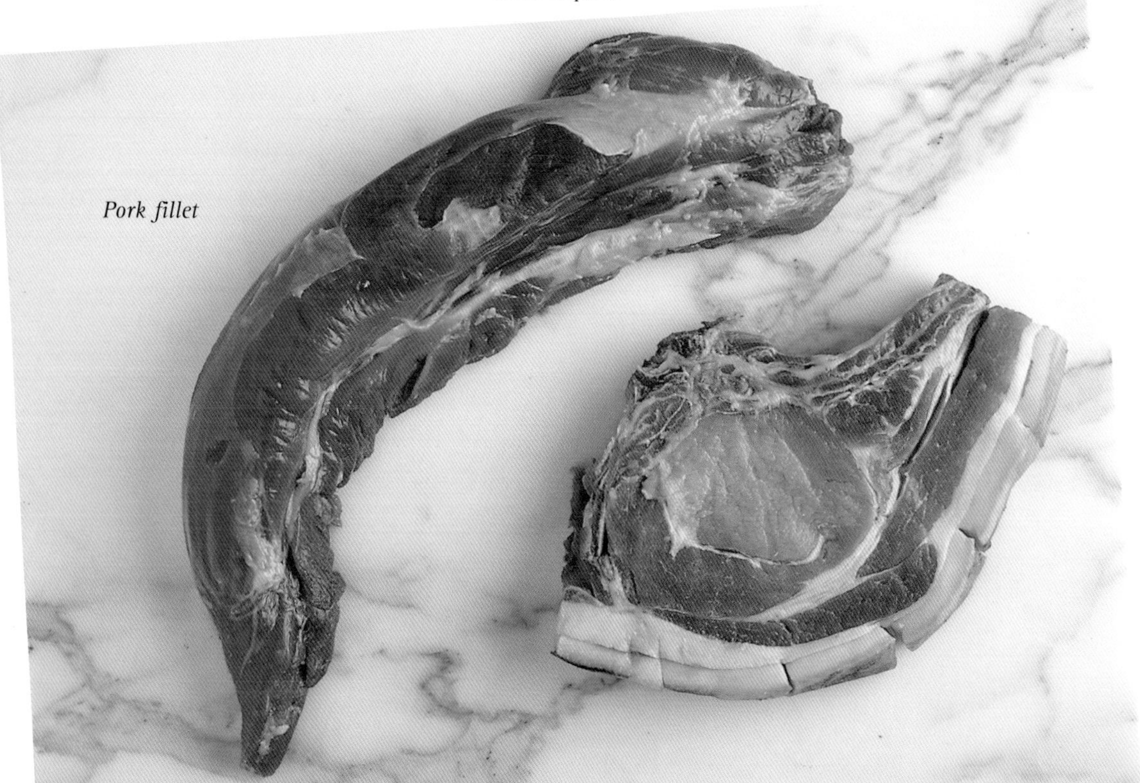

Pork fillet

Pork chop

A boneless smoked loin (sometimes referred to in the U.S. as Canadian bacon) is also popular. One of its classic uses is as a component of eggs Benedict.

HAM (Leg)

Primal, Steaks, Cured, Prosciutto, Stewing, Ground (minced)

This primal cut is often referred to as the ham, regardless of whether or not it has been cured. Fresh pork roasts or hams are quite different in flavor and texture from cured hams.

Ham (gammon) steaks (available fresh, cured or smoked) are popular breakfast items; they also have a place on lunch and dinner menus.

Cured or smoked hams are occasionally fully cooked and ready to eat. These items may benefit from simmering, or they may be roasted to enhance tenderness and flavor. Others, including hams such as prosciutto, need not be cooked after curing.

Stewing meat and ground (minced) pork are also produced from lean trimmings of smaller cuts taken from this primal.

CURED PORK AND PORK BY-PRODUCTS

Bacon, Fatback (streaky), Jowl (knuckle end), Hocks, Pigs' feet, Knuckles, Liver, Heart, Kidney

It has often been said that you can use everything on the pig except its grunt. This has given rise to a number of specialty items produced from the pig.

Bacon is made by curing and/or smoking the belly. This classic breakfast item may be sold as slab bacon (bacon joint), with or without the rind, or sliced. Special types of bacon such as Italian pancetta are produced by different cuisines. Bacon and other cured meats may contain nitrites which, in excess, can react in the stomach to form cancer-causing chemicals called nitrosamines. Bacon is also usually high in salt, so it should be eaten cautiously by those with high blood pressure.

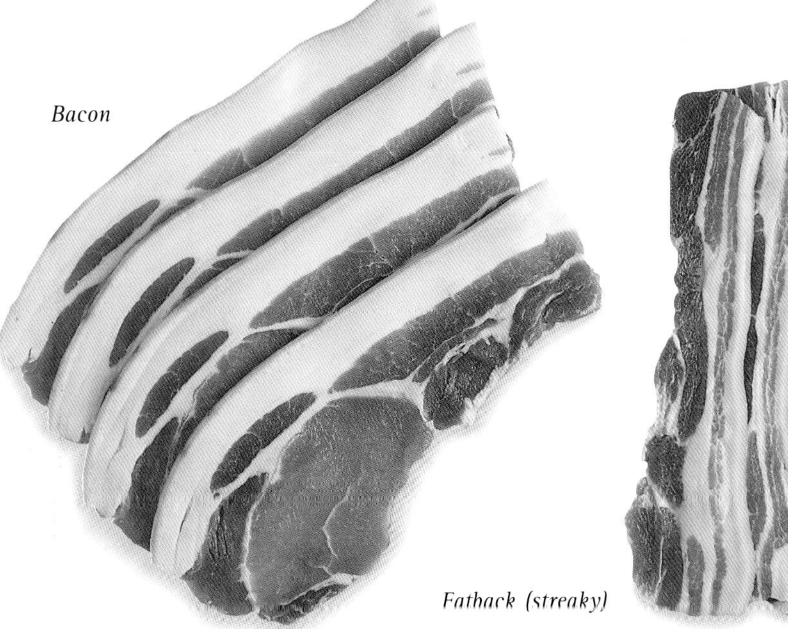

Bacon

Fatback (streaky)

Fatback (streaky) bacon is used for barding (covering) poultry to prevent it from drying out during roasting and for lining pâté and terrine molds. It comes from the clear fat along the animal's back. It is referred to as clear fat to distinguish it from the belly fat, sometimes known as streak of lean, an apt description of bacon's composition. Jowl bacon (knuckle end) is not well suited for cooking as strips (rashers) but is excellent as a flavoring ingredient.

Ham hocks, pigs' feet, knuckles and even snouts are used to produce a variety of regional and ethnic dishes. These items are available fresh, cured and smoked.

Pigs' liver, heart and kidneys are sometimes available, but their use is limited largely because of consumer resistance.

SPARERIBS

Spareribs are similar to short ribs, breast of veal and breast of lamb. This cut has more bone than meat but is immensely popular. Some cuisines include trademark preparations that feature this succulent cut. Spareribs are sold whole or cut into portions. Baby back ribs and country-style ribs are also available.

PORK	*FAT(g)*	*SFA(g)*	*Vit A(mcg)*	*FOLAT(mcg)*
Pork chops, loin, broiled (grilled), loin with fat and bone *64 calories (portion 100g)*	5.62	3.26	–	5.92
Sausage, pork, broiled (grilled) *237 calories (portion 20g)*	4.92	1.90	–	0.60
Kidney, pig's, stewed *153 calories (portion 100g)*	–	–	46.00	43.00

Lamb and Mutton

Lamb is slaughtered when still quite young, so it is tender. Most cuts can be cooked by any method. Spring lamb and hot-house lamb are not fed grass or grain because these things make the flesh lose some of its delicacy. As the animal ages, the flesh darkens in color, taking on a slightly coarser texture and developing a more pronounced flavor. Any sheep slaughtered over the age of one year must be labeled mutton.

Lamb's liver is also available. As with other livers it is high in vitamin A and vitamin B_{12}.

LOIN

A tender cut from the back, loin is sold with the bone in or out. Loin of lamb is well suited to roasting.

LAMB	FAT(g)	SFA(g)	Vit A(mcg)	FOLAT(mcg)
Lamb, loin chops, broiled (grilled), lean *149 calories (portion 70g)*	7.49	3.43	0.00	4.20
Lamb, breast, roasted, lean *246 calories (portion 90g)*	16.65	7.74	0.00	5.40
Lamb, shoulder, whole, frozen, roasted, lean *226 calories (portion 90g)*	14.04	6.39	0.00	4.50
Liver, lamb's, fried *237 calories (portion 100g)*	12.90	–	22,680.00	260.00
Heart, lamb's, roasted *226 calories (portion 100g)*	–	–	0.00	2.00
Sweetbread, lamb, raw *131 calories (portion 100g)*	–	–	0.00	13.00

LAMB CUTS

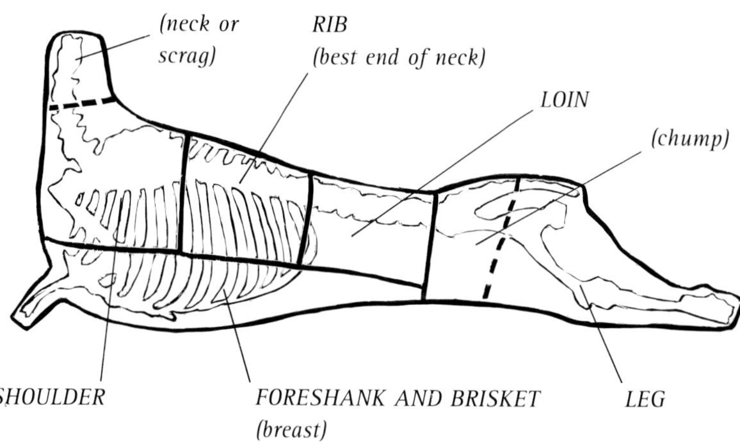

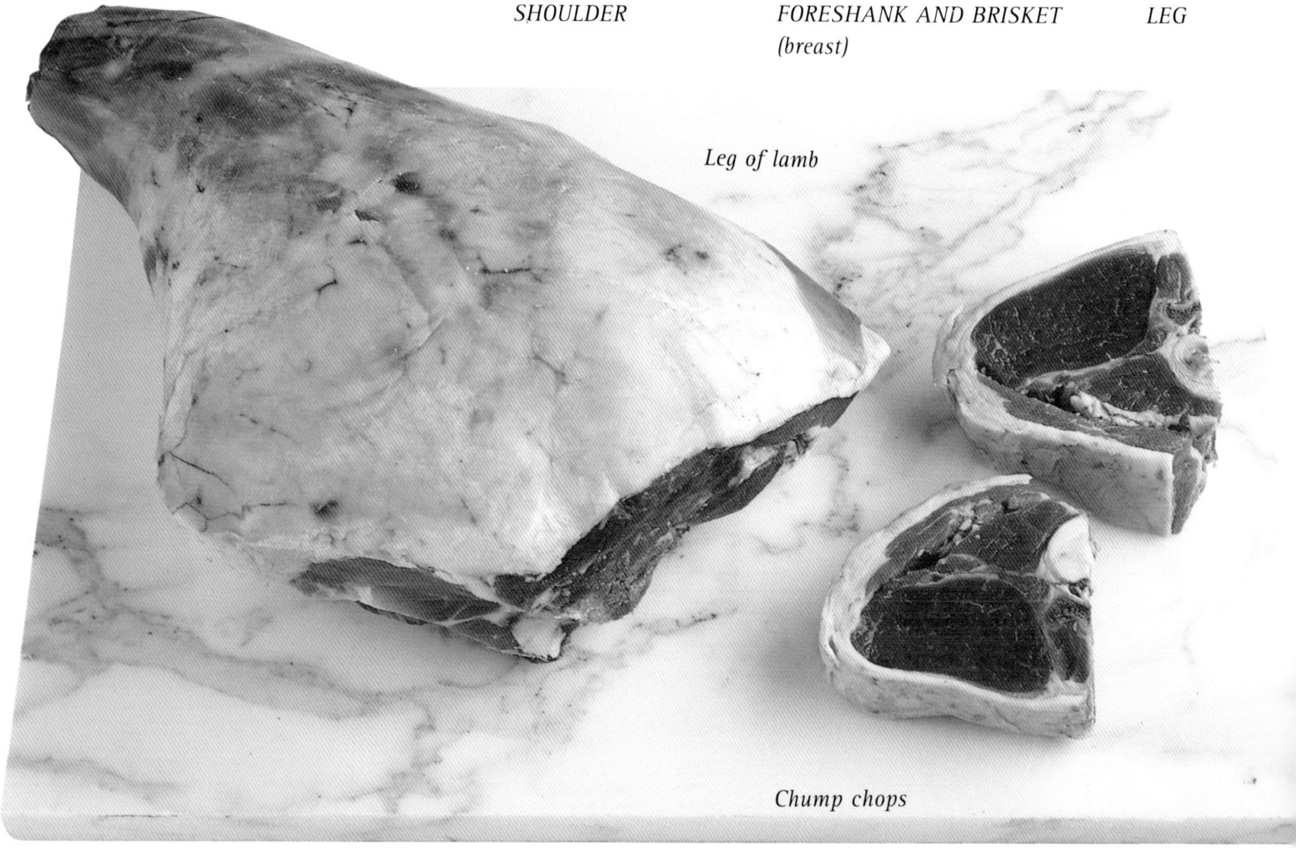

Leg of lamb

Chump chops

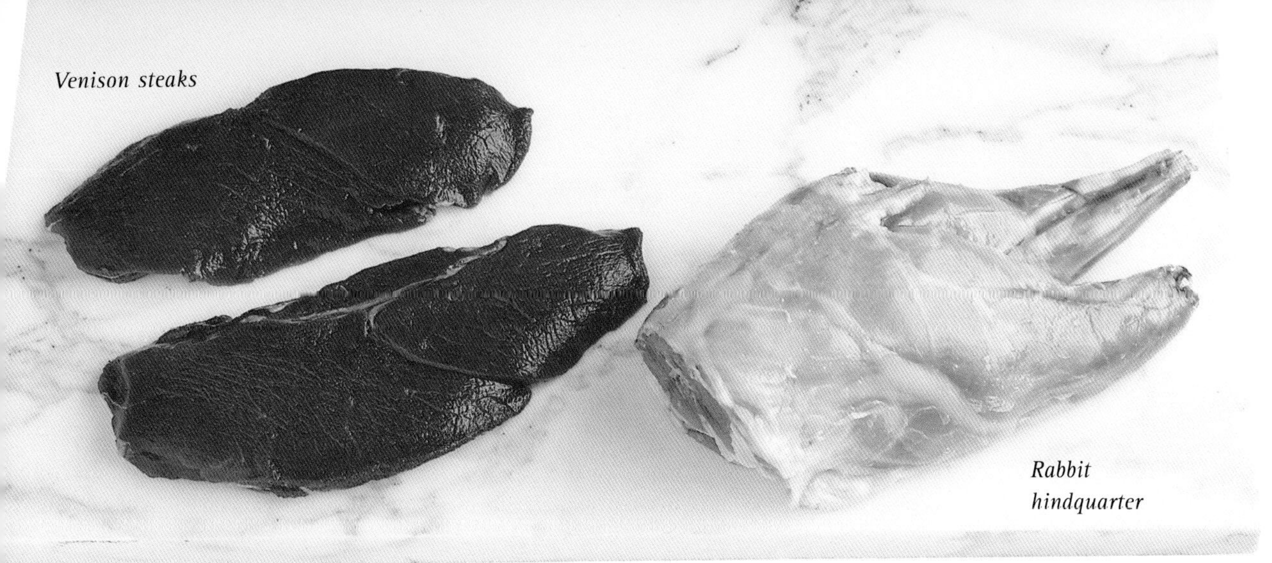

CHUMP CHOPS

Chump chops are cut from between the leg and loin. They can be grilled or fried.

LEG

Leg of lamb is one of the most popular roasting joints. The tender cut is often divided into fillet and shank. Boned and rolled legs can also be casseroled.

LAMB'S LIVER

Lamb's liver, like other types of liver, is a particularly rich source of iron and vitamin A. It is strongly flavored and can be grilled, fried or stewed.

Venison and Large Game

Farm-raised (fallow) deer have lean, tasty meat with less intramuscular fat and cholesterol than beef. The loin and the ribs are quite tender and can be suitable for most cooking techniques, especially roasting, broiling (grilling) and sautéing. The haunch and legs are more exercised and therefore tougher, so they are best prepared by moist-heat or combination techniques.

In the U.S., depending upon area, other types of game–including wild boar, elk and bear–may be available. They should be prepared in the same way as beef.

Cuts from less-exercised portions of the animal may be prepared by any technique and are frequently paired with dry-heat methods such as broiling (grilling) or roasting.

Well-exercised areas of the animal such as the leg (or haunch), shank and shoulder are best cooked by moist-heat or combination methods. These cuts are also used for preparing pâtés and other charcuterie items. They tend to have a lot more intramuscular fat and are therefore less healthy.

Rabbit

Rabbit, raised domestically, is available throughout the year. The loin meat is delicate in flavor and color but has a tendency to dry out if it is not handled carefully. Traditional preparation methods include roasting, braising and jugging, which preserves the meat by cooking and storing it in fat. The loin and legs are often prepared by two separate techniques–the loin is roasted or sautéd, and the legs, which are more exercised, are cooked by stewing or braising.

VENISON AND RABBIT *all values per 100g*	*PROT(g)*	*FAT(g)*	*Fe(mg)*	*Se(mcg)*
Venison, roasted *165 calories*	35.60	2.50	5.10	–
Rabbit, stewed, meat only *114 calories*	21.20	3.20	1.10	16.00

Poultry

Poultry production is now a big business, with breeding, care and feeding all scientifically controlled. Poultry used to be regarded as an expensive treat, but intensive rearing and management of birds have made their meat cheap and accessible.

Today, chicken, turkey and farmed game birds can be found that are sold as free-range and/or organic. Some cooks prefer birds raised in a free-range environment as the birds have been allowed at least some exercise outside, rather than spending their entire lives in cages. Organically raised birds may also be free of chemical growth enhancers and steroids, but it is important to read the labels and ask questions about any organic product you buy.

Removing the skin before serving poultry will remove half of the fat content as well as a sizeable number of calories. It is not essential to do this before cooking, unless you are steaming or poaching the bird.

The younger the bird, the more tender its flesh will be.

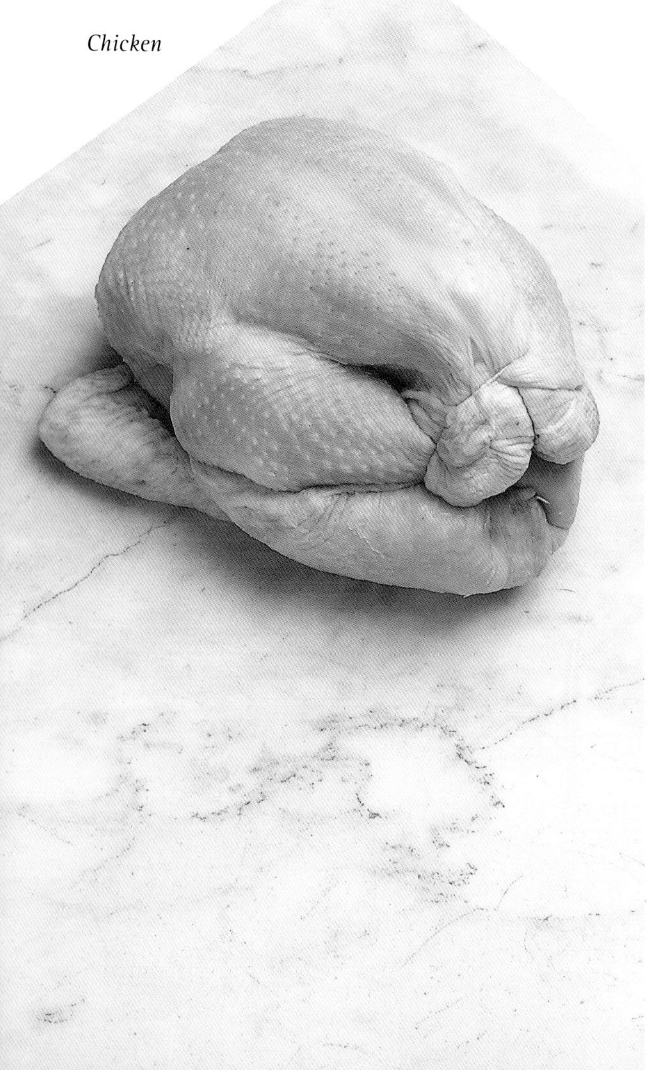

Chicken

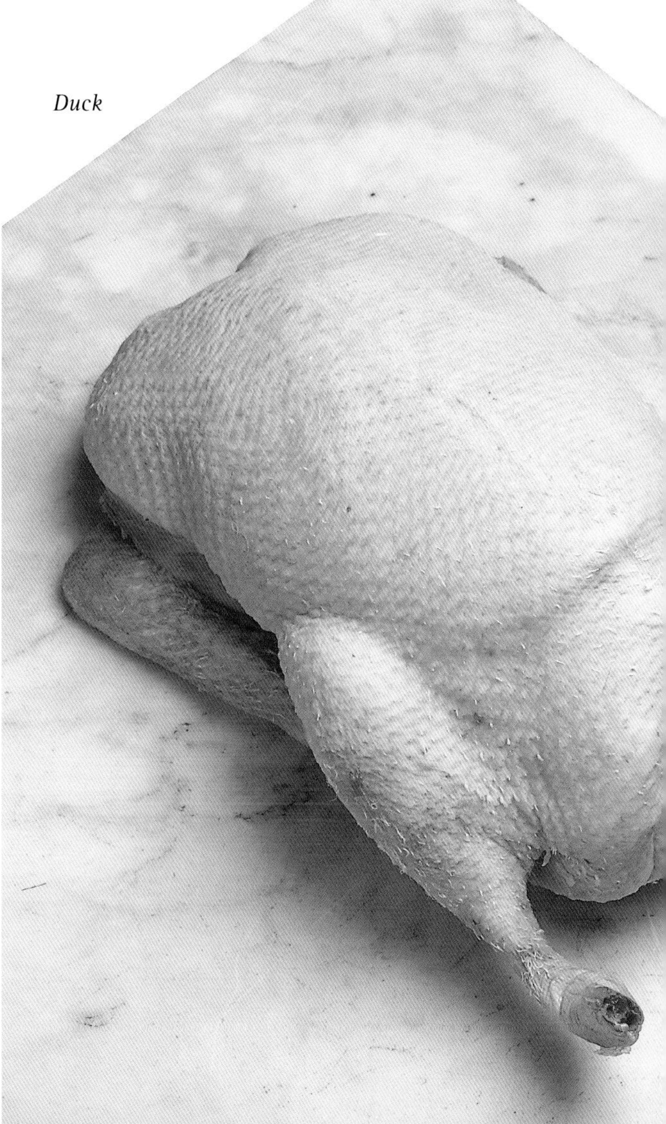

Duck

Domestic Poultry

In domestically raised birds there is a distinction between the nutritional value of breast (or white) meat as opposed to dark (or leg) meat. The white meat is generally lower in fat, while the dark meat has a greater supply of iron and other minerals.

CHICKEN, TURKEY, GOOSE AND DUCK	*FAT(g)*	*PROT(g)*	*Zn(mg)*	*B_6(mg)*
Chicken breast, broiled (grilled), without skin *192 calories (portion 130g)*	2.86	41.60	1.04	0.82
Chicken thighs, skinned, casseroled *135 calories (portion 75g)*	6.45	19.20	1.57	0.14
Turkey breast, fillet, broiled (grilled), meat only *140 calories (portion 90g)*	1.53	31.50	1.53	0.57
Turkey, dark meat, roasted *159 calories (portion 90g)*	5.94	26.46	3.06	0.40
Goose, roasted, meat only *287 calories (portion 90g)*	19.80	26.37	2.34	0.38
Duck, roasted, meat only *361 calories (portion 185g)*	19.24	46.81	4.81	0.46

CHICKEN

Chickens are usually available as broilers, fryers or roasters in the U.S. and as roasters or boilers in the U.K. They may be roasted, broiled (grilled), baked in pieces, sautéd, pan-fried or deep-fried. However, any form of fried chicken is very high in fat. Very small chickens, called poussins, are available and usually served whole.

Stewing (boiling) hens or fowls are more mature birds and are best simmered, stewed or braised. They are excellent for soups.

Chicken livers, gizzards, hearts and necks (known collectively as giblets) are sold with the bird and are particularly useful for making stock or gravy. Schmaltz, or rendered chicken fat, is an important component in kosher cooking.

DUCKS AND GEESE

Ducklings (ducks under one year old) are generally roasted. Full-grown ducks may be roasted but are also braised, stewed or made into *confit* (preserved in their own fat). Long Island duck, moularde duck and Muscovy duck are

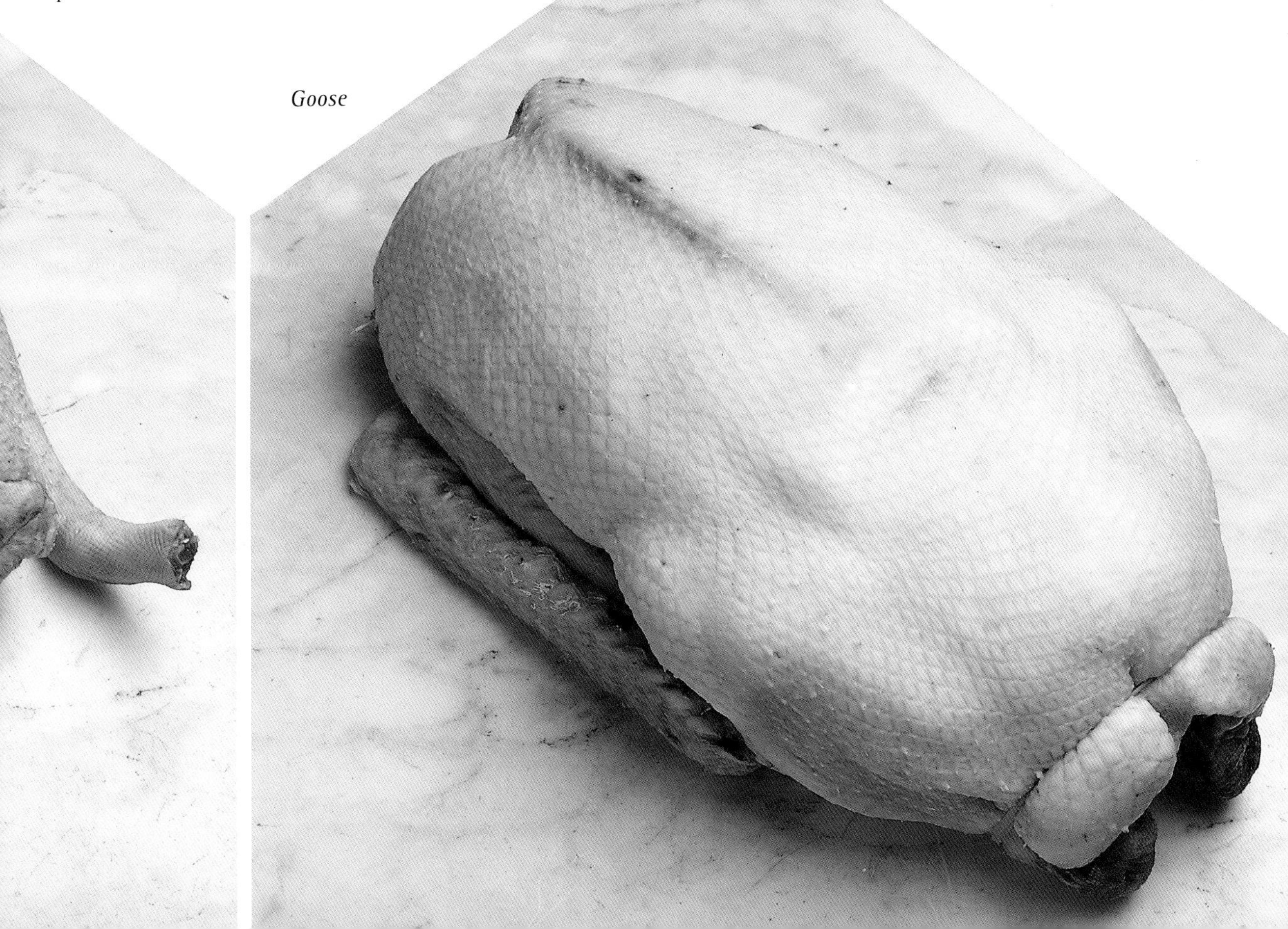

Goose

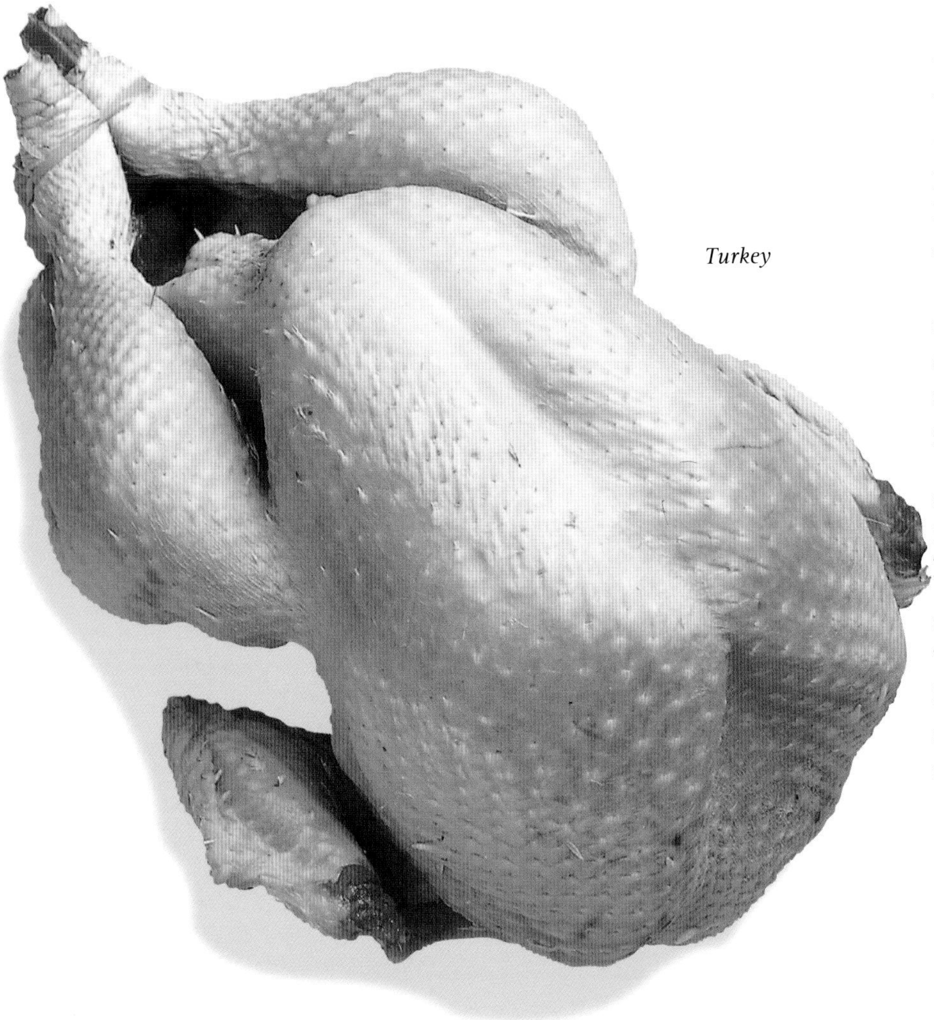

Turkey

common breeds of duck in the U.S. but Aylesbury duck is the most common British variety. Duck eaten with the fat and skin has up to three times more fat than the lean meat alone.

It is possible to purchase duck portions, including the liver. The breast is often sautéd, broiled (grilled) or pan-seared. Legs are typically slow-roasted or braised. The fattened liver of the moularde duck, known as *foie gras*, is now produced commercially outside France, so it is more easily available as a fresh product.

Geese are generally suited to roasting. Those over one year old may be better stewed or braised. Goose meat contains more than 20 percent fat.

CORNISH GAME HEN/ ROCK CORNISH GAME HEN

These small, relatively plump birds are the result of careful breeding. They have more breast meat than leg meat in relation to their overall size and composition. These birds are ideal for roasting.

TURKEY

This large bird has gained in popularity over the years, and turkey products are finding their way on to the menu all year round, instead of just at Thanksgiving and Christmas. In general, the meat-to-bone ratio is best at weights over 12 lb (5.5 kg).

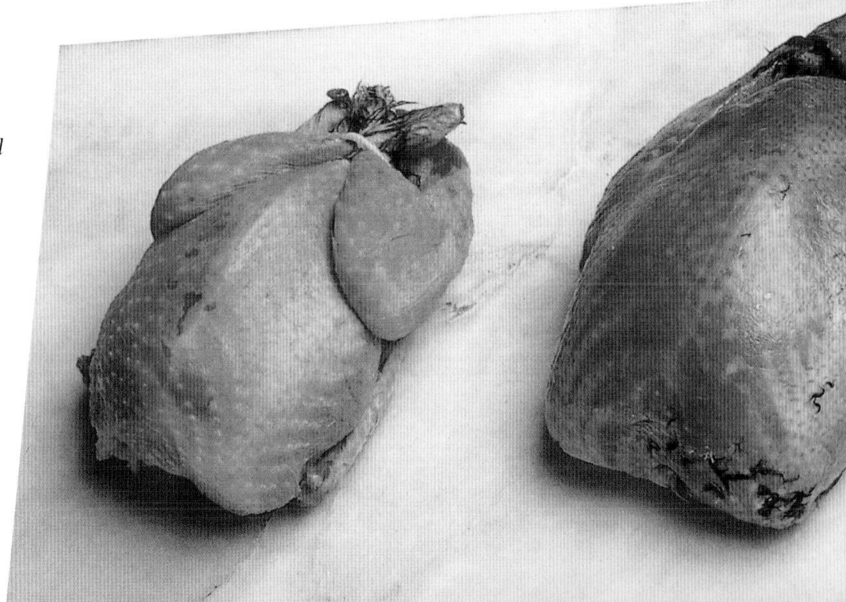

Quail

Grouse

Turkey is increasingly available in individual portions. It has a more distinct flavor than chicken, so it may be preferred by some consumers. Whole turkeys are usually roasted. Smaller portions are often cooked in a casserole.

FEATHERED GAME *all values per 100g*	*PROT(g)*	*FAT(g)*	*NAeq(mg)*	*Fe(mg)*
Pheasant, roasted, meat only *220 calories*	27.90	12.00	15.20	2.20
Partridge, roasted, meat only *212 calories*	36.70	7.20	–	7.70
Grouse, roasted, meat only, with bone *59 calories*	12.70	0.90	7.50	2.10

Game birds are an excellent source of iron. Other good sources include liver (12.2 mg per 100 g), mussels and cockles (8–10 mg/portion), red meats and curries.

Wild Game Birds

Game birds are wild species, but some are now farm-raised. Most birds, especially free range birds, are at their best from October through December or January, but the season varies for each bird.

Young game birds should have soft, smooth, pliable skin; the breastbone should be flexible, as it is for domestic fowl. Most are hung for several days to increase their flavor. They have about the same amount of fat as lean steak.

QUAIL

Quail is the smallest of the game birds and should be eaten fresh. It is traditionally spit-roasted or poached.

SNIPE AND WOODCOCK

Snipe and woodcock are hard to come by unless you are a good shot. They are traditionally roasted ungutted.

WILD DUCK

Wild duck (teal) is considered a delicacy. As wild duck ages, the flesh may take on a fishy or oily taste.

PHEASANT

Pheasant is one of the meatiest game birds and is usually roasted or braised. Domestically raised pheasant will not have a pronounced flavor unless it is hung for several days.

GROUSE

The grouse season is from August to December, and the bird is often frozen for the festive season. One plump roasted bird serves two people. Grouse can be hung or eaten freshly killed.

PARTRIDGE

Partridge flesh is white, fine and sweet, and one bird feeds one person. Partridge is best cooked plainly with just a little butter rubbed in the skin before roasting.

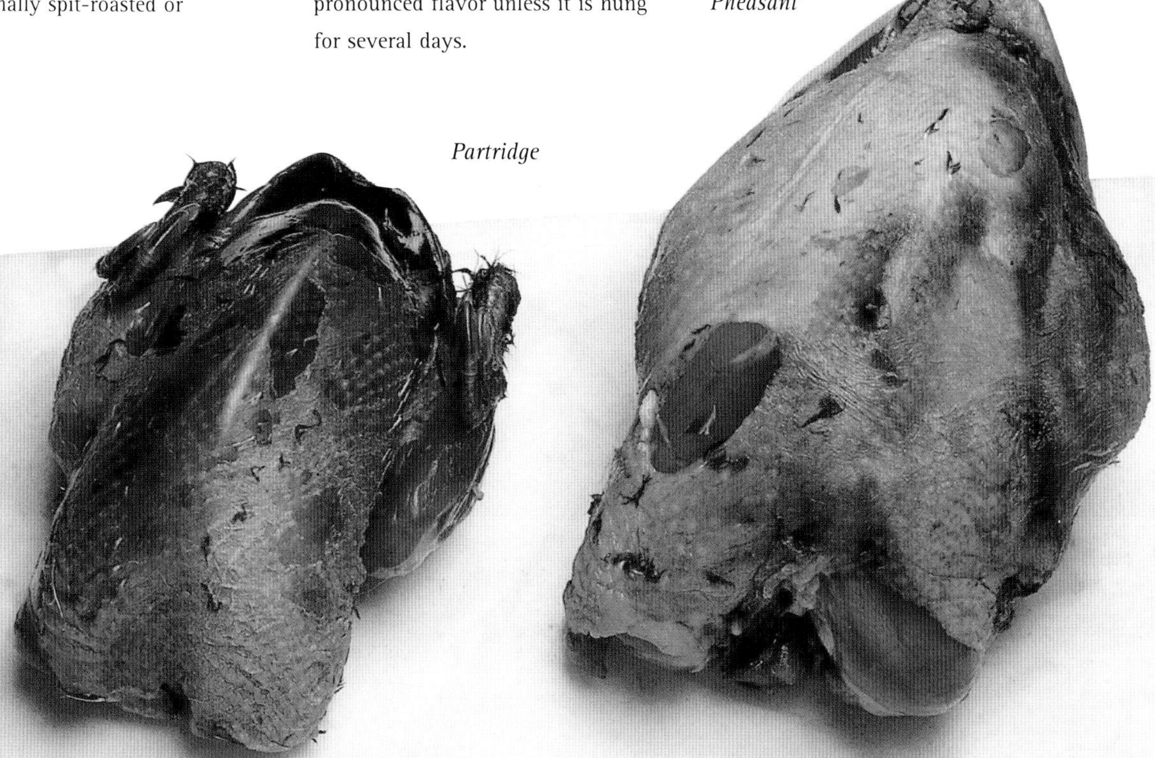

Partridge

Pheasant

Fish and Shellfish

Fish were once plentiful and inexpensive, but overfishing has caused demand to outstrip supply. At the time of writing, regulations have been passed by a number of countries restricting commercial fishing concerns to an ever-smaller percentage of the best fishing waters. Farmed fish is therefore becoming more popular. Nutritionally, there is little difference between farmed fish and wild fish.

Aquaculture, or farm-raising fish, is growing in importance as fish farms become one of the few reliable sources of fresh fish. Today trout, salmon, tilapia (St. Peter's Fish), catfish, oysters, mussels and clams are found easily because they are farmed.

Fish, especially oily fish such as mackerel, is the best source of omega-3 fatty acids. These compounds help reduce the stickiness of the blood, and the consumption of two to three servings of fish a week is related to a lower risk of heart attack.

Shellfish cause concern because some contain relatively high amounts of cholesterol. In the majority of people, however, the body adapts to the cholesterol in seafood and other food by reducing the amount it manufactures in the liver.

CHOOSING FISH

Select absolutely fresh fish of the best quality. The fishmonger should properly handle, ice and display the fish and should be able to answer any questions regarding its origin and qualities: lean or oily, firm-textured or delicate, whether appropriate for oven, steamer or broiler (grill). To ensure that fish are of the best quality, apply as many as possible of the following tests.

- **Smell the fish.** It should have a fresh, clean, "sea" aroma. Very strong odors are a clear indication that the fish is aging or has been improperly handled or stored.
- **Feel the skin.** It should feel slick and moist. The scales, if any, should be firmly attached.
- **Look at the fins and tail.** They should be moist, flexible and full, not ragged or dry.
- **Press the flesh.** It should feel firm and elastic and retain no visible fingerprint when you lift your finger away.
- **Check the eyes.** They should be clear and full. As the fish ages, the eyes begin to lose moisture and sink back into the head.
- **Check the gills.** They should have a good red to maroon color with no traces of gray or brown and should be moist and fresh-looking. The shade of red will depend on the fish type.
- **Check the belly.** There should be no sign of "belly burn," which occurs when the guts are not removed promptly; the stomach enzymes begin to eat the flesh, causing it to come away from the bones. There should also be no breaks or tears in the flesh.
- **Check live shellfish for signs of movement.** Lobsters and crabs should move about. Clams, mussels and oysters should be tightly closed; as they age, they start to open. Any shells that do not snap shut when tapped should be discarded; the shellfish are dead.

STORAGE

Buy only the amount of fish needed for a day or two at most, and store it properly. Fresh fish should be loosely wrapped in paper and kept in the coolest part of the refrigerator. Shellfish should be kept in a bag or box. Frozen fish or shellfish should be kept frozen.

Commonly Available Fish

Some fish are naturally lean, while others are more oily; some have extremely delicate and subtle flavors, while others are robust and meaty. The best way of deciding how to cook a particular fish is to consider the flesh. Oily fish such as mackerel and bluefish are often prepared by dry-heat techniques such as broiling (grilling). Fish with moderate amounts of fat (salmon and trout) adapt to any cooking method, with the possible exception of deep-frying. Very lean fish such as sole or flounder are most successfully prepared by poaching, sautéing, pan-frying or deep-frying.

OILY FISH

Trout, Salmon, Mackerel, Tuna, Herrings, Sardines

Oily fish have their oils spread throughout their flesh rather than concentrated in the liver as do white fish. They are rich sources of omega-3 fatty acids, which may help reduce the risk of heart attack.

Trout are farm-raised in large quantities. Rainbow trout and brown trout, the most commonly available species, are excellent when pan-fried, roasted or poached.

Salmon is a firm, moderately oily fish with a distinctively colored flesh, ranging from pale pink to a deep orange-pink. A number of different species are available, including coho, king and Atlantic. Salmon may be obtained fresh, smoked or cured as "gravlax."

Mackerel is an oily, soft-textured fish, the flesh of which flakes easily when cooked. Mackerel is best when prepared with dry-heat cooking techniques and is commonly broiled (grilled).

Tuna's flavor is unique, and the flesh's color ranges from a deep pinkish beige to a dark maroon. A member of the mackerel family, tuna has a distinctive strip of darker colored flesh along its back. Tuna is often roasted or cut into steaks and grilled. Also popular is canned tuna – although some of the omega-3 fatty acids are destroyed in the canning process.

Herrings are small fish that can be stuffed, baked or grilled. Their extreme oiliness makes them ideal for curing as well, for example, rollmops.

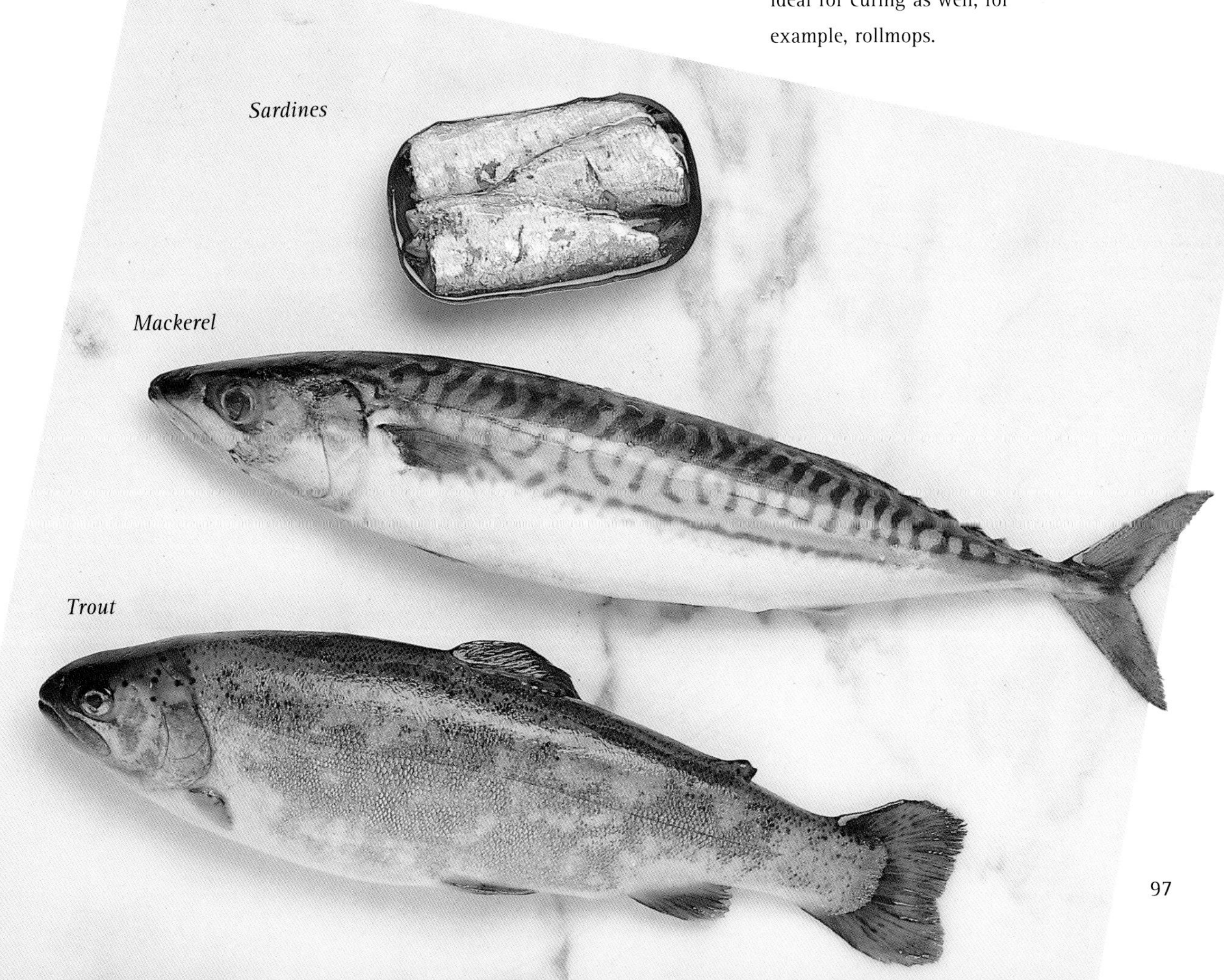
Sardines

Mackerel

Trout

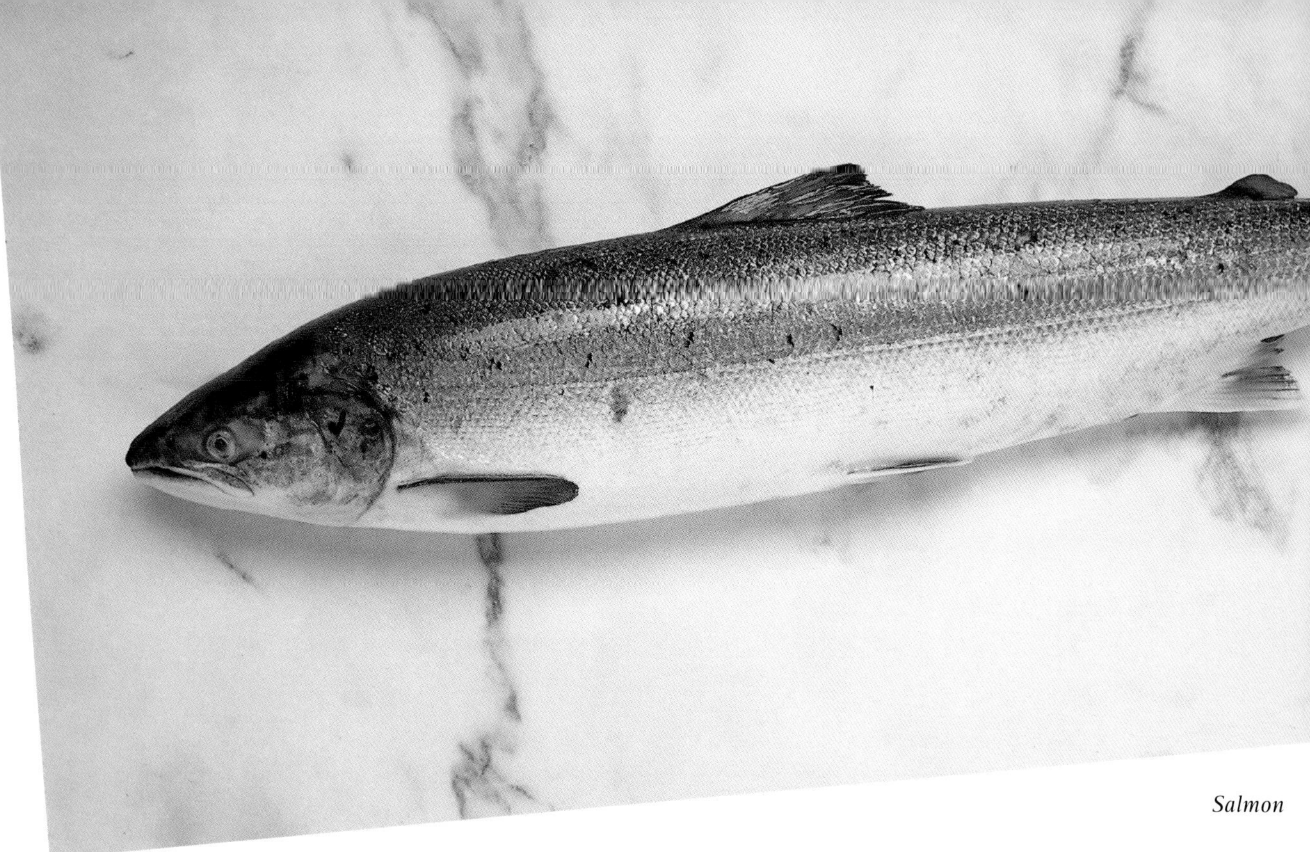

Salmon

Sardines are strong-tasting oily fish that are sold fresh and canned in oil, brine or tomato sauce. Large sardines (still very small) are called pilchards; three or four makes one portion.

WHITE FISH

Catfish (rockfish), Bass, Cod, Monkfish, Snapper, Dover sole, Halibut

White fish have nonoily flesh and contain very little fat. They are a wonderful source of digestible protein, as well as B vitamins. Because they are dry, they lend themselves to being cooked with sauces.

Catfish (rockfish) are raised in farms or ponds. They have a firm-textured, slightly sweet flesh and must be skinned before cooking (ideally by your fishmonger).

Bass are available in several varieties. Black sea bass feed primarily on shrimp (prawns), crabs and mollusks. They have firm, well-flavored flesh that responds well to all cooking techniques. They average 1 to 3 lb (450 g to 1.4 kg) in weight, but may be larger in fall. Similar varieties, such as striped bass, sea bass and pike may be cooked in similar ways.

Cod has lean, white flesh which may be poached, steamed, deep-fried or used in chowder (fish stew). A salted form, known as *bacalão*, is also available. Haddock, whiting, hake and pollack are all members of the cod family.

Monkfish is known by a number of names, including angler fish, goosefish, lawyer fish and belly fish. The French name is *lotte*. It is available as the fillet from the tail. Monkfish has a firm, dense texture and sweet taste. Suitable for any cooking technique, it is commonly used in fish stews such as *bouillabaisse*.

OILY FISH

	FAT(g)	*PUFA(g)*	*Vit A(mcg)*	*Vit D(mcg)*
Trout, brown, steamed *209 calories (portion 155g)*	6.97	2.33	60.45	–
Salmon, grilled *176 calories (portion 82g)*	10.74	3.36	13.12	7.87
Salmon, pink, canned in brine, drained *185 calories (portion 121g)*	7.99	2.30	37.51	20.57
Tuna, canned in oil, drained *85 calories (portion 45g)*	4.05	2.16	–	1.35
Sardines, canned in brine, drained *172 calories (portion 100g)*	9.60	–	6.00	4.60
Herring, grilled *215 calories (portion 119g)*	13.33	2.74	40.46	19.16

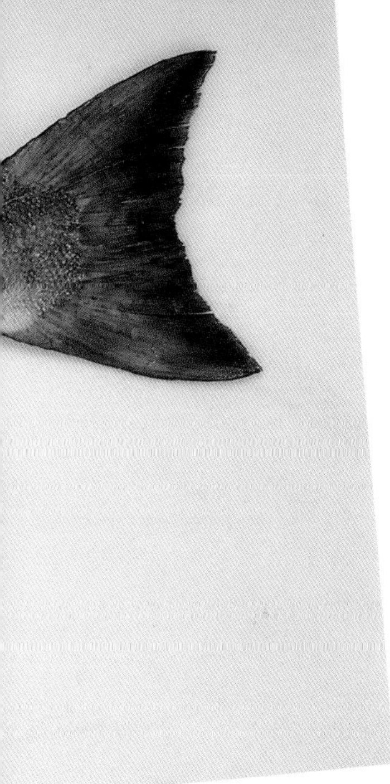

WHITE FISH	PROT(g)	FAT(g)	Se(mcg)	I(mcg)
Cod, baked *168 calories (portion 175g)*	37.45	2.10	59.50	227.50
Fish sticks (fish fingers), cod, grilled *56 calories (portion 28g)*	4.00	2.49	6.44	30.80
Haddock, grilled *125 calories (portion 120g)*	29.16	0.96	42.00	384.00
Hoki (Japanese flat white fish), grilled *230 calories (portion 190g)*	45.79	5.13	114.00	–
Plaice (flat white fish), grilled *125 calories (portion 130g)*	26.13	2.21	58.50	52.00

Red snapper is one of the most popular varieties of snapper, of which there are many: vermillion, silk, mutton, mangrove, gray, beeliner, pink and yellowtail.

The flesh is firm, moist and finely textured and responds well to all cooking methods.

Dover sole, one of the few true species of sole, is a flat fish with a compact, oval shape and firmly textured, delicately flavored flesh. It is so highly esteemed that hundreds of recipes have been devised around it.

Halibut has delicately flavored, firm, white flesh which can be cut into steaks or fillets. A halibut of 10 to 40 lb (4.5 to 18 kg) is considered small as this species can grow to be over 200 lb (90 kg).

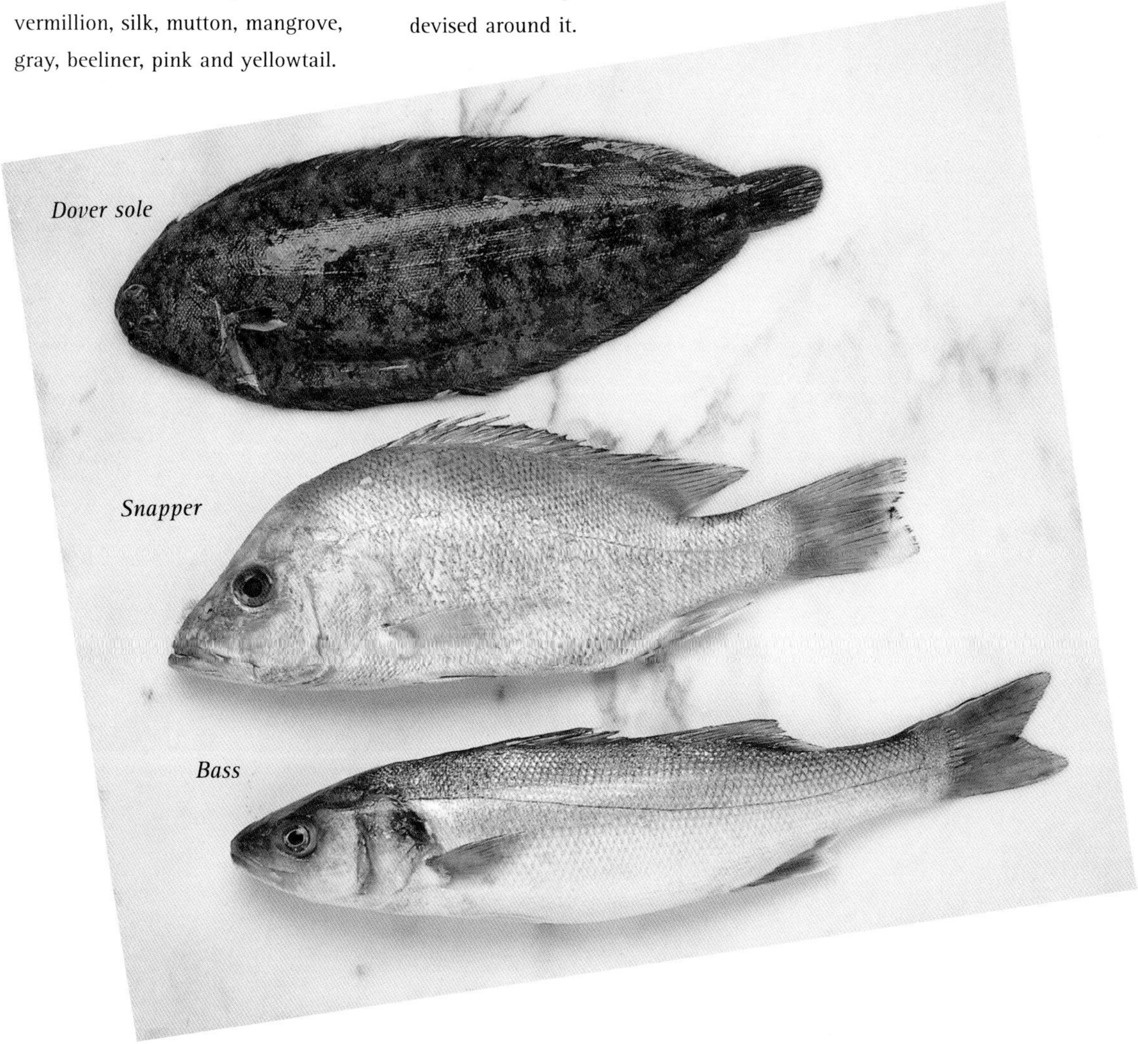

Dover sole

Snapper

Bass

Seafood

Seafood is the general term given to shellfish and sea creatures other than fish.

MOLLUSKS

Oysters, Scallops, Clams, Mussels

Clams are available in the shell, shucked (shelled and possibly frozen) and canned. Clams sold live should have tightly closed shells, which indicates that they are alive. They should have a sweet smell. There are various sizes and types of clam. Littlenecks are small, hardshell clams often eaten raw on the half shell. Cherrystones are the next largest in size and are also commonly eaten raw. If hardshell clams are more than 3 in (7.5 cm) in diameter, they are generally referred to as quahogs and used for chowder or fritters.

Most commercially available mussels are farm-raised and sold live in the shell. They should be debearded before cooking. A popular method of preparation is *à la marinière* (steamed with wine, garlic and lemon).

Oysters are sold live in the shell or shucked (shelled). They are frequently eaten raw on the half shell and in stews and omelets.

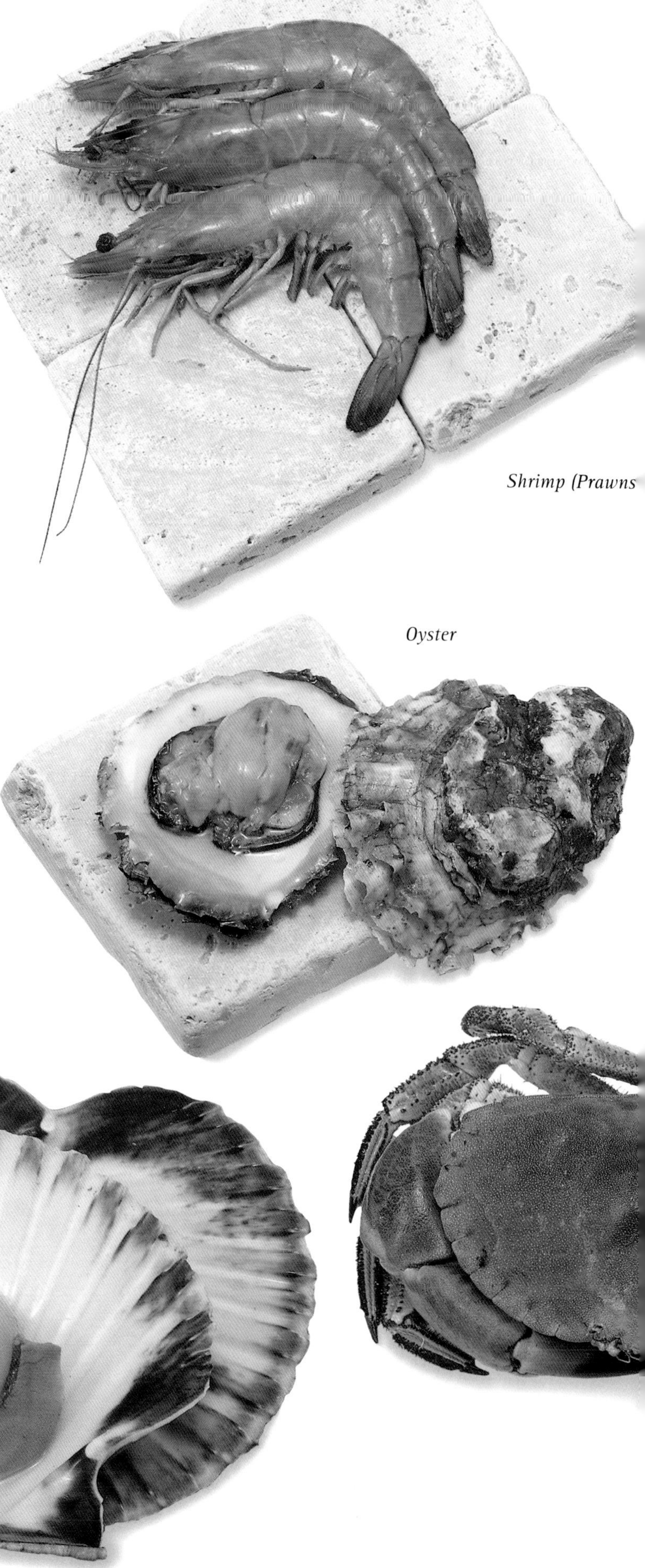

Shrimp (Prawns

Oyster

Scallop

Oysters Rockefeller is a special dish that includes spinach and Pernod, an aniseed-flavored aperitif.

Three species of scallop are of commercial importance: bay scallops, sea scallops and calico scallops. Sea scallops can become quite large (2 to 3 in [5 to 7.5 cm] in diameter), bay and calico scallops are smaller. Bay scallops are generally considered superior to calicos.

Most scallops are sold shucked (shelled). Occasionally, farm-raised scallops in the shell are available.

MOLLUSKS AND CRUSTACEANS	*Na(mg)*	*Fe(mg)*	*Se(mcg)*	*B_{12}(mcg)*
Mussels, boiled *42 calories (portion 40g)*	144.00	2.72	17.20	8.80
Oysters, raw *78 calories (portion 120g)*	612.00	6.84	27.60	20.40
Crab, boiled *51 calories (portion 40g)*	168.00	0.64	6.80	–
Lobster, boiled *88 calories (portion 85g)*	280.50	0.68	110.50	2.55
Scallops, steamed *83 calories (portion 70g)*	126.00	0.77	35.70	6.30
Shrimp (prawns), boiled *59 calories (portion 60g)*	954.00	0.66	13.80	4.80

CRUSTACEANS

Crab, Lobster, Shrimp

Common kinds of crab include blue, Dungeness, king and spider. Softshelled crabs, available from spring through late summer, are commonly pan-fried or sautéd. Hardshelled crabs may be boiled or steamed. The meat may be removed and used in a variety of preparations, including crab cakes, a famous American specialty.

Lobster is available live or cooked and canned, and it has firm and succulent meat. Varieties include the American lobster, northern lobster and rock lobster (often sold as frozen tails). Dublin Bay prawns, also known as scampi in the U.K., are other famous members of the lobster family.

Shrimp (prawns) are probably the most popular crustacean. They are most commonly available frozen as fishermen generally remove the heads and flash-freeze them on the boat in order to preserve flavor and quality. Fresh shrimp (prawns), of which there are saltwater and freshwater species, should be eaten the day they are bought. The flesh has a sweet flavor and a firm, almost crisp texture.

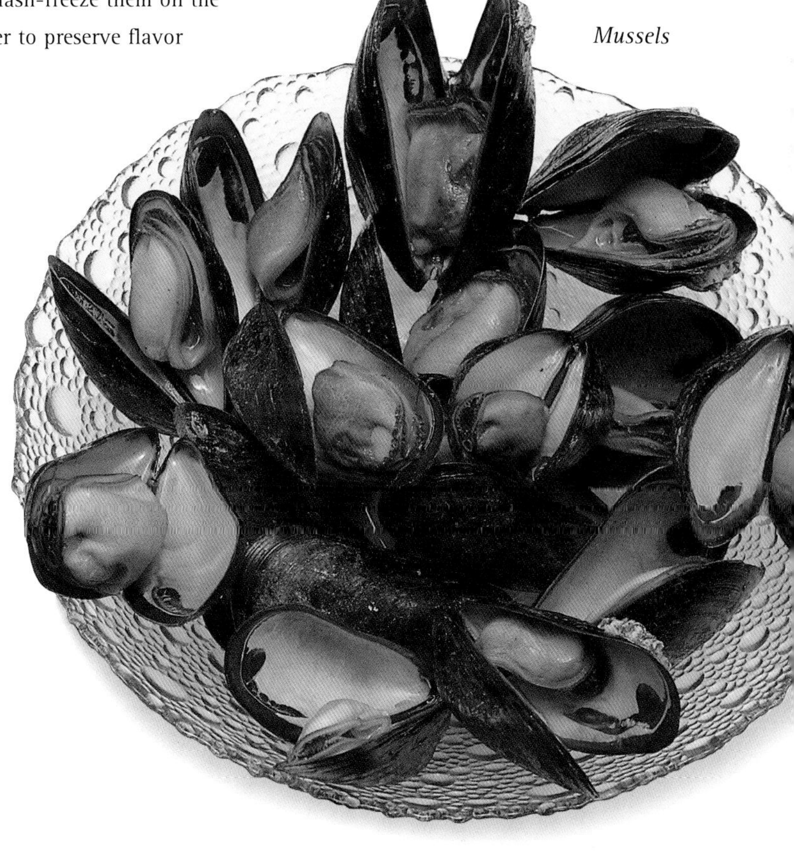

Mussels

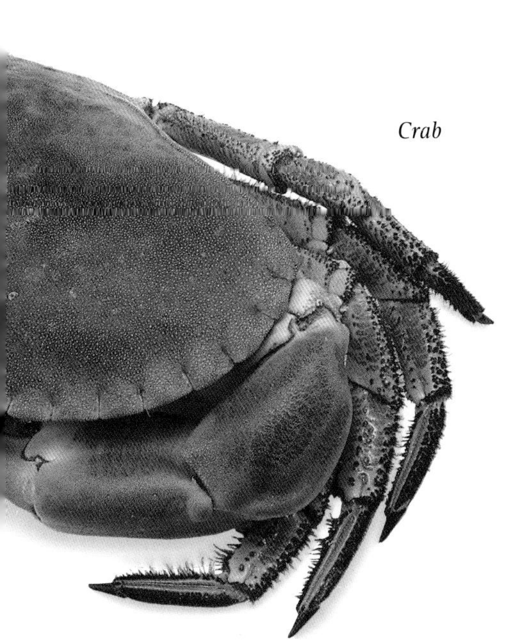

Crab

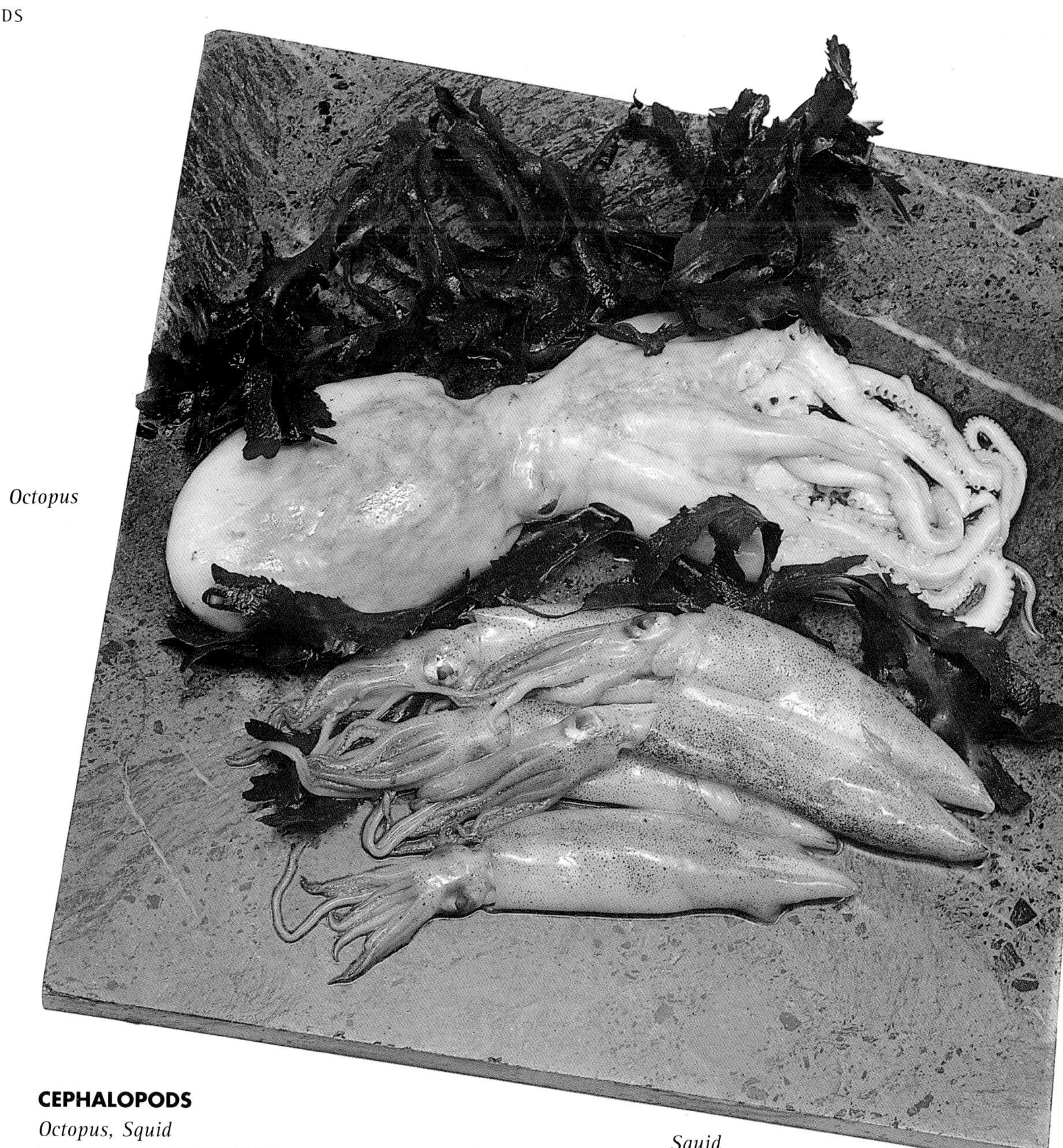

CEPHALOPODS

Octopus, Squid

Octopus is firmly textured with a sweet marine flavor. It is generally sold fresh, cleaned of its ink and beak, but it is also available frozen. Octopus features in many dishes, including seviche, chowders and salads.

Squid have long been part of Mediterranean and Oriental cuisines and are continuing to gain popularity in the U.S. and Britain. Small squid are frequently stuffed and cooked whole in a sauce, whereas large squid are cut into rings, dipped in batter and deep-fried.

CEPHALOPODS AND MISCELLANEOUS SEAFOOD

all values per 100g	*FAT(g)*	*Na(mg)*	*I(mcg)*	*Se(mcg)*
Octopus, raw *83 calories*	1.30	–	20.00	75.00
Squid, raw *81 calories*	1.70	110.00	20.00	66.00
Cuttlefish, raw *71 calories*	0.70	370.00	–	65.00
Caviar, bottled in brine, drained *92 calories*	5.40	2,120.00	–	–

Seafood can contain large amounts of sodium – one 5-ml teaspoon of table salt contains approximately 2,000 mg of sodium.

FROGS' LEGS

Prized for their delicate texture, the flesh of frogs' legs tastes something like chicken. Only the hind legs of certain frogs are used. Mostly sold ready-prepared, frogs' legs can be canned, frozen or fresh. They can be battered or deep-fried, or sautéd. Around four pairs are normally served per person.

CAVIAR

A great delicacy, caviar is the roe (eggs) from the Sturgeon fish. The finest beluga caviar is very expensive indeed. Caviar is quite salty in taste. It is often served simply with champagne. Gout sufferers should avoid caviar as it has a high content of purines that could exacerbate their condition.

SALMON ROE

Salmon roe is eaten in the same way as caviar, and is sometimes referred to as caviar. However, this word really only applies to the more expensive and high-quality sturgeon roe. Salmon roe is orange whereas caviar is black.

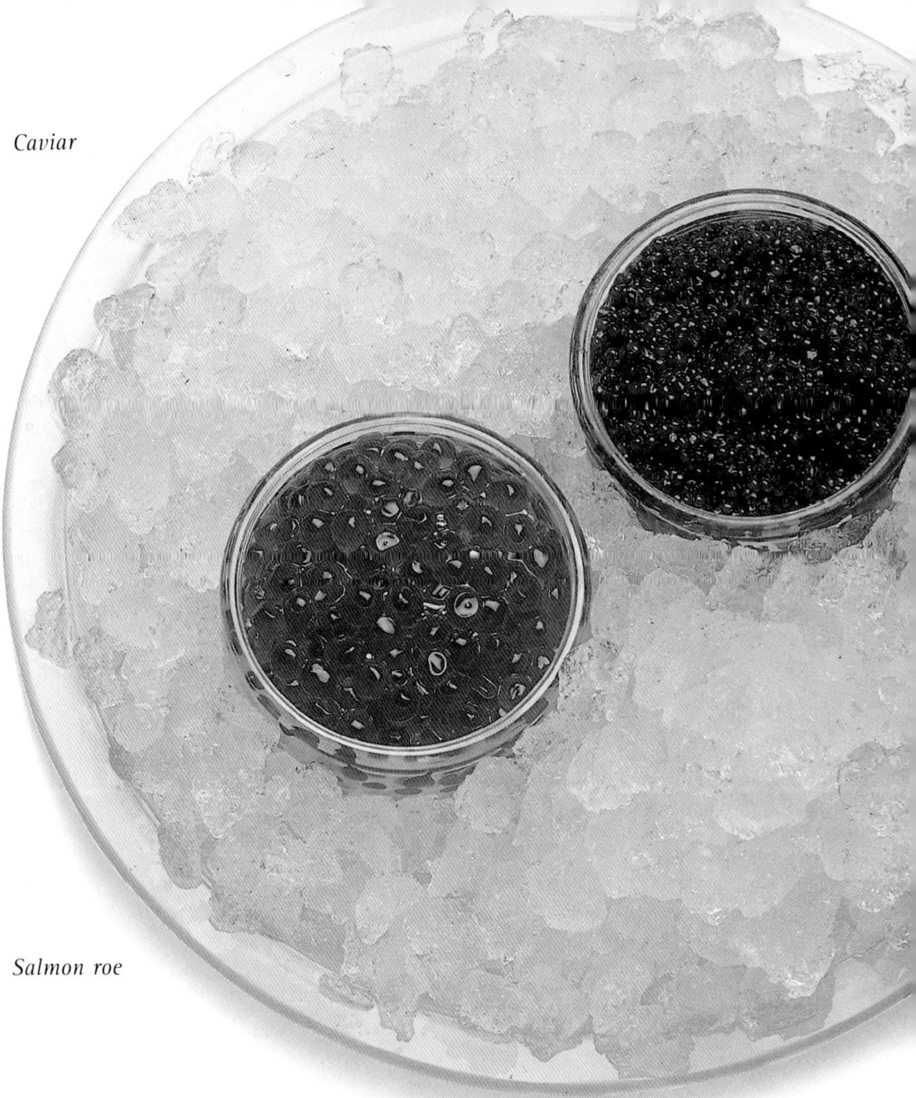

Caviar

Salmon roe

Frogs' legs

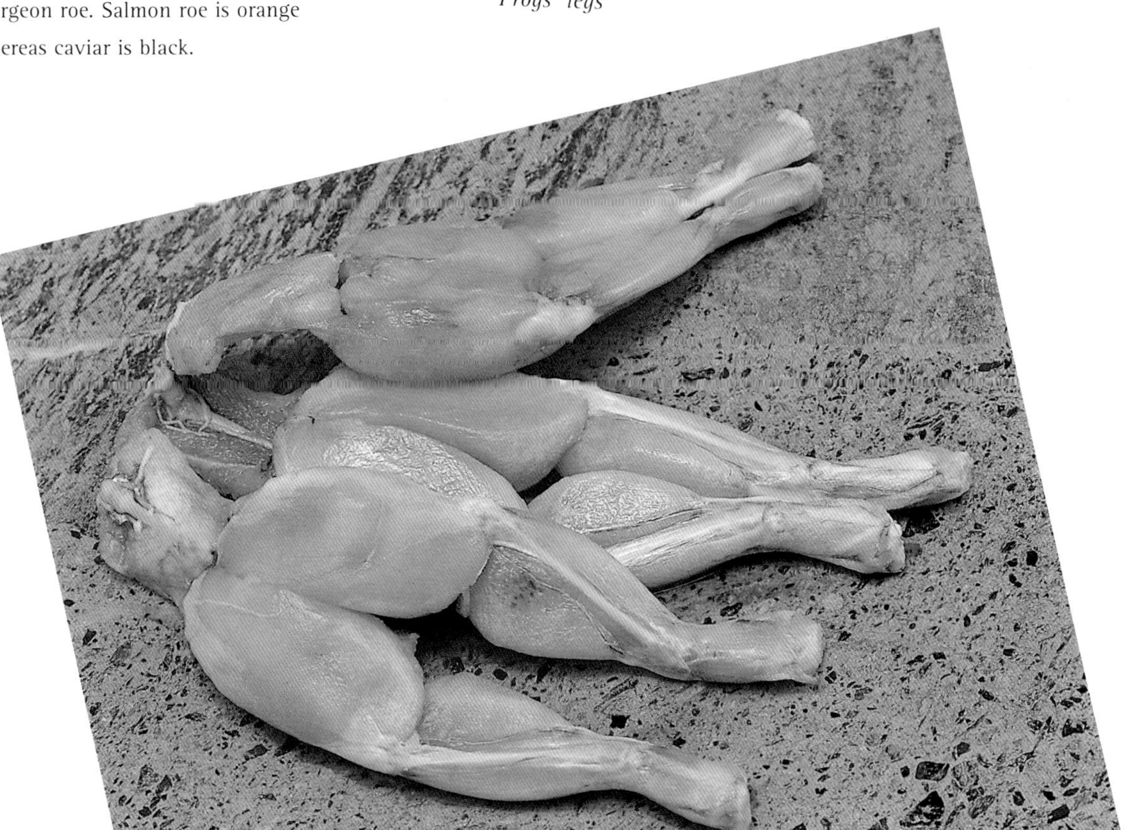

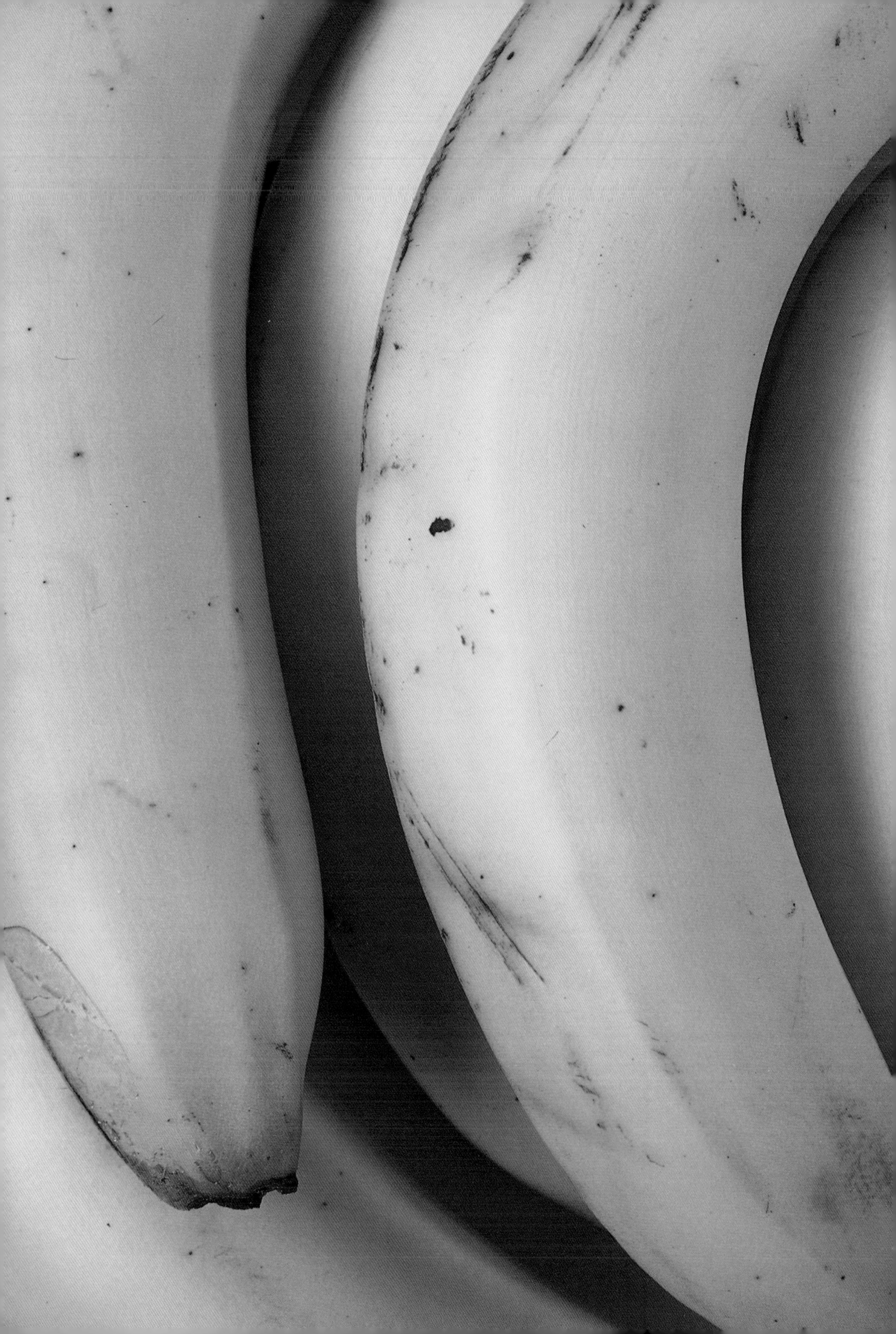

VITAMINS AND MINERALS

Despite the fact that we only need vitamins and minerals in tiny amounts, they are vital to our life and well-being.
This section includes analysis charts to help you compare certain foods containing each relevant vitamin or mineral, and charts which indicate the recommended daily allowances for each age group or those with special needs.

Vitamins and Minerals

Our knowledge about vitamins and minerals has increased enormously since the isolation of vitamin C, the first vitamin linked to a deficiency disease, scurvy. The primary function of vitamins and minerals is to regulate the body's metabolism, though some have other roles as components of bone (for example, calcium), or body fluids (such as potassium and sodium) or in hormonal activity (iodine, for example).

The amount of vitamins and minerals we each need depends on our state of health, our age, weight and height, physical activity level and our different physiological needs. However, scientists have calculated the approximate amount of vitamins and minerals that certain people need to eat to prevent developing diseases caused by deficiency. In the U.K. these amounts would cover the needs of almost all the population (97.5 percent), with 2.5 percent needing a little more or a little less. In the U.K. these figures are called the Reference Nutrient Intakes (RNIs).

In the U.S. these figures are called the Recommended Dietary Allowances (RDAs), and are intended to provide for individual variations among normal persons as they live in the U.S. under usual environmental stresses.

There are variations in the U.K. and U.S. figures (due to differences in interpreting scientific studies), which can be seen from the tables that follow in this section.

Where there is too little scientific data on record to set an RDA or RNI, a safe level of intake is suggested.

Supplementing Your Diet

While many publications have come out in favor of taking dietary supplements, you should use caution. Some vitamins, fat-soluble and water-soluble alike, can themselves reach toxic levels and you may begin to develop symptoms of a toxic disease. Depending upon the nature of the substance you are supplementing, you may compromise the absorption and metabolism of other important nutrients. Nutrients that are stored in the body's fat (such as vitamins A and D) are especially difficult to "flush out."

The body controls the amount of vitamins and minerals it obtains from food by absorbing as much as possible and excreting the extra, or by absorbing only the amount that is required. If these systems are overridden with the use of supplements, the body cannot easily control absorption, excess amounts pose a significant danger.

Minerals pose a special concern. Many are needed in minute quantities only and most interact in a very complicated fashion: if you take too much of one, it may hinder the absorption of another.

Self-medication with dietary supplements may not be harmful if it is done carefully. However, none of the information about vitamins and minerals that follows is a substitute for the advice of a trained professional.

IMPORTANT NOTE

Supplementation may make things worse rather than better if you have a serious medical condition, are of childbearing age or are pregnant, use alcohol, tobacco or street drugs.

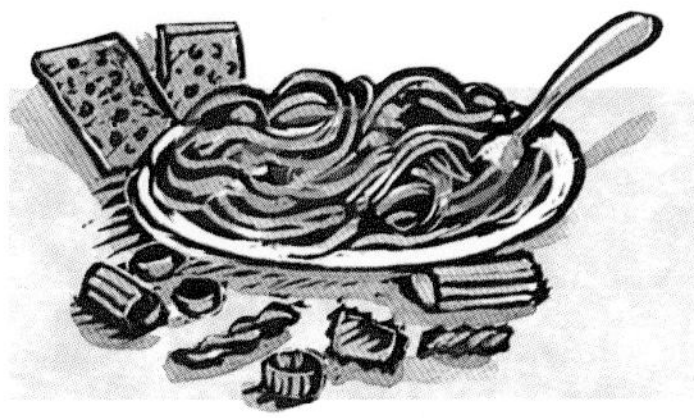

VITAMINS

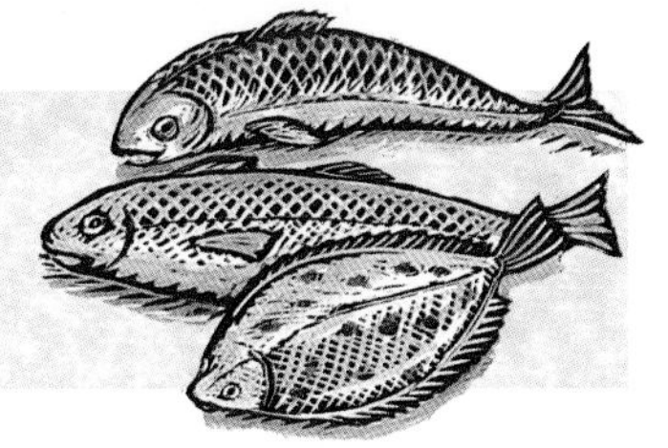

Vitamin A

(Retinol or Retinoic Acid)

Retinol (preformed vitamin A) is found in animal foods, while carotenes, including beta-carotene, are found in plant foods and are converted to retinol in the body.

Beta carotene appears to be an important antioxidant, and high levels of it in the diet have been linked to a reduced risk of lung cancer. Retinol is important in promoting good eyesight.

All epithelial tissues (including the cornea, the skin and the mucous linings of the lungs, intestines, vagina, bladder and urinary tract) rely on vitamin A to act as an effective barrier against infection and damage. It is this function that has led to continued studies on the role of vitamin A and carotenes in preventing certain cancers.

Deficiency of vitamin A may cause reproductive problems, but excess vitamin A during pregnancy can cause birth defects.

Intakes of 25,000 international units per day (i.u./day) (7,500 micrograms [mcg]/day) are thought to be nutritionally excessive.

In some countries, such as the U.K., pregnant women are advised not to eat liver and liver products because of the high levels of vitamin A they contain.

GOOD FOOD SOURCES

Fortified milk, cheese, cream, butter, eggs, and liver all contain the active form of vitamin A. The precursor, beta-carotene, is found in deep orange fruits and vegetables such as apricots, peaches, cantaloupes, carrots, sweet potatoes, squash, pumpkin and yams. Beta-carotene is also found in spinach and similar dark-green leafy vegetables, as well as in members of the cabbage family.

Vitamin A *mcg/day (micrograms per day)*

Age	*RDA*	*RNI*
0-12 months	375	350
1-10	400-700	400-500
11-14	800-1,000	600
15-18	800-1,000	600-700
19 plus	800-1,000	600-700
Pregnancy	800	700
Nursing	1,300-1,200[a]	950

© see below.
a Second six months.

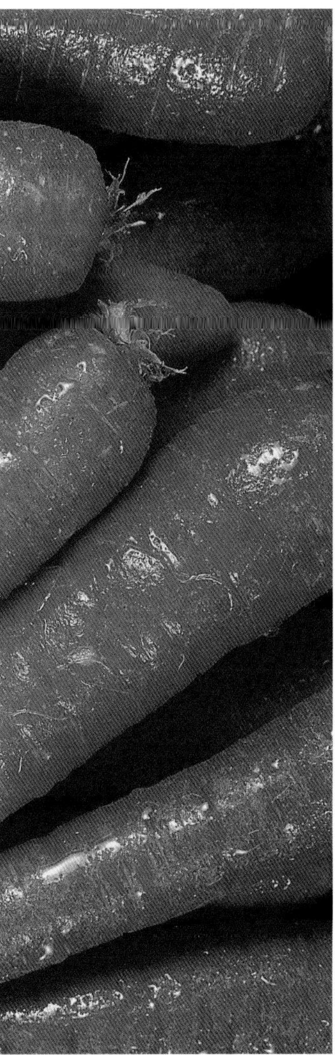

▲ *Carrots are the best source of beta carotene, which is the vegetable form of vitamin A.*

Analysis – Vitamin A *micrograms (mcg)*

	Portion	Amount
Pâté, liver	40g	2,932
Sweet potato, baked	130g	1,111
Carrots, raw	60g	811
Spinach, boiled	90g	576
Melon, canteloupe	150g	499
Eggs, scrambled with milk	120g	354

Analysed on Compeat 4.
Data rounded to one decimal place.

Vitamin B_1

(Thiamin)

Thiamin is used to generate energy from starchy foods, so a carbohydrate-rich diet needs more added thiamin.

In developing countries where the diet contains polished rice, a deficiency disease called beri-beri may occur. This disease (symptoms include stiffness, weakness or even paralysis) is the result of diets that rely on highly refined and processed grain products for their main carbohydrate source.

- Alcoholism is the main cause of thiamin deficiency in developed countries.
- Intakes of more than 3,000 milligrams (mg)/day can be toxic.

GOOD FOOD SOURCES

In some countries thiamin is added to wheat flour and, consequently, to breads, cereals and pastas. Breads, cereals, potatoes, milk and milk products, pork, wheat germ, brewer's yeast, green peas, greens, oranges and dried beans and peas are all good sources of thiamin.

Vitamin B_1 *mg/day (milligrams per day)*

Age	*RDA*	*RNI*
0–12 months	0.3–0.4	0.2–0.3
1–10	0.7–1.0	0.5–0.7
11–14	1.1–1.3	0.7–0.9
15–18	1.1–1.5	0.8–1.1
19 plus	1.1–1.5	0.8–1.0
Pregnancy	1.5	0.9[a]
Nursing	1.6	1.0

© see page 107.

a In last trimester only.

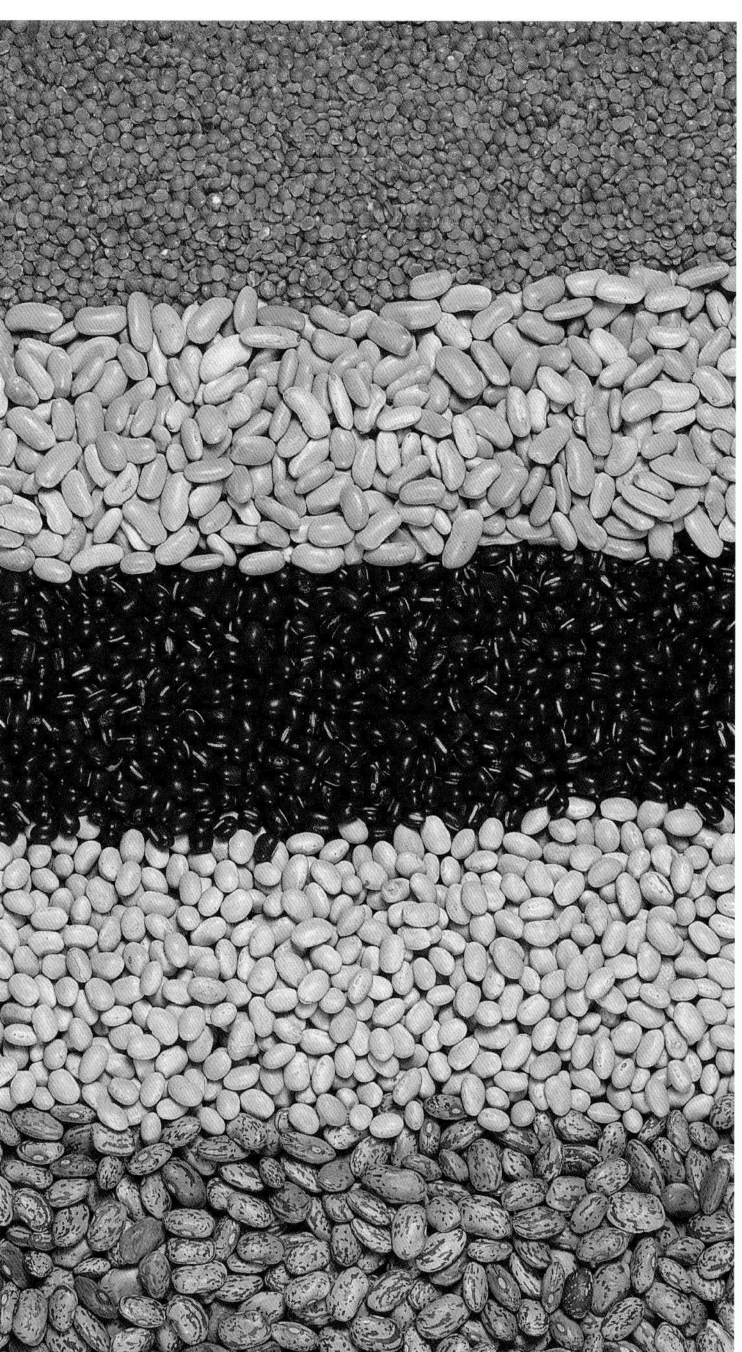

▲ *Legumes are an excellent source of thiamin.*

Analysis – Vitamin B_1 *milligrams (mg)*

	Portion	Amount
Pork fillet, grilled, lean	140g	2.2
Vegeburger, grilled	56g	1.3
Peas, boiled	70g	0.5
Potatoes, baked, flesh	160g	0.3
Milk, part skim	585ml	0.2
Bread, whole wheat	36g	0.1

© see page 107.

Vitamin B_2

(Riboflavin)

Riboflavin is used to metabolize energy from protein, fats and carbohydrates. It supports normal vision and general skin health. People lacking riboflavin may develop a sensitivity to light or cracks and fissures at the corners of their mouths.

Usually, the lack of riboflavin is accompanied by a similar lack of thiamin—with the thiamin deficiency often being severe enough to mask a B_2 deficiency.

Deficiency is most likely in people whose diets are low in meat and dairy products, especially vegans, who eat no animal products at all.

GOOD FOOD SOURCES

Dairy products (especially low-fat milk, cottage cheese and yogurt), mushrooms, fortified breakfast cereals and breads and dark green leafy vegetables all supply good amounts of riboflavin.

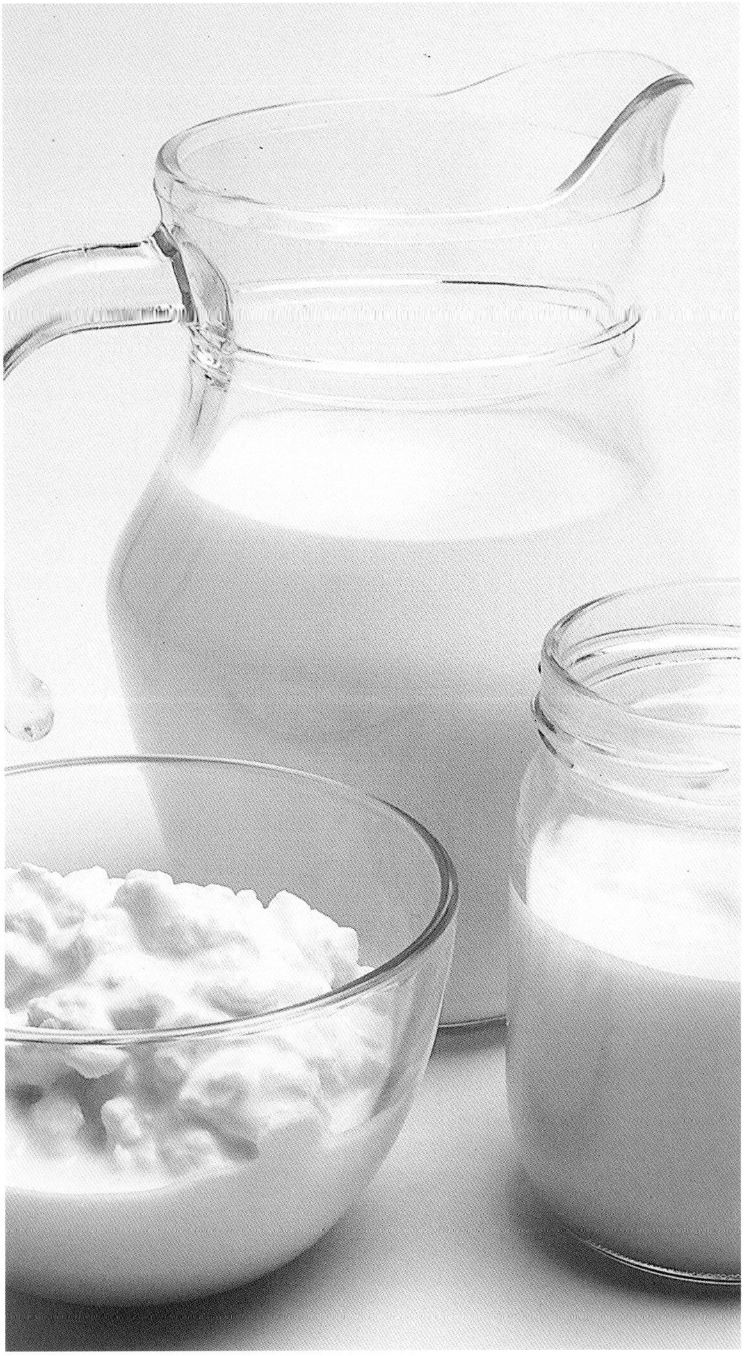

▲ *Include two servings of dairy products in the diet each day to ensure an adequate supply of riboflavin.*

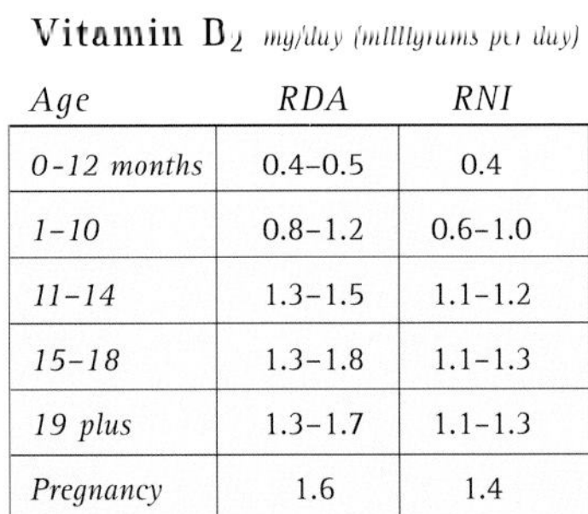

Vitamin B_2 *mg/day (milligrams per day)*

Age	RDA	RNI
0-12 months	0.4–0.5	0.4
1-10	0.8–1.2	0.6–1.0
11-14	1.3–1.5	1.1–1.2
15-18	1.3–1.8	1.1–1.3
19 plus	1.3–1.7	1.1–1.3
Pregnancy	1.6	1.4
Nursing	1.8–1.7[a]	1.6

© see page 107.
a Second six months.

Analysis – Vitamin B_2 *milligrams (mg)*

	Portion	Amount
Liver, lamb, fried	100g	5.65
Soy milk, plain	585ml	1.58
Milk, part skim	585ml	1.05
Duck, roast, meat only	185g	0.87
Hot oat cereal with milk	180g	0.90
Yogurt, Greek, cow's milk	100g	0.36

© see page 107.

Vitamin B_3

(Niacin)

Niacin, also known as nicotine acid/nicotinamide, helps release energy from foods. It can be made in the body from an amino acid (protein building block) called tryptophan (60 mg tryptophan = 1 mg niacin). In parts of the world where the diet comprises mainly corn (maize), the deficiency disease pellagra occurs. This is because the niacin is in a bound form.

The amount of niacin needed in the diet depends on calorie intake, but the normal diet usually supplies twice the amount required. High doses (3,000–6,000 mg/day) can cause liver damage.

GOOD FOOD SOURCES

Meat and meat products, fish and fortified breakfast cereals are good sources.

Wheat, rice, nuts and beans contain useful amounts of tryptophan for conversion into niacin.

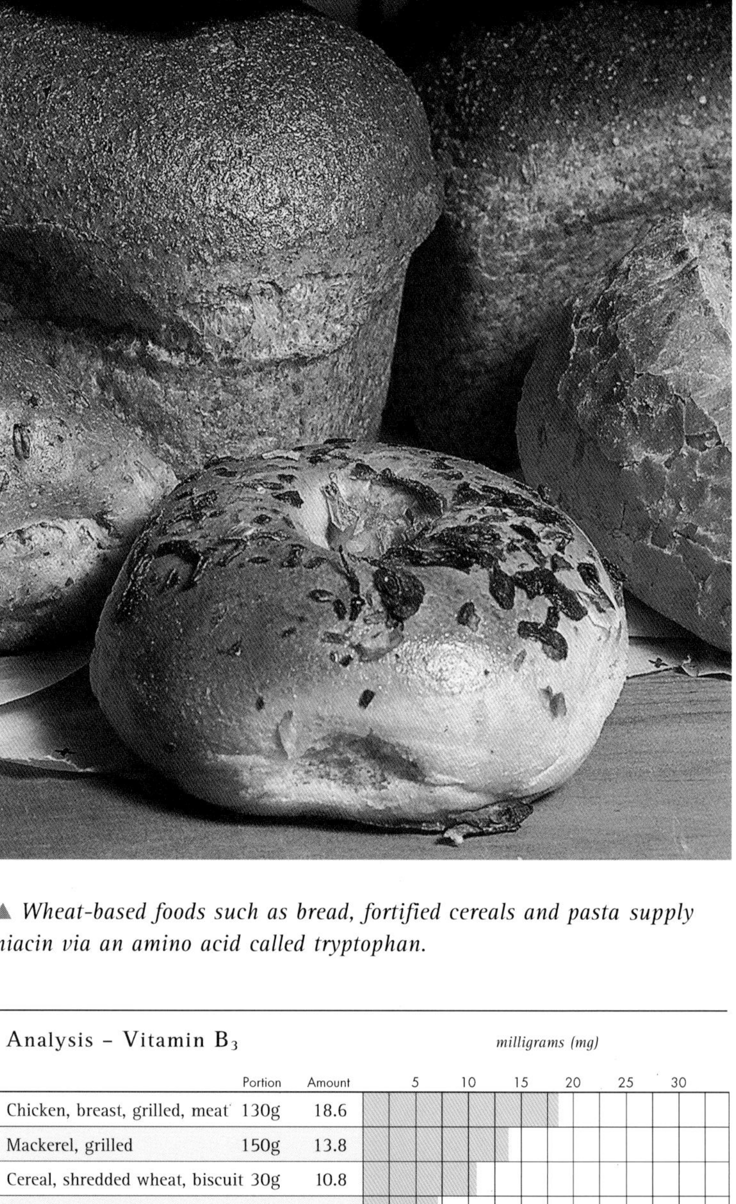

▲ *Wheat-based foods such as bread, fortified cereals and pasta supply niacin via an amino acid called tryptophan.*

Vitamin B_3 *mg/day (milligrams per day)*

Age	*RDA*	*RNI*
0–12 months	5–6	3–5
1–10	9–13	8–12
11–14	15–17	12–15
15–18	15–20	14–18
19 plus	15–19	13–17
Pregnancy	17	13
Nursing	20	15

© *see page 107.*

Analysis – Vitamin B_3 *milligrams (mg)*

	Portion	Amount
Chicken, breast, grilled, meat	130g	18.6
Mackerel, grilled	150g	13.8
Cereal, shredded wheat, biscuit	30g	10.8
Salmon, canned, red	120g	7.1
Fava (broad) beans, boiled	120g	3.6
Brown rice, boiled	150g	1.9

© *see page 107.*

Vitamin B_6

(Pyridoxine)

Vitamin B_6 is a mixture of pyridoxal, pyridoxine, pyridoxamine and related phosphates. It is essential for protein metabolism and for conversion of tryptophan to niacin (vitamin B_3) within the body.

Deficiencies of this vitamin have been linked to the use of oral contraceptives, but studies have failed to show this conclusively. However, supplements of B_6 may alleviate some of the side effects of oral contraceptives and appear to provide relief to some sufferers of premenstrual syndrome (PMS).

High intakes may cause a tingling sensation and loss of feeling in the fingers, and toxicity can occur at 2,000 mg/day.

GOOD FOOD SOURCES

Vitamin B_6 tends to be found in protein-rich foods including meat, poultry, fish, potatoes and dark-green leafy vegetables.

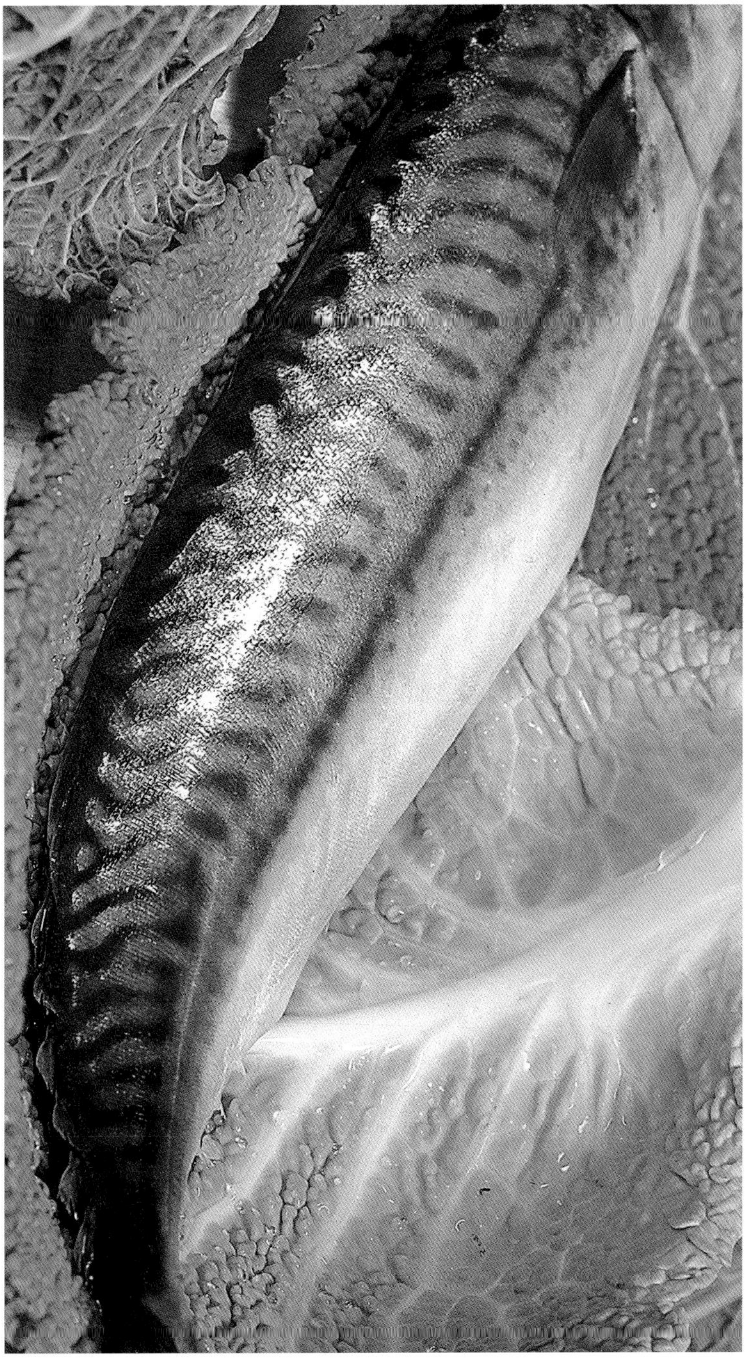

▲ *Fish is one of the richest sources of vitamin B_6.*

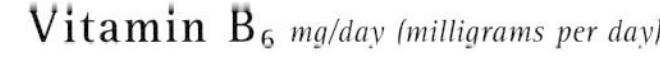

Vitamin B_6 *mg/day (milligrams per day)*

Age	*RDA*	*RNI*
0-12 months	0.3–0.6	0.2–0.4
1-10	1.0–1.4	0.7–1.0
11-14	1.4–1.7	1.0–1.2
15-18	1.5–2.0	1.2–1.5
19 plus	1.6–2.0	1.2–1.4
Pregnancy	2.2	1.2
Nursing	2.1	1.2

© see page 107.

Analysis – Vitamin B_6 *milligrams (mg)*

	Portion	Amount
Beef, fillet steak, grilled	168g	1.4
Salmon, grilled (with bones and skin)	170g	1.1
Chicken leg, roast meat and skin	190g	0.8
Chickpea curry	210g	0.3
Avocado	173g	0.6
Spinach, boiled	90g	0.1

© see page 107.

Vitamin B_{12}

(Cobalamin)

Vitamin B_{12} is essential for red blood cell formation; without it pernicious anemia can develop because DNA is not synthesized. Vitamin B_{12} is also involved in nerve maintenance.

Vitamin B_{12} is found almost exclusively in animal foods, though some algae and bacteria can make it. Vegans (those who eat no animal products) are therefore at risk of deficiency and should take a daily supplement.

The most common cause of vitamin B_{12} deficiency is not dietary but is due to a lack of "intrinsic factor." This essential stomach secretion is needed to bind vitamin B_{12} to other compounds for absorption in the intestine.

Some drugs, including cholestyramine and oral contraceptives, interfere with B_{12} absorption.

GOOD FOOD SOURCES

Liver, meat, eggs, milk and milk products are all good sources of vitamin B_{12}. Vegans may find it difficult to obtain adequate supplies of this vitamin from foods and should be sure to include brewer's yeast or B_{12}-fortified products such as soy milk, yeast extract and fortified breakfast cereals. They should also take supplements in their diets.

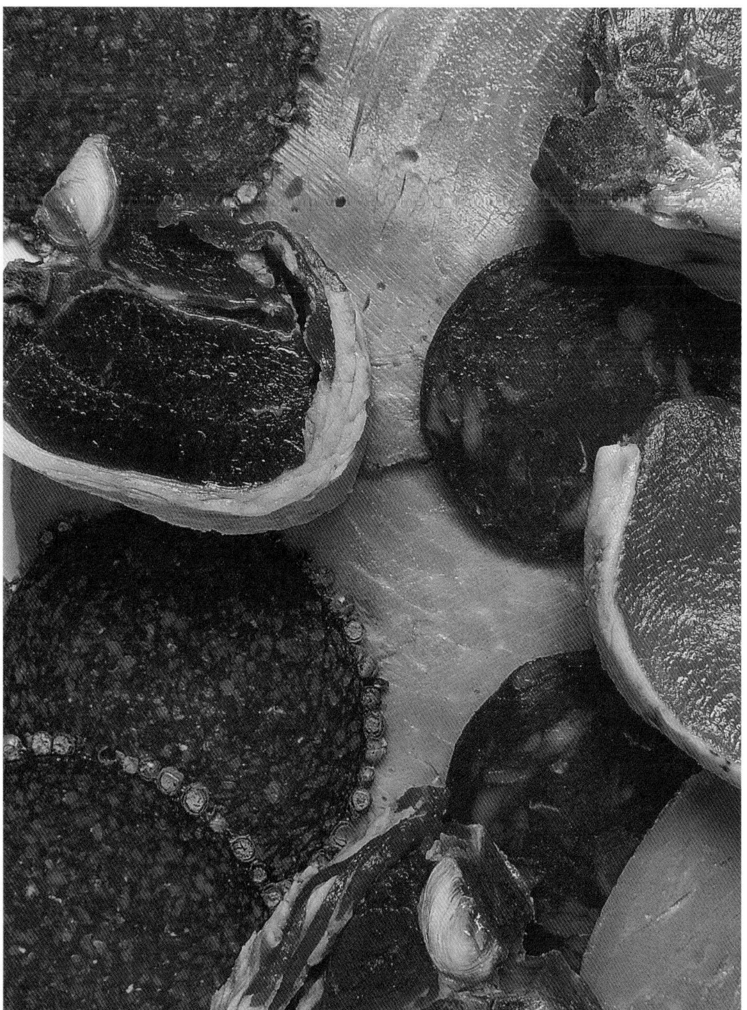

▲ *Animal foods provide the only naturally occurring sources of vitamin B_{12}. Liver and other organ meats are exceptionally rich sources of this important vitamin.*

Vitamin B_{12} *mcg/day (micrograms per day)*

Age	*RDA*	*RNI*
0-12 months	0.3–0.5	0.3–0.4
1–10	0.7–1.4	0.5–1.0
11–14	2.0	1.2
15–18	2.0	1.5
19 plus	2.0	1.5
Pregnancy	2.2	1.5
Nursing	2.6	2.0

© *see page 107.*

Analysis – Vitamin B_{12} *micrograms (mcg)*

	Portion	Amount
Liver, lamb, fried	100g	83.0
Sardines, canned in oil	100g	23.0
Trout, grilled	230g	9.2
Salmon, canned in brine	120g	4.8
Beef, rump steak, grilled	145g	4.3
Cornflakes (fortified)	30g	0.5

© *see page 107.*

Vitamin C

(Ascorbic Acid)

This vitamin is water-soluble, which makes it highly susceptible to loss when fruit and vegetables containing it are cut, cooked and stored. Once vitamin C is exposed to light, air or heat, levels are diminished. Because of vitamin C's important function as an antioxidant, it is vital to take in a good supply of it. This supply needs to be replenished each day since it is excreted along with bodily fluids.

Ascorbic acid, as vitamin C is also known, is important for promoting the growth of connective tissues, as well as for protecting tissues against destruction from free radicals (this is its anti-oxidant role). People who chronically lack vitamin C may be at risk of developing scurvy, a disease that is manifest in bleeding gums and sores that will not heal. If people are under severe stress, their supplies of this important vitamin are depleted since it is used up in the release of stress hormones. Smokers are also often in need of greater amounts of vitamin C, usually at least double the daily amount. As always, look to the diet first. Although vitamin C is water soluble, making it relatively easy for the body to excrete any excess, high intakes may result in diarrhea and are unsuitable for people with kidney stones.

Drugs such as aspirin, tetracyclines and oral contraceptives can increase the excretion of vitamin C.

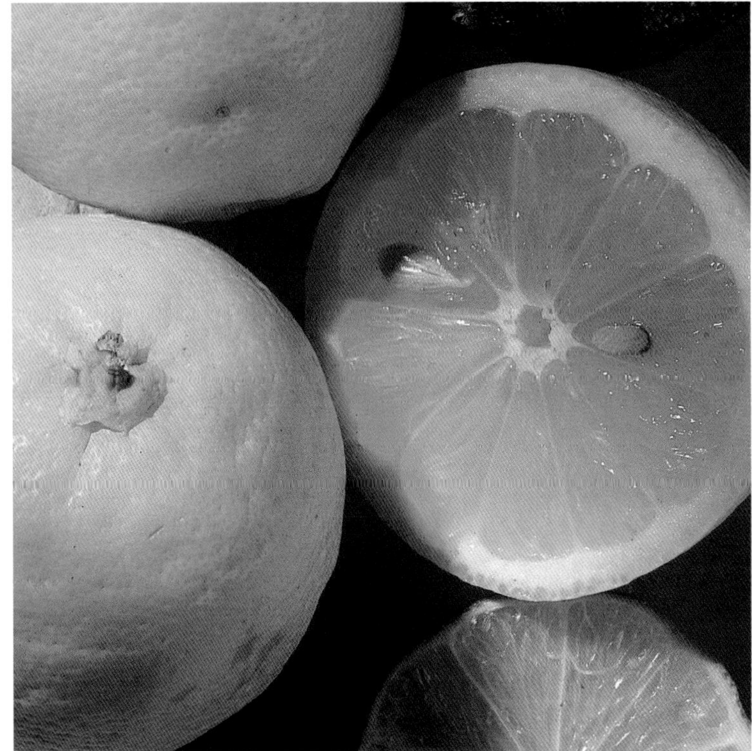

▲ *Citrus fruits are among the best sources of vitamin C. However, a variety of other fruits and vegetables also supply this important vitamin.*

GOOD FOOD SOURCES

Many foods are good sources of vitamin C: citrus fruits, melons, strawberries, tomatoes, broccoli and other members of the cabbage family, dark-green leafy vegetables, potatoes, peppers and chilies. Try to eat these foods as close to their natural states as possible. If you do cook them, try stir-frying, steaming or microwaving them to help preserve their vitamin C content.

Vitamin C *mg/day (milligrams per day)*

Age	*RDA*	*RNI*
0–12 months	30–35	25
1–10	40–45	30
11–14	50	35
15–18	60	40
19 plus	60	40
Pregnancy	70	50
Nursing	95–90[a]	70

© *see page 107.*
a Second six months.

Analysis – Vitamin C *milligrams (mg)*

	Portion	Amount
Guava, raw	90g	207
Black currants, with sugar	140g	161
Oranges	160g	86
Spring greens, boiled	90g	69
Broccoli, green, boiled	90g	39
New potatoes, boiled in skin	175g	26

© *see page 107.*

Vitamin D

(Ergocalciferol or Cholecalciferol)

This vitamin is sometimes known as the "sunshine vitamin." We do not necessarily have to consume it in order to maintain adequate levels because it is made by ultraviolet irradiation of a derivative of cholesterol.

Vitamin D increases the blood levels of calcium and phosphorus, permitting these minerals to perform their functions in strengthening and maintaining healthy bones and teeth.

Insufficient vitamin D results in little calcium being absorbed and the poor development of bones which can lead to rickets. This can be a problem for those who get little exposure to sunlight, for example, housebound individuals or those living in northern latitudes. It can also be a problem for vegans. Young children and pregnant women are often given supplements if they are at risk of deficiency.

Vitamin D can easily build to toxic levels in the body, and the consequences of long-term overdosing can be serious. In early stages of toxicity, an individual will suffer headaches and nausea. Unchecked, toxic levels of vitamin D can cause calcium deposits to build up in the soft tissue, ultimately leading to death. Since this is a fat-soluble vitamin, it is difficult to excrete once absorbed into the body.

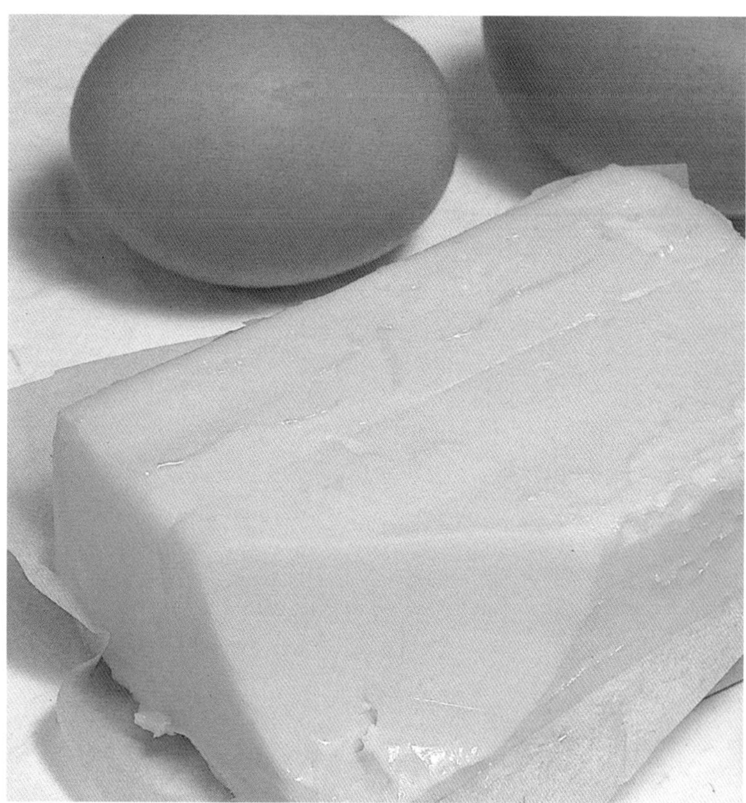

▲ *Fat-soluble vitamin D helps to form strong bones. It is found in foods such as butter and eggs.*

GOOD FOOD SOURCES

Food sources of vitamin D include fatty fish such as mackerel, herring, tuna and sardines and fish oils (which is why doses of cod-liver oil were often administered to growing children). Butter, cream, egg yolks and organ meats, such as liver, also contain vitamin D. In some countries, it is added to milk, margarines and low-fat spreads.

Vitamin D *mcg/day (micrograms per day)*

Age	*RDA*	*RNI*
0-12 months	7.5–10	8.5–7
1-10	10	7[a]
11-14	10	b
15-18	10	b
19 plus	10–5[c]	b
Pregnancy	10	10
Nursing	10	10

© see page 107.
a Up to age 3.
b No figures set.
c After age 25.

Analysis – Vitamin D *micrograms (mcg)*

	Portion	Amount
Kipper, baked	130g	32.5
Salmon, pink, canned	120g	20.6
Sardines, canned in tomato sauce	100g	8.0
Eggs, scrambled with milk	100g	1.9
Lamb stew, lean	260g	1.6
Polyunsaturated margarine	7g	0.6

© see page 107.

Vitamin E

(Alpha Tocopherol)

Vitamin E has been heralded as a virtual cure-all, probably in response to its highly vaunted role as an anti-oxidant. The vitamin is available in small amounts in a variety of foods, and an absolute deficiency is unlikely to occur in healthy individuals.

Vitamin E is thought to protect against cancer by boosting the immune system, mopping up free radicals and converting nitrites in the stomach. Higher levels of vitamin E are also thought to inhibit the development of atherosclerosis and reduce the risk of a heart attack.

If your diet is extremely low in fats, or if you suffer from an impaired ability to absorb fats, you may need to supplement your diet.

GOOD FOOD SOURCES

Plant oils offer the richest source of vitamin E: Wheat germ, soybeans, tofu, corn oil (and other vegetable oils), avocados, nuts and seeds are all excellent sources. Dark-green leafy vegetables and whole grains also contain useful amounts of vitamin E.

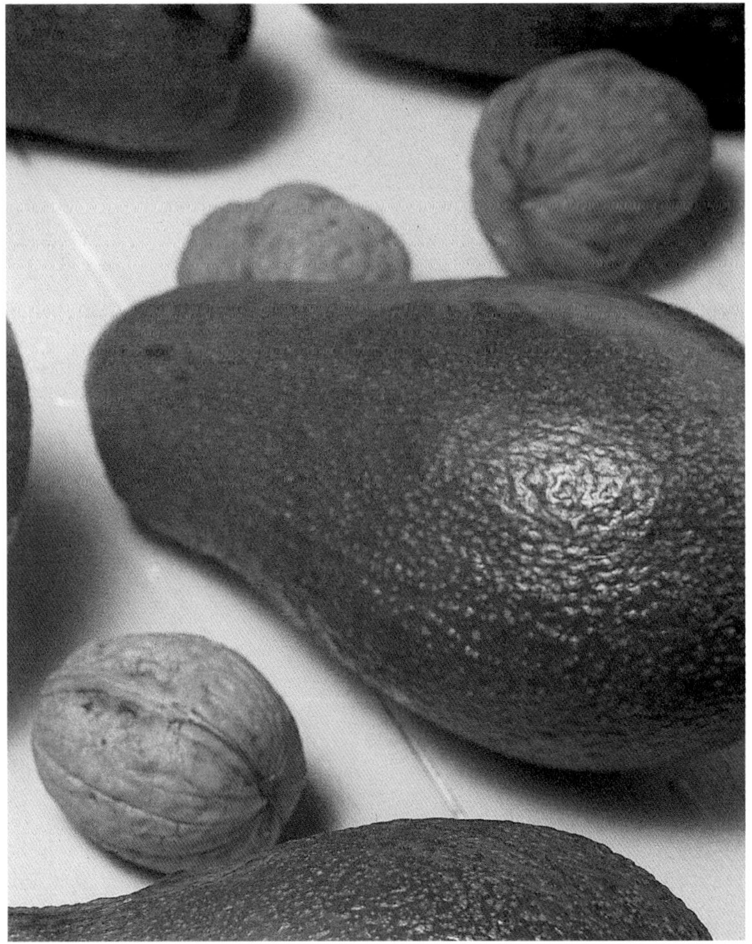

▲ *Vitamin E, an essential anti-oxidant, is found in vegetable oils and foods such as avocados, nuts and wheat germ. Ensuring a good daily supply may lower your risk of developing cancer and heart disease.*

Vitamin E *mg/day (milligrams per day)*

Age	*RDA*	*RNI*
0–12 months	3–4	*a*
1–10	6–7	*a*
11–14	8–10	*a*
15–18	8–10	*a*
19 plus	8–10	*a*
Pregnancy	10	*a*
Nursing	12–11[b]	*a*

© see page 107.
a No UK RNI set. Daily intake of 3mg for women, 4mg for men thought to be safe.
b Second six months.

Analysis – Vitamin E *milligrams (mg)*

	Portion	Amount
Popcorn, plain	75g	8.3
French fries (chips), fried in corn oil	165g	8.1
Sunflower seeds	16g	6.0
Sweet potato, steamed	130g	5.7
Avocado	173g	5.5
Sunflower oil	11g	5.4

© see page 107.

Vitamin K

(Phylloquinone)

This fat-soluble vitamin plays a part in blood clotting, and helps other complex reactions take place in the body. Deficiency is rare, but it sometimes occurs within two months of birth in exclusively breastfed babies. To prevent this hemorrhagic disease of the newborn, vitamin K is often administered at birth.

Phylloquinones are the most common form of vitamin K, although bacteria in the digestive system can synthesize menaquinones.

GOOD FOOD SOURCES

Dark-green leafy vegetables are the richest sources of vitamin K, although dairy products, fruits, fortified cereals, vegetable oils and some vegetables contain significant amounts.

Vitamin K *mcg/day (micrograms per day)*

Age	*RDA*	*RNI*
0-12 months	5-10	*a*
1-10	15-30	*a*
11-14	45	*a*
15-18	55-65	*a*
19 plus	60-70	*a*
Pregnancy	65	*a*
Nursing	65	*a*

© see page 107.
a No U.K. RNI but 1.0mcg per kilogram body weight thought to be a safe daily intake for adults. Infants may safely have 10mcg per day.

Please note: Information to create a comparative chart is unavailable.

Biotin

This little known B vitamin is important in the metabolism of fats, carbohydrates and the breakdown of proteins. The only likely cause of deficiency is eating large quantities of raw egg whites, which contain a substance that binds biotin.

GOOD FOOD SOURCES

Organ meats (such as liver), fish, nuts, eggs, milk and milk products, cereals, fish, fruits and vegetables all contain biotin.

Biotin *mcg/day (micrograms per day)*

Age	*RDA[a]*	*RNI*
0-12 months	10-15	*b*
1-10	20-30	*b*
11-14	30-100	*b*
15-18	30-100	*b*
19 plus	30-100	*b*
Pregnancy	*c*	*b*
Nursing	*c*	*b*

© see page 107.
a No RDA but an estimated safe and adequate daily dietary intake.
b No U.K. RNI but 10-200mcg/day are regarded as safe.
c No data available.

Analysis - Biotin *micrograms (mcg)*

	Portion	Amount
Kidney, pig, fried	140g	180
Chicken livers (for paté)	40g	68
Peanuts, roasted, salted	50g	57
Eggs, scrambled with milk	120g	20
Cod roe, fried	116g	17
Milk, most types	585ml	11

© see page 107.

Folic Acid

There are several types of folate, or folacin, compounds that all incorporate the folic acid molecule.

Women of childbearing age are now urged to keep up their intakes of folic acid. When folic acid is in short supply in mothers, there can be serious consequences for the fetus, including neural tube defects such as spina bifida.

In the U.K., a daily folic acid supplement of 400 mcg is recommended from the time of planning a pregnancy until 12 weeks into the pregnancy.

Folic acid is known to play a part in the production of genetic material in cells as well as in the production of amino acids.

Low folic acid levels are linked to an increased risk of heart disease through an increase in homocysteine. People who drink significant amounts of alcohol and those who take anticonvulsants, aspirin and oral contraceptives may need to be vigilant about getting enough folic acid.

Pantothenic Acid

Pantothenic acid helps break down foods to provide energy, and deficiency is unlikely due to the widespread distribution of the vitamin.

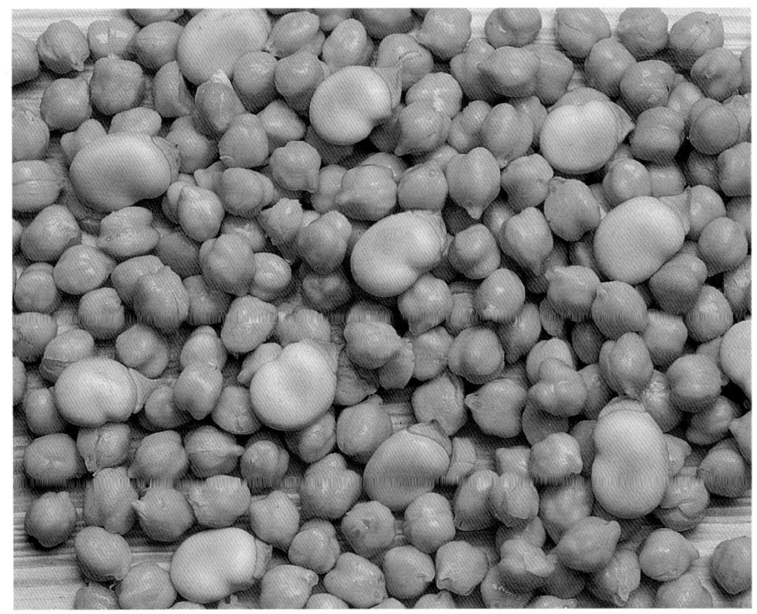

▲ *Pantothenic acid, which is an important B vitamin, is quite widely distributed in the diet.*

GOOD FOOD SOURCES

Liver, legumes, especially fava (broad) beans, meats, milk and cereals are good sources. Ale-type beer (not lager) contains seven times more pantothenic acid than liver.

Pantothenic Acid *mg/day (milligrams per day)*

Age	RDA[a]	RNI
0-12 months	2-3	*b*
1-10	3-5	*b*
11-14	4-7	*b*
15-18	4-7	*b*
19 plus	4-7	*b*
Pregnancy	*c*	*b*
Nursing	*c*	*b*

© see page 107.
a No RDA but an estimated safe and adequate daily dietary intake.
b No U.K. RNI but 1.7mg/day are felt to be safe for babies and 3-7mg/day for adults.
c No data available.

Analysis – Pantothenic Acid *milligrams (mg)*

	Portion	Amount
Liver, lamb, fried	100g	8.0
Fava (broad) beans, boiled	120g	4.6
Lamb, stewed	260g	3.4
Milk, skim (long-life/UHT	585ml	1.9
Eggs, scrambled with milk	120g	1.5
Chickpeas, dried, boiled	35g	0.1

© see page 107.

GOOD FOOD SOURCES

Liver is the richest food source, though some believe this is unsuitable for pregnant women due to the high levels of vitamin A it contains.

Brussels sprouts, broccoli, cauliflower, spinach and black-eyed peas (beans) are good sources. Fortified breakfast cereals and yeast extract contain varying but useful amounts.

Folate *mcg/day (micrograms per day)*

Age	RDA	RNI
0-12 months	25-35	50
1-10	50-100	70-150
11-14	150	200
15-18	180-200	200
19 plus	180-200	200
Pregnancy	400	300[a]
Nursing	280-260[b]	260

© see page 107.
a Plus a 400mcg tablet for first 12 weeks of pregnancy.
b Second six months.
Folic acid is one of the most common types of folate.

Analysis – Folate *micrograms (mcg)*

	Portion	Amount
Liver, lamb, fried	100g	140
Spinach, raw	90g	135
Black-eyed beans, dried, boiled	60g	126
Broccoli, boiled	85g	119
Brussels sprouts	90g	99
Oranges	160g	50

© see page 107.

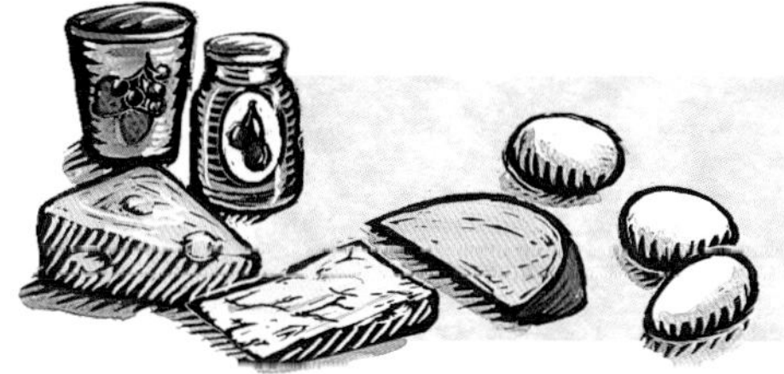

MINERALS

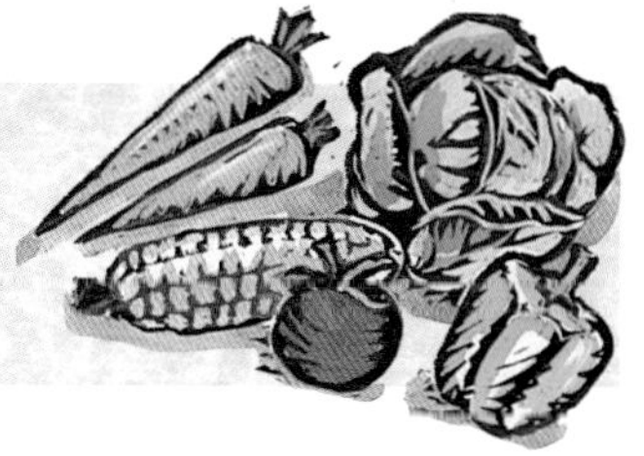

Calcium

Calcium is the most abundant mineral in the body. It helps keep the skeleton strong. Ninety-nine percent of the calcium found in our bodies is located in the bones and teeth, where it is an essential structural component. An equally important role of calcium is regulating metabolic processes; blood clotting, nerve transmission and muscle contraction all rely on calcium.

An individual's ability to absorb calcium from foods is directly related to that person's specific calcium needs and the availability of vitamin D. Vitamin D helps the uptake of calcium from the intestines. During times of great growth, recovery from illness and pregnancy, more calcium and vitamin D can be absorbed from foods.

Regular exercise and a diet rich in calcium during childhood, adolescence and early adulthood can help optimize peak bone mass. This is usually reached around the age of 30 and after this time bone mineral density decreases, leading to more brittle bones in later life. The higher the peak bone mass, the longer it takes for calcium loss to reach a level where brittle bones may break (osteoporosis).

Although calcium supplements are available, they are not recommended for people with kidney stones.

▲ *Shrimp (prawns), mussels and certain other types of seafood and fish make tasty alternatives to the more usual dairy sources.*

GOOD FOOD SOURCES

The following foods should be eaten to get a good supply of calcium: dairy products such as reduced-fat milk, cheeses, cottage cheese, fromage frais, yogurt, and so on; canned fish such as salmon and sardines, which contain the small bones found in these fish; dark-green leafy vegetables such as spinach, broccoli, green cabbage and watercress; lime-processed corn tortillas (made with masa harina—a flour made from cassava root); seafoods, especially oysters and shrimp (prawns); sesame seeds, dried figs and almonds.

Calcium *mg/day (milligrams per day)*

Age	*RDA*	*RNI*
0–12 months	400–600	525
1–10	800	350–550
11–14	1,200	800–1,000
15–18	1,200	800–1,000
19 plus	1,200–800[a]	700
Pregnancy	1,200	700
Nursing	1,200	1250

© *see page 107.*
a Drop to 800 after age 25.

Analysis – Calcium *milligrams (mg)*

	Portion	Amount
Fortified milk	585g	994
Skim/part skim milk	585g	702
Sardines, canned in oil	100g	500
Cheese, cheddar, low-fat	40g	336
Yogurt, plain, low-fat	150g	285
Figs, ready to eat	55g	126

Chart scale (mg): 250 500 750 1000 1250 1500

© *see page 107.*

Sodium

Sodium, along with potassium, is one of the minerals that control blood pressure. It accomplishes this by maintaining the proper electric charge between cells. Sodium is a positively charged ion that remains outside the cell. It is offset by the ions within the cell. When levels are out of sync, either through sodium excess or as a result of a particular malfunction of an individual's metabolism, high blood pressure (hypertension) is the typical result.

Other roles played by sodium include transmitting nerve impulses and signalling for muscle contractions.

Deficiencies are rare in most parts of the world. Instead, the concern for most cultures is keeping sodium intake at lower levels to reduce the risk of developing hypertension.

An average adult needs only 1,600 mg (1.6 gram) of sodium a day, but the amount consumed often exceeds this.

GOOD FOOD SOURCES

Sodium chloride is the chemical name for table salt. Apart from being added to food at the table, salt is also used in cooking. Processed foods often contain high levels of sodium; unprocessed foods generally contain very little.

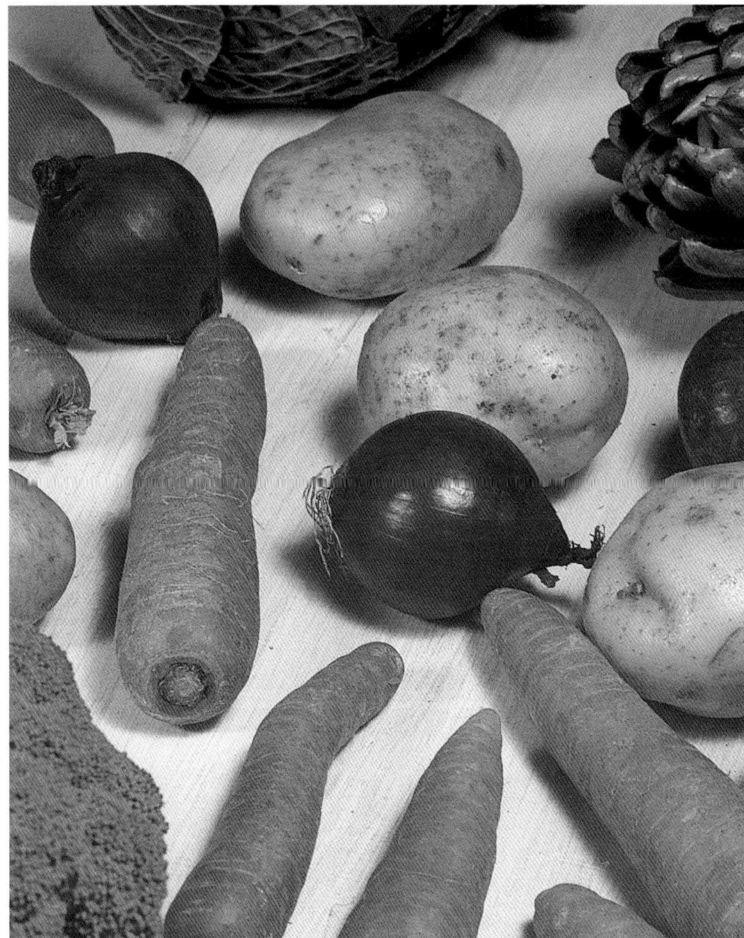

▲ *Vegetables and other unprocessed foods provide sodium in small amounts. They are the best foods to choose to ensure that sodium levels in the body are adequate but don't rise too high.*

Sodium *mg/day (milligrams per day)*

Age	*RDA*	*RNI*
0–12 months	*a*	210–350
1–10	*a*	500–1,200
11–14	*a*	1,600
15–18	*a*	1,600
19 plus	*a*	1,600
Pregnancy	*a*	1,600
Nursing	*a*	1,600

© *see page 107.*
a No RDA. Required by the body but adequate amounts are supplied by the diet.

Analysis – Sodium *milligrams (mg)*

Food	Portion	Amount
Ham (gammon), boiled	170g	1,887
Chicken curry (bought)	350g	1,610
Haddock, smoked, steamed	150g	1,485
Feta cheese	55g	792
Cheddar cheese	40g	268
Potato chips (crisps) (1 bag)	30g	252

© *see page 107.*

Iron

Iron is an essential nutrient involved in many reactions in body cells. It is found in many forms in the body. One of the most important is hemoglobin in red blood cells, which transport oxygen around the body. Hemoglobin levels are generally used to indicate iron status, though low ferritin (stored iron) levels are also indicative of iron deficiency.

Iron deficiency leads to anemia, which first shows up as tiredness and shortness of breath. Iron deficiency anemia is the most common nutritional disorder in the world. Those most at risk are babies who are fed only breast milk for more than six months, bottle-fed babies who are given cow's milk as a main drink before one year of age, toddlers, adolescents and women in their reproductive years. Deficiencies in babies and toddlers can affect mental and physical development.

Iron is found as heme (haem) iron in animal foods, and as nonheme iron in plant foods. Heme iron is well absorbed from foods while nonheme iron needs the presence of vitamin C to be more efficiently absorbed.

Some foods contain substances that prevent iron from being absorbed. This means that although a food may contain iron, not much of this may be available for use in the body or that these substances can prevent iron present in another food from being absorbed. These substances include phytate, which is found in bran, oats, leafy vegetables, nuts, soy protein and corn products, and polyphenols, which are found in tea, coffee and leafy vegetables. Other minerals such as calcium, manganese and copper (especially in supplement form) can also hinder iron absorption.

A few genetically susceptible people can suffer from iron overload, but generally deficiency is more of a problem than excess. High levels from supplements can be dangerous, especially to children.

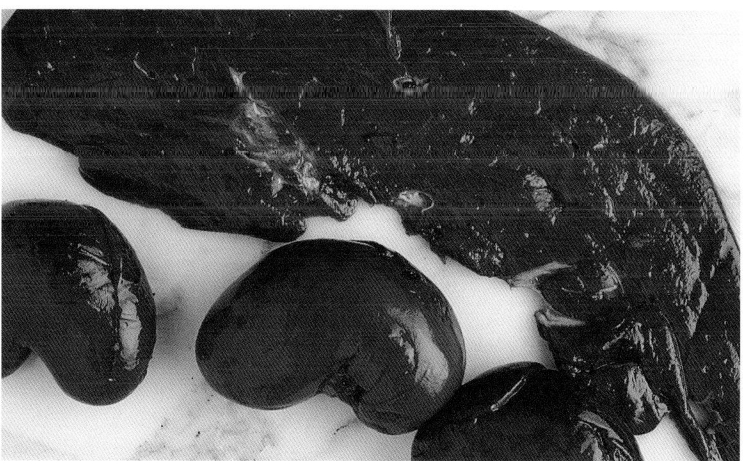

▲ *The best, most well-absorbed forms of iron are animal foods, particularly organ meat such as liver and kidney and red meat. It is worth trying to occasionally incorporate these foods into the diet.*

GOOD FOOD SOURCES

Animal iron is found in beef, lamb; organ meats (such as liver, kidney, hearts); cockles, mussels and sardines.

Plant iron is found in dried fruits, lentils and baked beans, fortified breakfast cereals, breads and dark-green leafy vegetables.

Iron *mg/day (milligrams per day)*

Age	*RDA*	*RNI*
0–12 months	6–10	1.7–7.8
1–10	10	6.9–8.7
11–14	12, 15[a]	11.3, 14.8[a]
15–18	12, 15[a]	11.3, 14.8[a]
19 plus	10, 15[a]	8.7, 14.8[a]
Pregnancy	30	14.8
Nursing	15	14.8

© *see page 107.*
a Higher figure for women.

Analysis – Iron *milligrams (mg)*

	Portion	Amount
Liver, lamb, fried	100g	10.9
Chickpea curry	210g	8.4
Beef, steak, lean	168g	6.0
Bran breakfast cereal	40g	4.8
Sardines, canned in tomato sauce	100g	3.1
Spinach, boiled	90g	1.4

© *see page 107.*

Molybdenum and Manganese

Both of these trace minerals play a role in general metabolic processes. Molybdenum is involved in iron metabolism in the body, while manganese is a component of an anti-oxidant enzyme system and is needed for sex hormone synthesis and healthy joints, bones and nervous system. Manganese appears to have the ability to aid in the proper metabolism of carbohydrates (the body's preferred source of energy).

Remember that trace minerals are needed in very small amounts, so it should be easy to get an adequate supply by eating a good, varied diet that includes whole, fresh foods and limits highly processed items. Deficiencies, which can cause serious consequences, are unlikely as it is easy to build up toxic levels of these trace minerals. Supplements are not normally necessary unless you have specific extra needs or a medical condition that requires a higher intake.

GOOD FOOD SOURCES

Grains, pasta, legumes, berry fruits and vegetables are good sources of manganese. Molybdenum is found in organ meats, legumes, cereals and potatoes. Whole-grain and unprocessed plant foods contain more than processed ones.

Molybdenum *mcg/day (micrograms per day)*

Age	*RDA[a]*	*RNI*
0-12 months	15-40	*b*
1-10	25-150	*b*
11-14	75-250	*b*
15-18	75-250	*b*
19 plus	75-250	*b*
Pregnancy	c	*b*
Nursing	c	*b*

© see page 107.
a No RDA but an estimated safe and adequate daily dietary intake.
b No U.K. RNI but a safe daily intake of 50-400mcg for adults is recommended. For children, babies and adolescents a safe daily intake of 0.5-1.5mcg per kilogram of body weight.
c No data available.

Manganese *mg/day (milligrams per day)*

Age	*RDA[a]*	*RNI*
0-12 months	0.3-1.0	*b*
1-10	1.0-3.0	*b*
11-14	2.0-5.0	*b*
15-18	2.0-5.0	*b*
19 plus	2.0-5.0	*b*
Pregnancy	c	*b*
Nursing	c	*b*

© see page 107.
a No RDA but an estimated safe and adequate daily dietary intake.
b No U.K. RNI but a safe daily intake of 1.4mg for adults. For infants and children 16mcg a day is regarded to be safe.
c No data available.

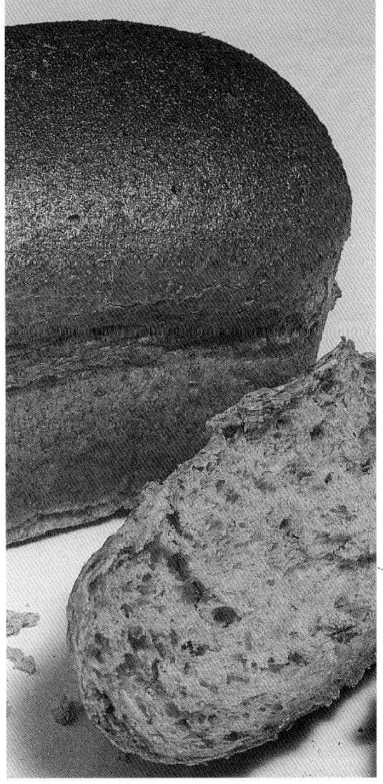

▲ *Whole wheat bread is a good source of many trace nutrients including the minerals manganese and molybdenum. Despite only being needed in small amounts, these trace minerals are essential to the functioning of many body systems.*

Analysis – Molybdenum *micrograms (mcg)*

	Portion	Amount
Liver, lamb, fried	100g	150
Peas, boiled	70g	91
Kidney, lamb, fried	100g	70
White rice, boiled	180g	18
Potatoes, old, boiled	175g	12
White bread	36g	8

Data from Briony Thomas (ed), Manual of Dietetic Practice *(2nd edition), Blackwell Scientific Publications, 1994.*

Analysis – Manganese *milligrams (mg)*

	Portion	Amount
White rice, boiled	180g	7.0
Chickpea curry	210g	2.3
Spaghetti, whole wheat (wholemeal)	200g	1.8
Blackberries	140g	1.7
Whole wheat (wholemeal) bread	36g	0.7
Tomatoes, grilled	85g	0.3

© see page 107.

Iodine

Iodine is an important part of the hormone thyroxine. This and similar hormones, produced and released by the thyroid gland are necessary for controlling the rate at which the body burns food (metabolic rate). Iodine deficiency diseases are common in parts of the world where there is little iodine in the soil and where imported foods are rare. Deficiency can lead to the development of a goiter—or swollen thyroid gland—decreased fertility and abnormalities at birth. Severe deficiency in early pregnancy leads to poor brain development and babies born with cretinism (irreversible muscle and nerve damage).

Some foods (turnips, cabbage, cassava, millet, corn, bamboo shoots, lima [butter] beans and sweet potatoes) contain substances that interfere with iodine metabolism.

High intakes of iodine can be toxic.

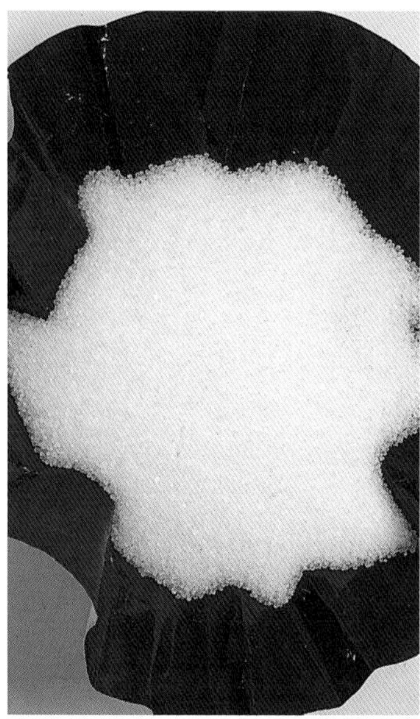

▲ *In some countries, iodine is added to table salt to ensure a good supply in the daily diet.*

GOOD FOOD SOURCES

Seafood and foods grown in parts of the world that were once under water are all good sources of iodine. Milk is a significant source of iodine because livestock are often fed food supplemented with iodine. In some countries iodine is routinely added to all types of table salt. In others labels indicate if iodine is present.

Iodine *mcg/day (micrograms per day)*

Age	*RDA*	*RNI*
0–12 months	40–50	50–60
1–10	70–120	70–110
11–14	150	130
15–18	150	140
19 plus	150	140
Pregnancy	175	140
Nursing	200	140

© *see page 107.*

Analysis – Iodine *micrograms (mcg)*

	Portion	Amount
Haddock, grilled	130g	390
Haddock, steamed	128g	320
Yogurt, plain, low fat	150g	94
Milk (all)	585ml	87
Eggs, scrambled without milk	100g	57
Potatoes, new, boiled	175g	5

© *see page 107.*

Magnesium

Magnesium is required for proper nerve function and the transmission of nerve impulses. It also plays a role in muscle contraction. Low levels of dietary magnesium can affect the body's use of calcium since the functions of the two minerals are linked.

Deficiency is not common but is usually associated with absorption disorders, alcohol abuse, and poorly controlled diabetes. A lack of magnesium might be responsible for weakness, confusion, PMS symptoms, involuntary twitching or other uncontrollable muscle contractions.

Fluoride

Fluoride, like calcium is of critical importance to the formation, growth, repair and restoration of bones and teeth. Based on studies done in the 1940s, many communities have opted to treat their municipal water sources with fluoride. Dental caries (the formation of cavities) and osteoporosis have both been shown to occur at lower levels in communities with fluoride treatment

GOOD FOOD SOURCES

Nuts and very dark chocolate are excellent sources of magnesium. Green vegetables are also a good source of it, as are wheat flour, bread, fortified breakfast cereals dried beans, peas, seafood, milk and meats.

Magnesium *mg/day (milligrams per day)*

Age	*RDA*	*RNI*
0–12 months	40–60	55–80
1–10	80–170	85–200
11–14	270–280	280
15–18	300–400	300
19 plus	280–350	270–300
Pregnancy	320	270
Nursing	355–340[a]	320

© see page 107.
a Second six months.

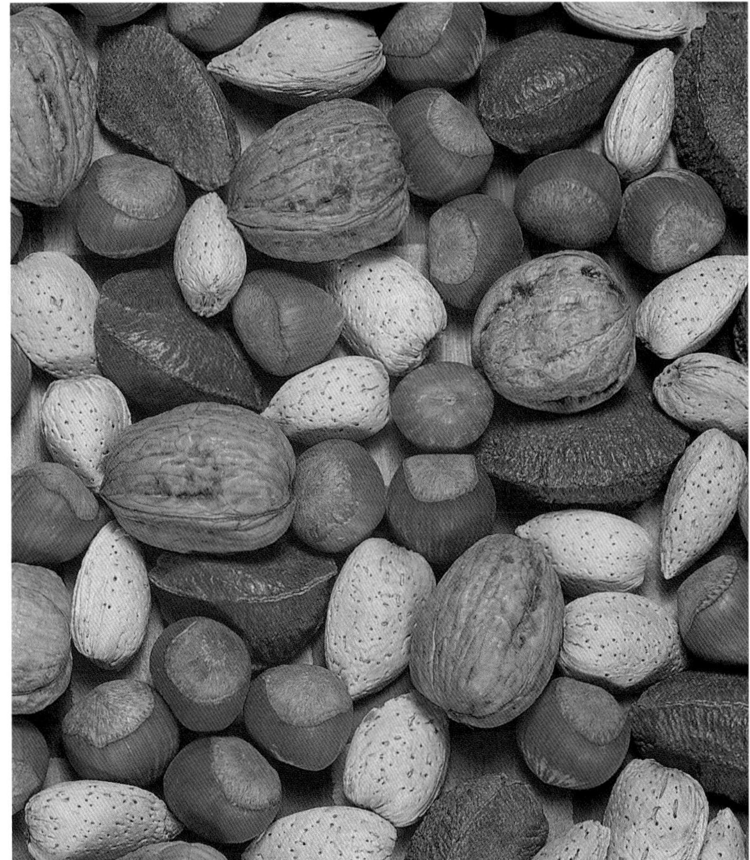

▲ *If you want to ensure a good source of magnesium in your diet, include a selection of nuts and seeds. Green vegetables also provide useful amounts of this important dietary mineral. Magnesium is essential for a healthy nervous system.*

Analysis – Magnesium *milligrams (mg)*

	Portion	Amount
Plantain, fried	200g	108
Peanuts, roasted, salted	50g	90
Dark (plain) chocolate	50g	44
Spinach, boiled	90g	31
Whole wheat bread, toasted	31g	27
Tomatoes, grilled	85g	17

© see page 107.

programs as well as in individuals who either supplement their diets or select fluoride-rich foods.

However, too much fluoride can cause teeth to become discolored, and excess can affect the skeleton. Parents of young children should note that too much fluoride may affect permanent teeth and should limit the amount used for brushing teeth and ensure none is swallowed.

GOOD FOOD SOURCES

Many communities treat their water sources with fluoride, to one part per million, making it relatively easy for local inhabitants to receive adequate supplies. Tea and seafood are good dietary sources for those who live in areas without a fluoride treatment program or whose water is fluoride-free.

Fluoride *mg/day (milligrams per day)*

Age	*RDA[a]*	*RNI*
0–12 months	0.1–1.0	*b*
1–10	0.5–2.5	*b*
11–14	1.5–2.5	*b*
15–18	1.5–2.5	*b*
19 plus	1.5–4.0	*b*
Pregnancy	*c*	*b*
Nursing	*c*	*b*

© see page 107.
a No RDA but an estimated safe and adequate daily dietary intake.
b There is no U.K. RNI. A safe daily intake of 0.05mg per kilogram body weight is given for babies under one year.
c No data available.

Potassium

Potassium, along with sodium, is an important electrolyte. This mineral is the major positive ion inside cells and is in balance with sodium outside the cells. This balancing process is fundamental to many body functions such as the transmission of nerve impulses, rhythmic heart contractions, production of protein and enzymes required by the body and the balance of fluids and electrolytes.

Deficiency can lead to depression, irregular heartbeat and poor kidney function. Toxicity problems are only likely from megadoses (more than 17.6 g/day of supplements) – the symptoms include disturbance in the body's water balance and nervous system.

GOOD FOOD SOURCES

Potassium is widely distributed in foods. Vegetables and fresh fruits, especially bananas, offer the greatest supply of potassium because of the quantity consumed.

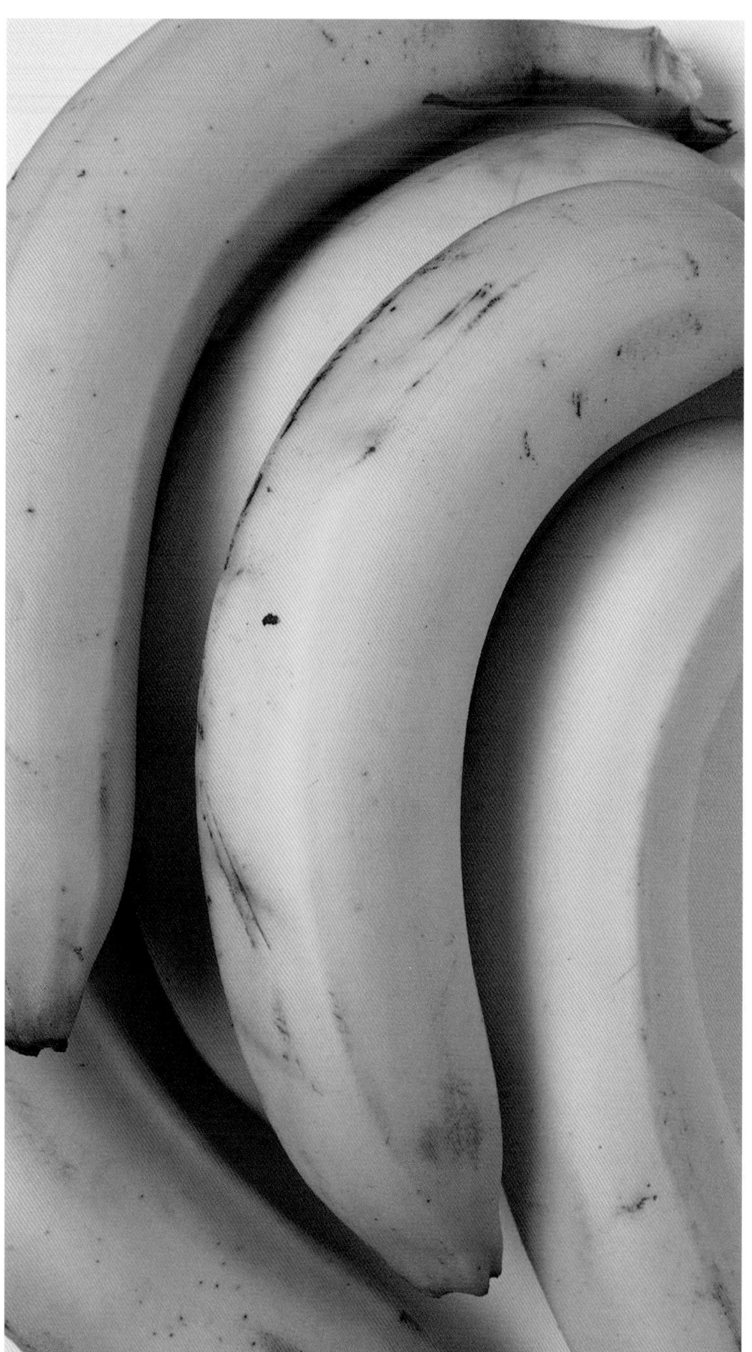

▲ *Bananas are a favorite source of the essential mineral potassium.*

Potassium *mg/day (milligrams per day)*

Age	*RDA*	*RNI*
0-12 months	*a*	800–700
1-10	*a*	800–2,000
11-14	*a*	3,100
15-18	*a*	3,500
19 plus	*a*	3,500
Pregnancy	*a*	3,500
Nursing	*a*	3,500

© see page 107.
a No RDA. Required by the body but adequate amounts are available in a well-balanced diet.

Analysis – Potassium *milligrams (mg)*

	Portion	Amount
Potatoes, baked, with skin	180g	1,134
Milk, part skim	585ml	877
Avocado	175g	813
Pork fillet, grilled	140g	728
Yam, baked	130g	663
Bananas	100g	400

© see page 107.

Chromium

Chromium is an important part of "glucose tolerance factor", which assists insulin in the control of blood sugar levels. Adults who are deficient in chromium may experience a diabetic-like condition, including fluctuating blood sugar levels. When exercising, the body excretes more chromium than usual, so an adequate dietary supply is required by physically active people.

Analysis – Chromium *micrograms (mcg)*

	Portion	Amount
White wine	125ml	15.0
Mixed nuts	50g	5.0
Lamb, roast	90g	3.6
Banana	100g	3.0
Milk chocolate	50g	3.0
Golden raisins (sultanas)	30g	3.0

See note page 121.

GOOD FOOD SOURCES

Chromium is not found in most processed foods, although milk chocolate and white wine are luxury sources of it.

Meats, organ meats fish and poultry are good sources of chromium. Almost all unprocessed foods contain some chromium, and vegetarians can find good supplies in nuts and golden raisins (sultanas), and some in whole-grain cereals and vegetables.

Chromium *mcg/day (micrograms per day)*

Age	*RDA*[a]	*RNI*
0-12 months	10–60	*b*
1-10	20–200	*b*
11-14	50–200	*b*
15-18	50–200	*b*
19 plus	50–200	*b*
Pregnancy	*c*	*b*
Nursing	*c*	*b*

© see page 107.
a No RDA but an estimated safe and adequate daily dietary intake.
b No U.K. RNI but 25mcg a day are considered safe for adults and 0.1–1.0mcg per kilogram body weight a day for children and teenagers.
c No data available.

Copper

Copper aids the production of energy and is part of the mechanism that maintains connective tissues, especially blood vessels. It is also an important element in the metabolism of iron in the body. Your ability to produce hemoglobin is affected by the presence or absence of copper.

Copper deficiency leads to hair changes, raised blood cholesterol levels and anemia. In pregnancy deficiency can severely affect the development of the fetus.

Large doses of calcium, zinc and iron can hinder copper absorption.

GOOD FOOD SOURCES

The following foods all contain trace amounts of copper: meats, including organ meats such as liver; soybeans, tofu and lentils; nuts and golden raisins (sultanas); whole grains; chicken; oily fish; bananas and drinking water.

Copper *mg/day (milligrams per day)*

Age	*RDA*[a]	*RNI*
0-12 months	0.4–0.7	0.2–0.3
1-10	0.7–2.0	0.4–0.7
11-14	1.5–2.5	0.8
15-18	1.5–2.5	1.0
19 plus	1.5–3.0	1.2
Pregnancy	*b*	1.2
Nursing	*b*	1.5

© see page 107.
a No RDA but an estimated safe and adequate daily dietary intake.
b No data available.

Analysis – Copper *milligrams (mg)*

	Portion	Amount
Liver, lamb, fried	100g	13.5
Soy flour, low-fat	30g	0.9
Chick pea curry	210g	0.9
White rice, boiled	180g	0.6
Bulgur wheat	100g	0.6
Cashew nuts	30g	0.5

© see page 107.

Vanadium

Vanadium, along with tin, nickel, silicon and cobalt, is not considered to be essential but contributes to proper health, both physical and mental. The roles of these trace elements are still being established, but we do know that they are linked to numerous biological functions.

Please note: Information to create a comparative chart or a RDA/RNI chart is unavailable.

GOOD FOOD SOURCES

Choose a varied diet based as much as possible on whole, unrefined foods to be sure that you are receiving a full complement of these other trace minerals.

▼ *Wholesome, unprocessed foods are the best way to ensure a good intake of important trace minerals. Eat plenty of starchy foods such as potatoes, pasta, bread and grains since these are the richest sources.*

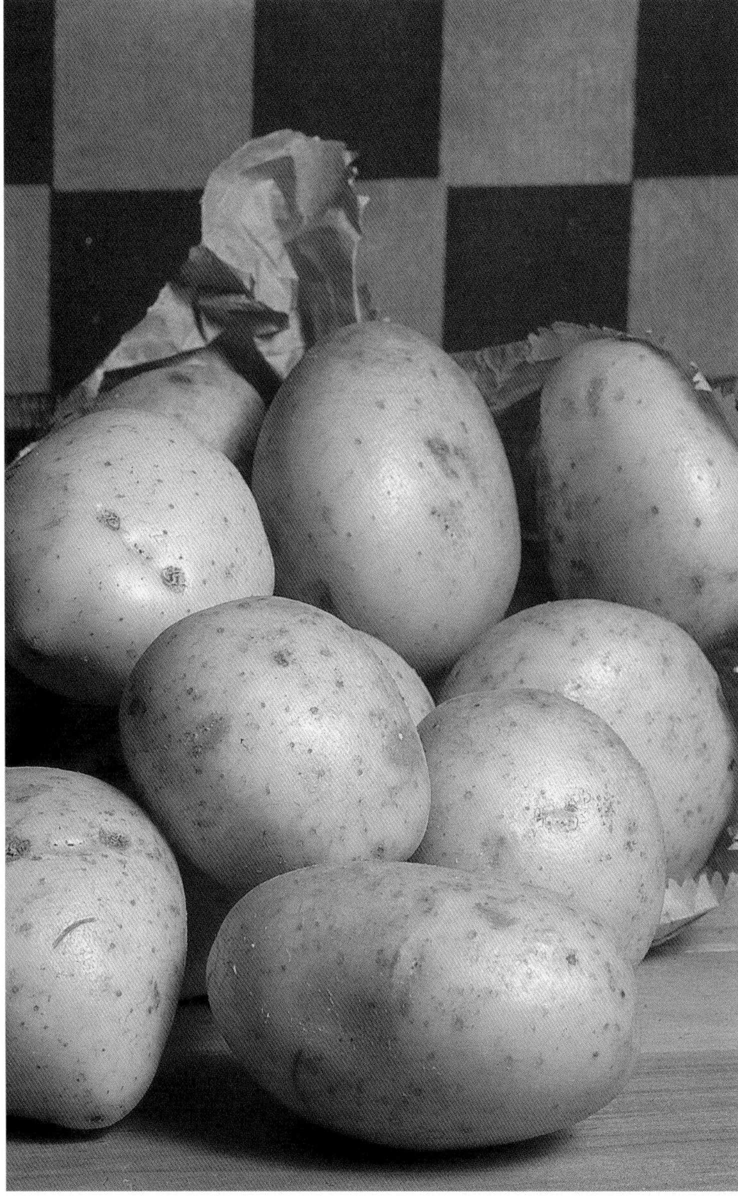

Selenium

As antioxidants become more and more a part of our nutritional collective conscience, we are looking for ways to optimize intake of these substances, which can help prevent tissues from becoming oxidized and the destruction of healthy cells. It is thought that selenium can act in a similar manner to vitamin E, and the two micronutrients appear to work together.

Low levels of selenium are linked to cancers. Extreme deficiency in locally grown foods in some parts of China has been linked to heart diseases.

It is also reported that a good selenium intake can help ease some symptoms of arthritis.

Zinc

There are so many ways in which a zinc deficiency might adversely affect the body that it is hard to believe that zinc is a trace mineral. It is found in more than 70 enzymes, which control a range of body functions. Zinc deficiencies are linked to a reduced sensitivity of taste, poor wound healing, impaired immune response, slow growth and wasting. Those most at risk are babies and children, the elderly and pregnant women.

Zinc can be found in a wide array of foods, but it appears that some foods contain compounds known as phytates (found in oats, bran and some leafy vegetables) that bind zinc and make it

GOOD FOOD SOURCES

High protein foods such as meats (especially kidney), fish and poultry contain selenium. Legumes such as lentils, nuts (particularly Brazil nuts) and whole-grain cereals also provide useful amounts of selenium. Dairy foods contain a small but significant quantity too.

Selenium *mcg/day (micrograms per day)*

Age	*RDA*	*RNI*
0–12 months	10–15	10–13
1–10	20–30	15–30
11–14	40–45[a]	45
15–18	50	60–70
19 plus	55–70	60–75
Pregnancy	65	60
Nursing	75	75

© see page 107.
a Higher figure for women.

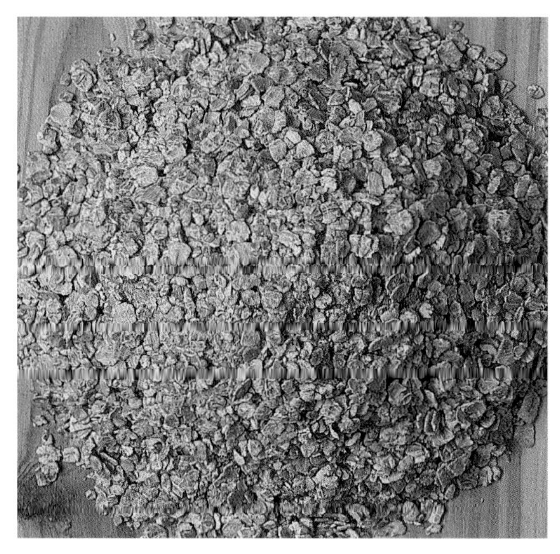

◀ *Wheat-based cereals and flour are the biggest contributors of the essential anti-oxidant selenium in our diets. The exact content of selenium depends on the soil in which cereals are grown.*

Analysis – Selenium *micrograms (mcg)*

	Portion	Amount
Kidney, pig, stewed	140g	350
Brazil nuts	10g	153
Mackerel, fried	160g	54
Salmon, canned	100g	25
Lentils, dried, boiled	40g	16
Milk (all)	585ml	6

© see page 107.

impossible for the body to absorb it properly.

Just as too little zinc can have dire consequences, so can levels even slightly above what is considered optimal.

The way zinc interacts with other minerals shows the fine balance of one nutrient against another and points to the dangers of unsupervised supplementation. When too much zinc from supplements is present, copper and iron are not properly absorbed from food. Conversely supplements of iron and calcium also inhibit zinc absorption from food.

In excess zinc is toxic in large amounts and can induce fever, nausea, vomiting and diarrhea.

GOOD FOOD SOURCES

Zinc is found in a wide range of foods, especially meats, fish and poultry. Grains, vegetables and nuts contain some zinc, but it may be bound with phytate. For this reason vegans risk deficiency.

Zinc *mg/day (milligrams per day)*

Age	*RDA*	*RNI*
0–12 months	5	4–5
1–10	10	5–7
11–14	12–15	9
15–18	12–15	7–9.5
19 plus	12–15	7–9.5
Pregnancy	15	7
Nursing	19–16[a]	13–9.5[b]

© see page 107.
a Second six months.
b After four months.

Analysis – Zinc *milligrams (mg)*

	Portion	Amount
Beef, stewed, lean	140g	11.9
Turkey, casserole, thighs	90g	4.8
Bran breakfast cereal	40g	2.7
Sardines, canned in oil	100g	2.5
Milk (all)	585ml	2.3
Cashew nuts, roasted, salted	25g	1.4

© see page 107.

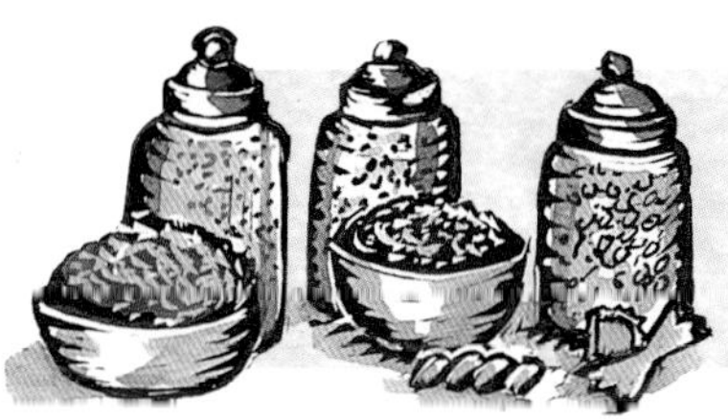

OTHER ORGANIC SUBSTANCES

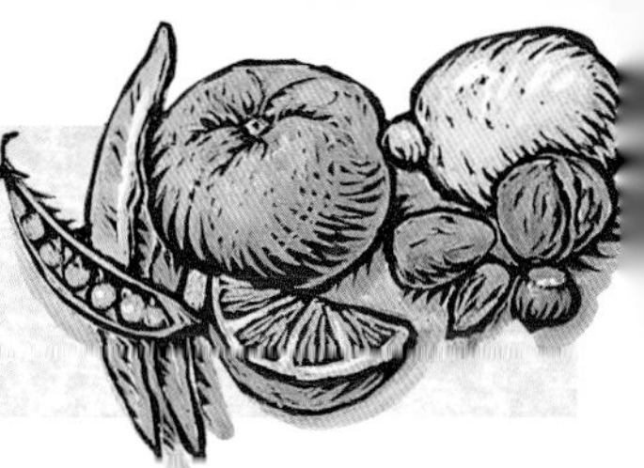

PABA

(Para-Aminobenzoic Acid)

PABA is the acronym for para-aminobenzoic acid; it is considered an essential nutrient. While it is not a vitamin itself, it has been shown to play an important role in the growth and reproduction of various life forms. Its application in human health and growth is still being researched. Like many other vitamins and minerals mentioned in this book, it is probable that a varied diet will supply adequate amounts of PABA. There are no known nutritional uses for PABA supplements.

GOOD FOOD SOURCES

Meats, fish, poultry, whole grains, nuts and seeds are good sources of PABA.

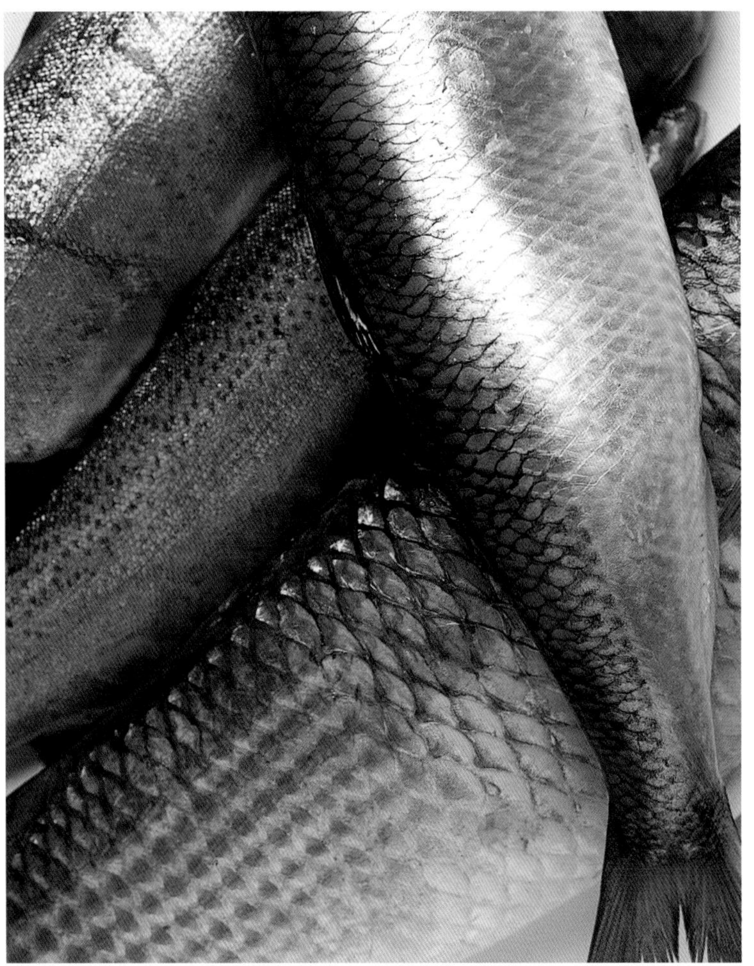

▲ *Fish provides PABA, the exact function of which is unknown in our bodies.*

Inositol

Inositol like choline is a vitamin B-like compound. It is not widely recognized in the scientific or medical communities as an essential nutrient.

Some claim that it lowers blood pressure, reduces hair loss, lowers blood cholesterol and improves brain function but these claims have not been proven.

It is, however, a nutrient that is recommended as important in infant formulas.

Choline

Choline is a compound similar to the B complex vitamins. It is not universally recognized as an essential nutrient. However, it is now considered essential for brain development and function. While your body can produce choline with the help of folic acid and vitamin B_{12}, a dietary source may be needed to keep the brain functioning at optimal levels.

GOOD FOOD SOURCES

Choline is often found in foods that contain significant quantities of lecithin a natural emulsifier found in egg yolks, wheat germ, organ meats , soybeans and tofu.

Please note: Information to create comparative charts or RDA/RNI charts are unavailable.

The American Academy of Pediatrics (AAP) lists inositol as a substance that should be included at levels equivalent to 4 mg per 100 calories of prepared formula.

GOOD FOOD SOURCES

Inositol is found in egg yolks, dairy foods, soybeans and tofu.

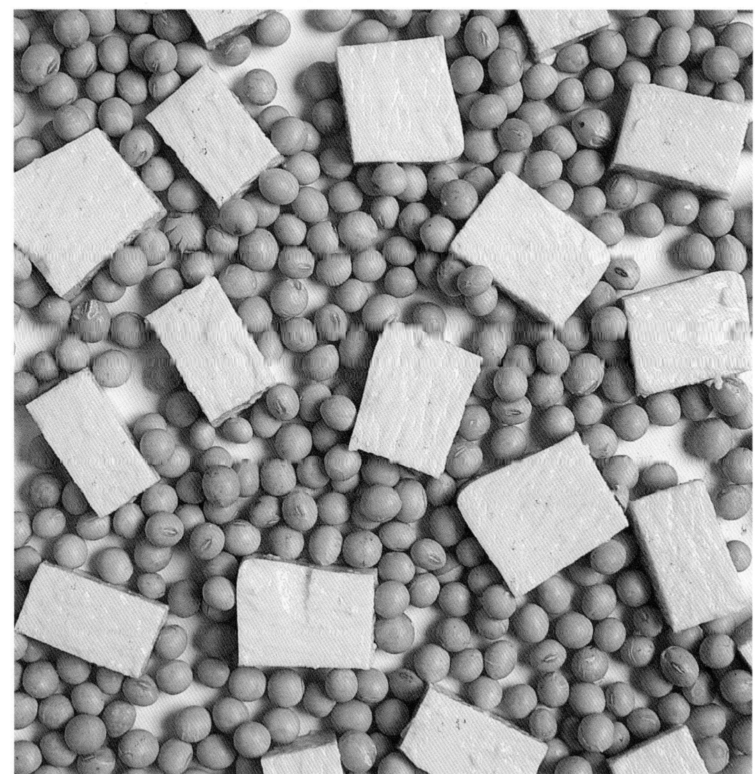

▶ *Inositol is similar in structure to B vitamins and is found in soybeans and tofu. It is thought to be an important factor in emulsifying fats and may keep cholesterol at a normal level.*

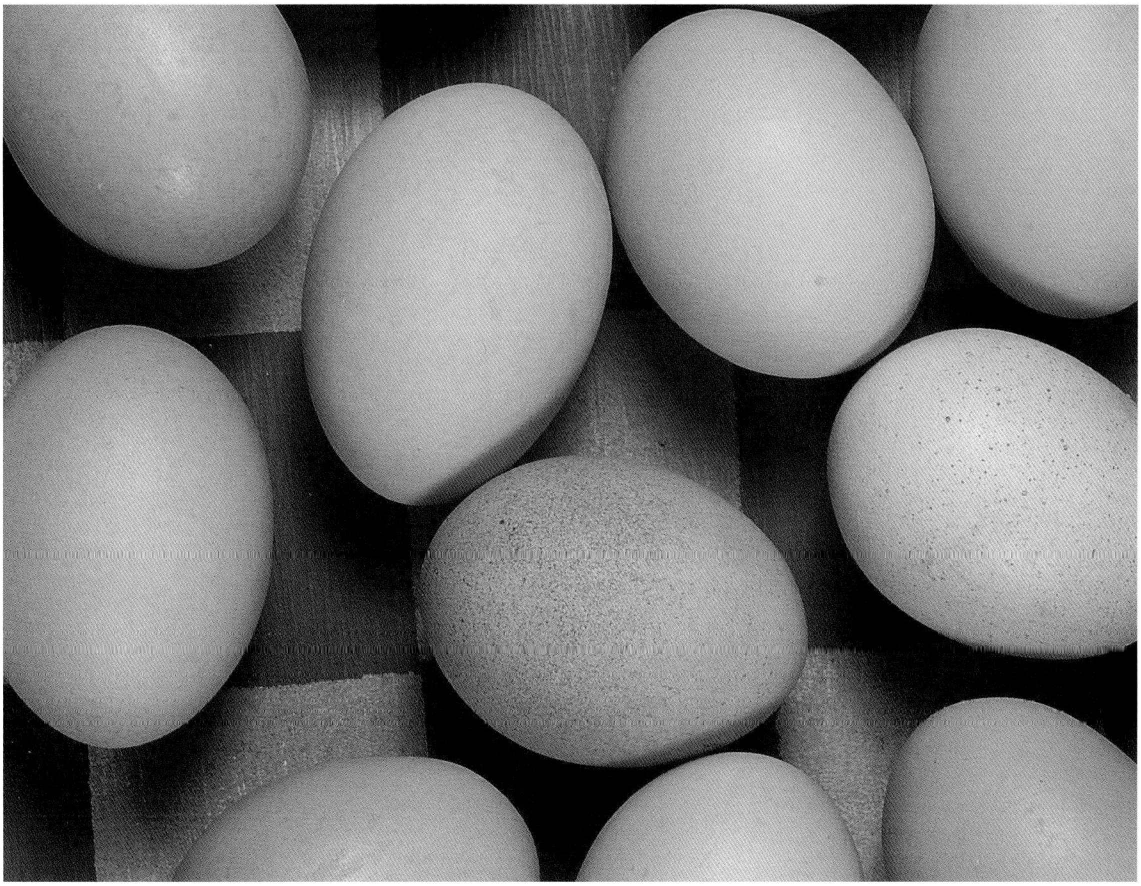

▲ *Choline is closely related to inositol, and they are both found in the lecithin component of egg yolks.*

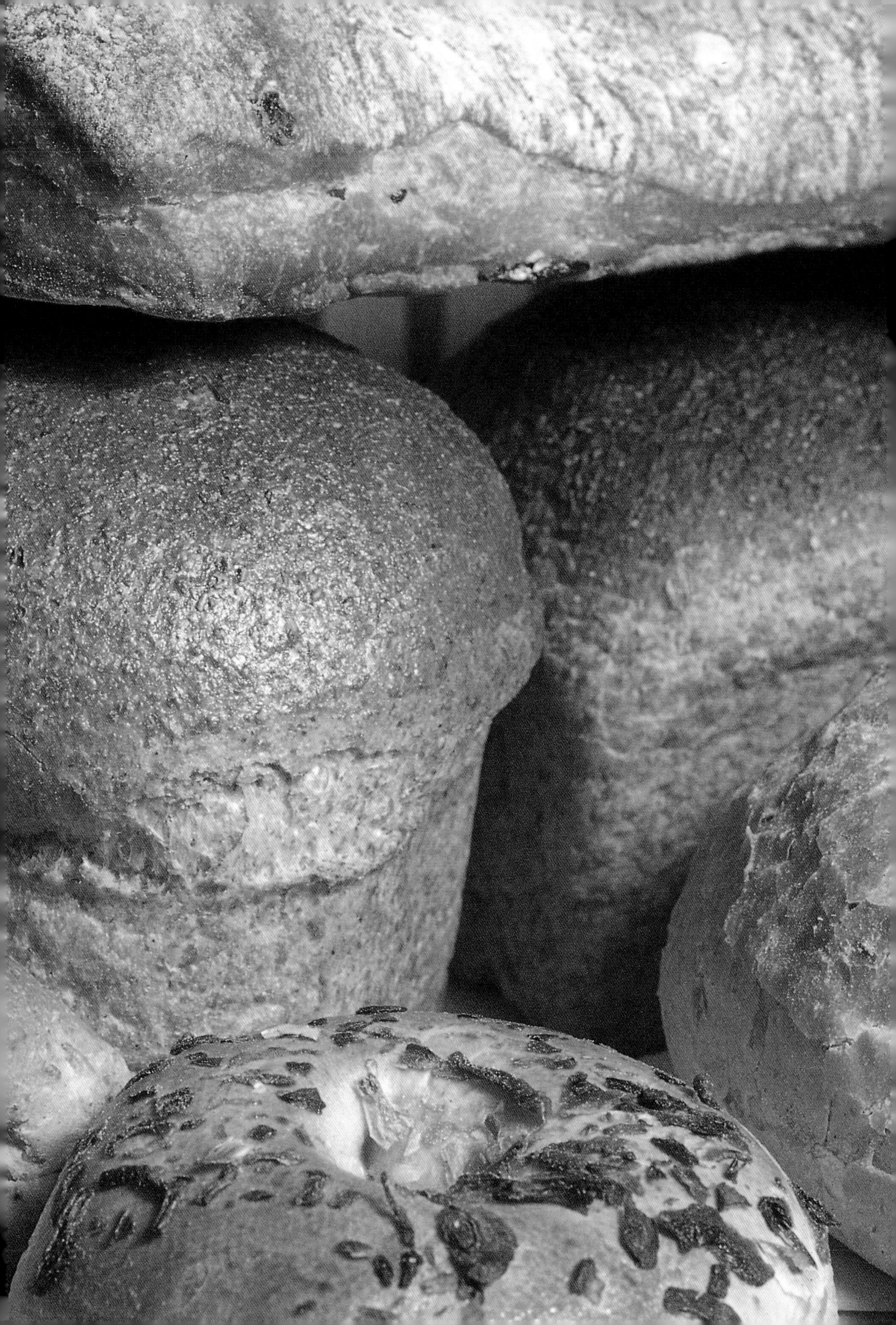

STAYING WELL WITH FOOD

What we eat or don't eat has a tremendous bearing on our health. Staying well with food is not just about using food as a necessity and an enjoyment. It is about using food as a tool to fend off or even treat the common diseases and conditions that ail us.

Staying Well with Food

If you want to look and feel your best, you need to supply your body with all the appropriate fuel: a diet providing the right balance of nutrients, plenty of exercise, sufficient sleep and a strategy for dealing with stress. However, even with the best of intentions, you can still become worn-out and run-down, it is useful to know that many common conditions can be eased or prevented by the food we eat.

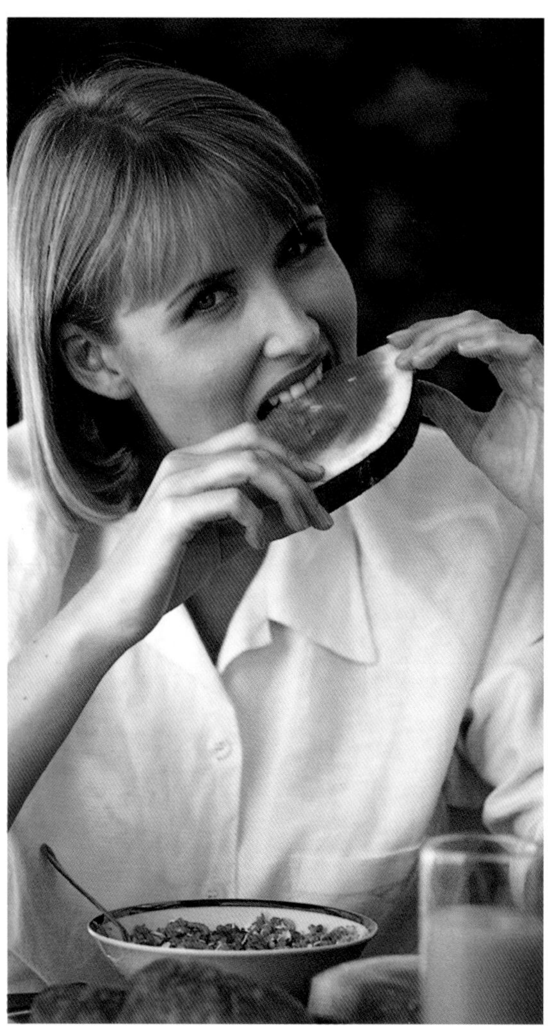

▲ *Eating healthily and staying well are closely linked. The food you eat has a large impact on whether you keep healthy or succumb to disease.*

Although we should always seek medical advice in the event of illness, this does not mean that our well-being is entirely in the hands of others. In Western cultures we all too easily relinquish rights over our own bodies and need to relearn how to control our own health and well-being. You live in your own body and should learn to recognize what it is telling you. Take the time to notice when you are feeling particularly well. What foods have you been eating? Which foods have you been avoiding? What kinds and amounts of exercise make up your daily routine? What is your emotional state? How well are you sleeping?

In a similar vein, pay attention to what your body is saying when you are not well. Has your regular routine been disrupted by something? Your physical environment can often offer clues. Have you changed an eating, exercise or sleeping routine? Have your relationships come under attack? Is the weather unusual in some way? Are you under an increased amount of stress? If you can begin to know how the answers to these questions affect your health, you are well on the way to becoming more in tune with your body. Realizing what makes your body tick means understanding how you can help to keep it in good health.

Remember that the lifestyle that works best for your own health may be totally foreign to others. Sleep needs, for instance, vary greatly

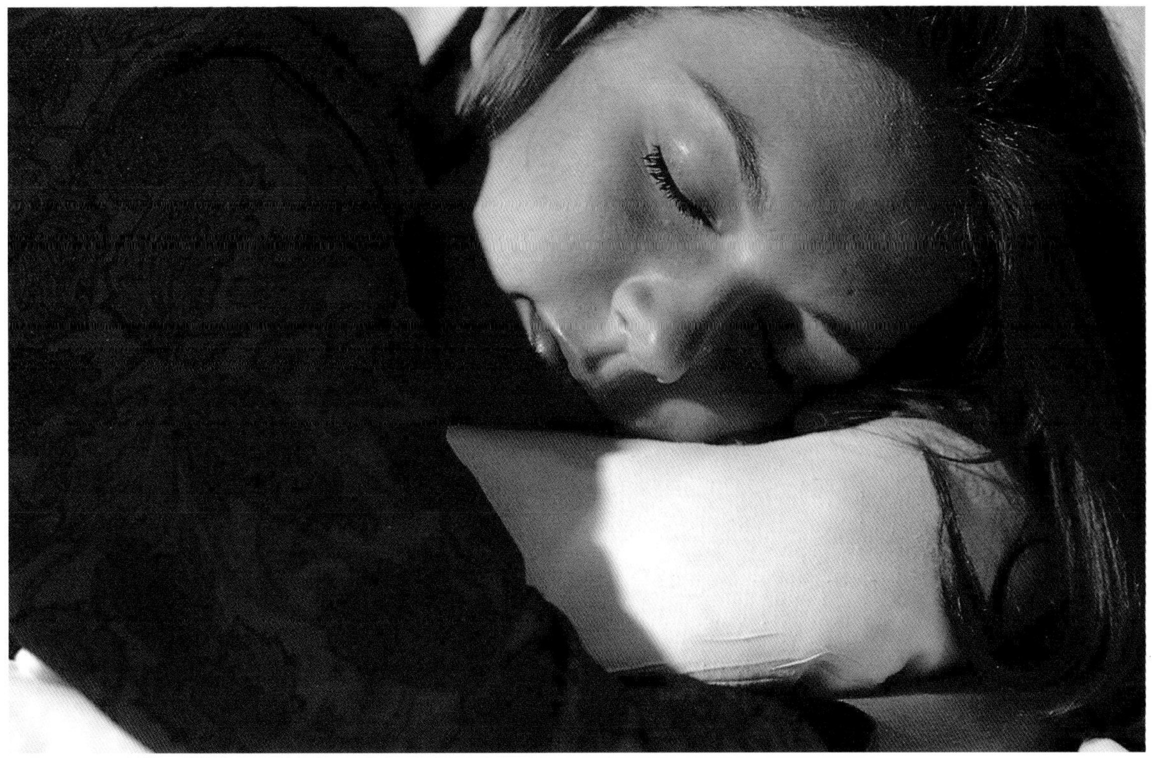

▲ *Late nights are sometimes inevitable, but getting the sleep your body needs is vital.*

from individual to individual. Don't berate yourself if you need nine or ten hours sleep each night to function well during the day. Conversely, don't crow if you can thrive on a high-stress lifestyle with fast food and little sleep. Surviving such a lifestyle depends on a whole host of circumstances individual to you, and a high-risk strategy that works for you today may turn against you tomorrow. It's worth remembering that nobody can abuse his or her body without paying for it in the long run. Whatever your current state of body and mind, looking after your health now will pay off in the future.

The information that follows in this section deals specifically with the dietary aspects of health and disease—explaining how the diet you eat can affect both your short- and long-term health. It is applicable whether you are bursting with health or less than well because it explains how nutrition affects the functioning of important body systems both in sickness and in health. This section also describes which groups of people may have extra nutritional needs and how these needs can be met. For example, the elderly may have reduced appetites but increased nutrient needs, so the concentration of highly nutritious foods in their diets needs to be high. Similarly, pregnant women require extra nutrients to meet the needs of developing fetuses. Children, too, have different dietary needs, including higher fat requirements than adults in the fast-developing years from birth to the age of five.

Of course, the information offered in the following pages is in no way meant to replace the suggestions, advice and guidelines of trained health professionals. If you are experiencing a specific condition that does not respond quickly to some of the commonsense dietary measures suggested, it is time to take medical advice. And remember: regardless of which health practice or system you subscribe to, self-medication, even with harmless substances, can be counter-productive. On the other hand, eating an appropriate healthy diet can only make you feel fitter. Food provides the energy and nutrients to heal and restore and, combined with other healthy lifestyle practices, is the ultimate weapon in ensuring good health.

Eating better really can make you feel a hundred times better. No wonder the philosopher Aristotle said, "Let food be your medicine and medicine be your food."

General Health and Well-Being

Health is more than just the absence of illness; it's about feeling fit and mentally alert, having lots of energy and looking good. Maintaining a healthy weight, altering your diet to accommodate your changing lifestyle, and understanding the impact of diet on your appearance will all help in improving your general well-being. Certain foods will particularly help towards a fitter and healthier you.

The Balance of Good Health

As this book has already explained, one of the keys to maintaining the body is to provide it with all of the nutrients we know it needs by adopting a diet built around a good variety of the following types of food:

- Bread, cereals and potatoes—base meals on them.
- Fruit and vegetables—aim for five servings daily.
- Meat, fish and alternatives (legumes, nuts, eggs)—two to three servings daily.
- Milk and dairy foods (preferably reduced fat)—eat two to three servings daily.
- Fatty and sugary foods—eat in small amounts.

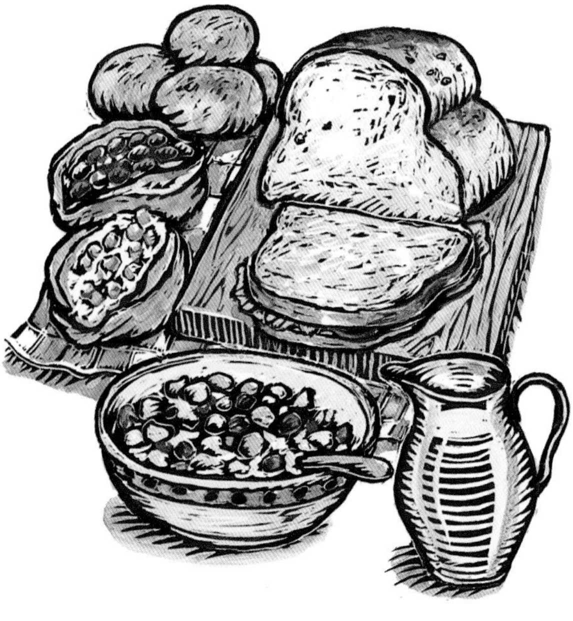

There is also growing evidence that alcoholic beverages taken in moderation (especially one to two glasses of red wine daily) can play a role in maintaining healthy blood cholesterol levels.

In many industrialized societies it has become increasingly difficult to avoid highly processed foods. However, avoiding such items as excess sodium (salt), sugar and fat is important. Too much sugar and fat can lead to problems such as excess weight and obesity, heart disease and diabetes. Excess salt has been shown to contribute to high blood pressure, which is a precursor to heart disease. And more than one-third of cancers could be prevented by reducing high fat, highly processed foods in the diet and replacing them with more starchy, high-fiber foods such as fruit and vegetables.

Particular Needs

At certain times our lifestyles may require us to pay more attention to what we eat in order to meet our nutritional needs. Women have increased requirements during pregnancy and lactation, and young children and the elderly also have special nutritional needs. People who smoke

SUPER FOODS FOR GENERAL GOOD HEALTH		
FOOD	**RICH IN**	**GOOD FOR**
Carrots	Beta-carotene	Mopping up harmful free radicals that damage cells
Cabbage family	Gluco-sinolates	Fighting cancer
Citrus fruits	Vitamin C	Boosting immune system
Red wine	Flavonoids	Reducing the risk of heart disease
Soy	Phyto-estrogens	Speeding estrogen metabolism—possibly reducing breast cancer risk
Onions and garlic	Sulfur compounds	Boosting immune function, fighting cancer and heart disease
Oily fish	Omega-3 fatty acids	Improving blood flow; easing joint pain
Oysters	Zinc	Healthy immune and reproductive systems
Oats and beans	Soluble fiber	Maintaining healthy cholesterol levels
Brazil nuts	Selenium	Reducing cancer risk
Wheat germ	Vitamin E	Lowering heart disease risk
Yogurt	Friendly bacteria	Helping maintain a healthy digestive system
Liver	Vitamin B_{12} and iron	Preventing anemia
Olive oil	Mono-unsaturated fats	Maintaining a healthy cholesterol balance

rob their bodies of valuable nutrients that need to be replaced, and highly active people also have greater nutritional needs. Vegetarians and vegans may need to plan their diets more carefully to ensure they achieve adequate nutrient intake.

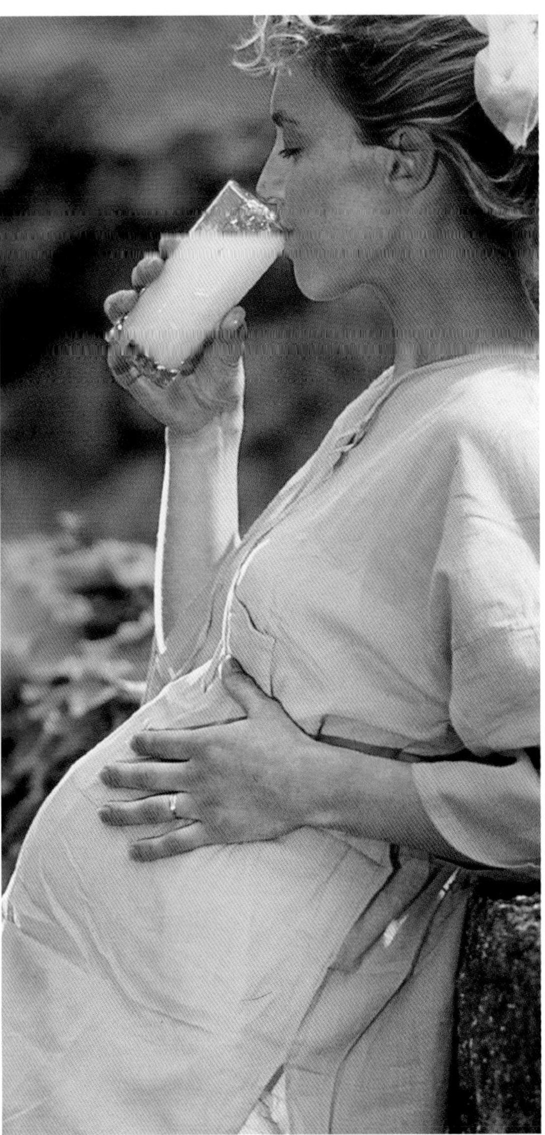

▲ *Pregnancy is a time to take special care of your diet. It is now known that a mother's nutrition can have far-reaching effects on her child's health.*

PREGNANCY

Pregnancy makes heavy demands on a woman's body, but most pregnant women can satisfy their needs and those of their growing fetus by eating a well-chosen diet that follows general healthy eating guidelines. The concept of "eating for two" is a well-worn excuse for eating excessively and gaining too much weight. In fact, for women who are not underweight at the beginning of their pregnancy, calorie requirements are not increased until the last three months, when up to 200 extra calories per day (equivalent to two to three slices of bread) may be required for the growing baby.

Before Conception

When trying to conceive, it is important that both partners eat a healthy diet and avoid drinking too much alcohol as this can adversely affect fertility. Research has proven that the B vitamin folic acid can reduce the risk of a baby being born with spina bifida or other similar birth defects, so foods rich in folic acid—such as green leafy vegetables, fortified breakfast cereals and potatoes—should be eaten regularly. In addition, all women should take 400 micrograms (mcg) of folic acid daily from before conception until 12 weeks into pregnancy.

Vitamins and Minerals

Needs for certain B complex vitamins (required for energy release) are increased in pregnancy, but including adequate amounts of grains, fish, milk and lean meat in the diet should cover these needs. Vitamin C requirements are also increased, but these can easily be met by eating citrus fruit every day. A dietary supply of vitamin D (which can also be supplied through sunlight) is essential in pregnancy to aid calcium absorption and the development of strong bones. This can be acquired by eating eggs (well-cooked), butter and especially canned fish. Vitamin A also needs to be increased by eating deep orange fruits and vegetables (such as apricots, peaches, carrots and pumpkin), dairy products or eggs. Liver is an extremely rich source of vitamin A, but it is not recommended in pregnancy because very large levels of the vitamin can harm the fetus.

Experts are divided about whether the need for iron is increased during pregnancy. The mineral is vital for creating the fetus's blood supply, and, if intakes are insufficient, the mother can become anemic. In the U.S. it is recommended that all women take an iron supplement during pregnancy, but in the U.K. it is generally felt that natural increases in the efficiency of iron absorption can cover the extra needs.

Whether your doctor advises you to take iron supplements or not, it is important to ensure an adequate dietary supply of the mineral. Good iron sources are red meat and liver, dark-green vegetables such as spinach and cabbage, dried fruit and fortified breakfast cereals (also see *Iron*, p. 120).

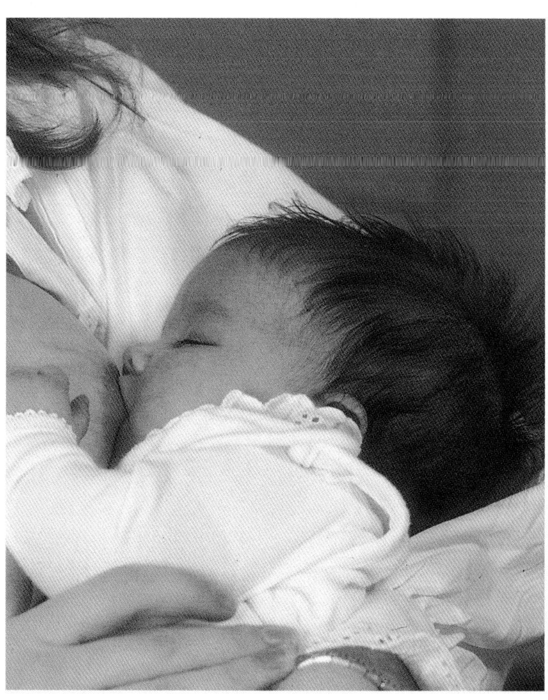

▲ *Breast milk is definitely best for a baby as long as the mother is healthy. Producing milk takes a lot of nutrients. This means that breast-feeding women need to pay special attention to their diet.*

EATING FOR PREGNANCY		
EAT PLENTY OF	**EAT LESS OF**	**AVOID**
Dairy foods	Fatty, sugary foods	Liver
Fish	Salt	Blue-vein, soft unpasteurized and mold-ripened cheeses
Green leafy vegetables	Alcohol (no more than a small glass of wine a day)	
Whole-grain cereals		
Fruit		

Pregnant women should ensure a good intake of calcium from dairy foods such as cheese, milk and yogurt. However, mold-ripened cheeses, such as Camembert, Brie, blue-veined and soft unpasteurized goat and sheep cheeses, should be avoided due to the risk of listeria infection.

Oily Fish

Scientists have found that omega-3 fatty acids present in oily fish, such as tuna, mackerel and sardines, are essential to early development of the fetal nervous system. Eating two or three portions a week of oily fish may be important for ensuring optimal brain development in the fetus.

BREAST-FEEDING WOMEN

Eating healthily is more important than ever after your child has been born. During breast-feeding, there are increased energy and protein requirements, as well as higher needs for many vitamins and minerals. Mostly these needs can be met by eating around 500 extra calories a day while adhering to healthy eating principles. As there are so many increased nutritional requirements during lactation, empty calories such as sugary foods should be avoided as much as possible. A modest multivitamin and mineral supplement may be a nutritional safeguard for busy breast-feeding mothers.

THE ELDERLY

Older people may experience a reduction in appetite or might find it more difficult to prepare and enjoy meals. Official tables often suggest that older people actually require fewer vitamins and minerals due to decreased energy expenditure, but in practice, requirements may be greater because of less efficient absorption. In particular, there is strong evidence that aging increases the requirements for vitamin D—needed for strong bones and the prevention of hip fractures—and certain B vitamins, which are particularly important for brain function and energy release. Liver is an excellent food that includes both these nutrients and should ideally be eaten by the elderly once a week.

It is not always easy for older people to change the dietary habits of a lifetime, but the following practices can easily be incorporated:

- Drinking a glass of fruit juice every day
- Starting the day with high-fiber, whole-grain breakfast cereal
- Eating meat or fish once a day
- Eating one or two servings of vegetables every day
- Taking a drink made with hot milk before bed (one that does not contain caffeine)

Older people should be encouraged to keep an emergency food supply for times of illness or bad weather. Some nutritious suggestions include canned soup, dried fruit, long-life milk, instant mashed potatoes, canned fish, breakfast cereals, cartons of fruit juice and crispbread or crackers.

▼ *Getting older doesn't mean you can give up eating healthily; in fact, a good diet can be the key to keeping fit and healthy until a ripe old age. However, elderly people may have special nutritional needs.*

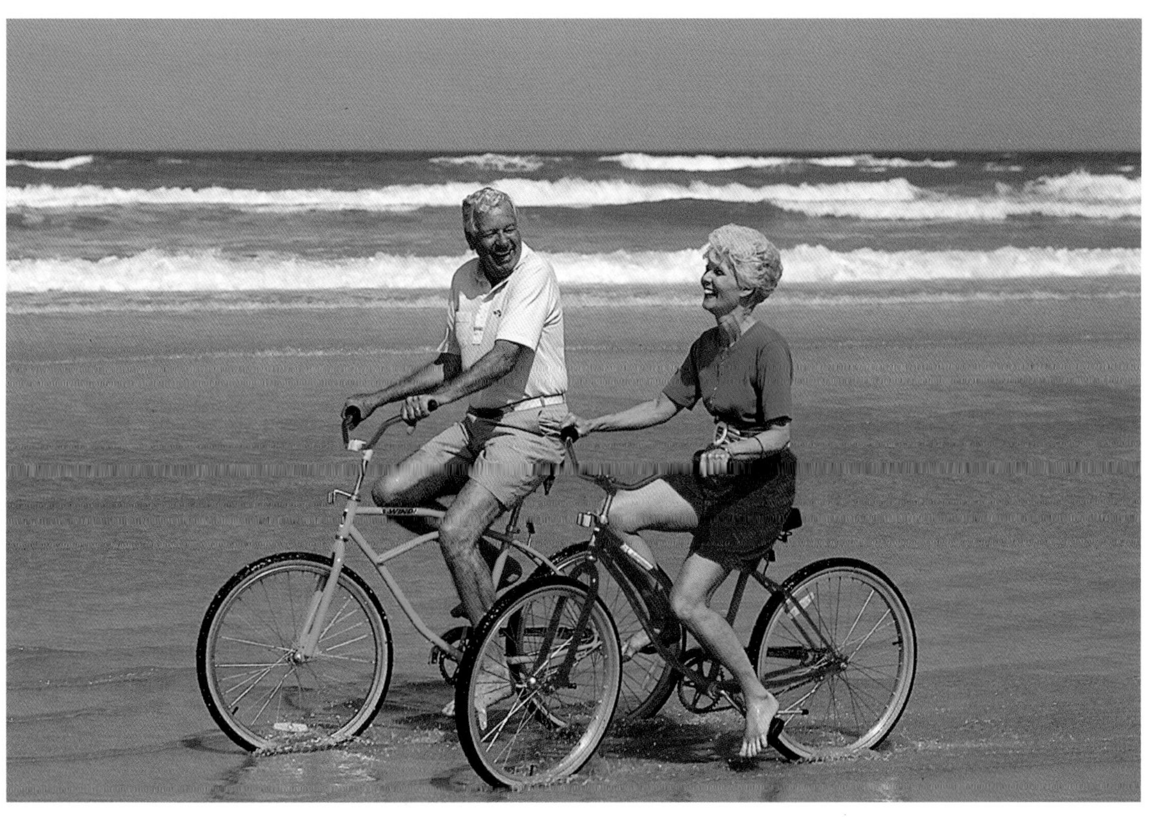

CHILDREN AND TEENAGERS

Preschool age children are developing rapidly and need to eat plenty of calories to support their growing bodies. Fat is a concentrated source of calories, and intake in preschoolers should not be restricted. Use full-fat dairy products for this age group, and avoid a very high-fiber diet as it may be too filling without supplying the right amount of calories. A combination of refined and whole grains is perfectly suitable, but avoid added bran or high-fiber breakfast cereals.

Recently, concerns have been expressed about low iron levels in the diets of both teenagers and younger children. Iron deficiency is associated with lower IQ scores and poor concentration. Including more lean red meat in the diet can help keep iron levels adequate and is especially important for preventing anemia in menstruating young females.

▼ *Children under five need full-fat foods to keep up their calorie intake. Dairy products are particularly important for developing bones and teeth.*

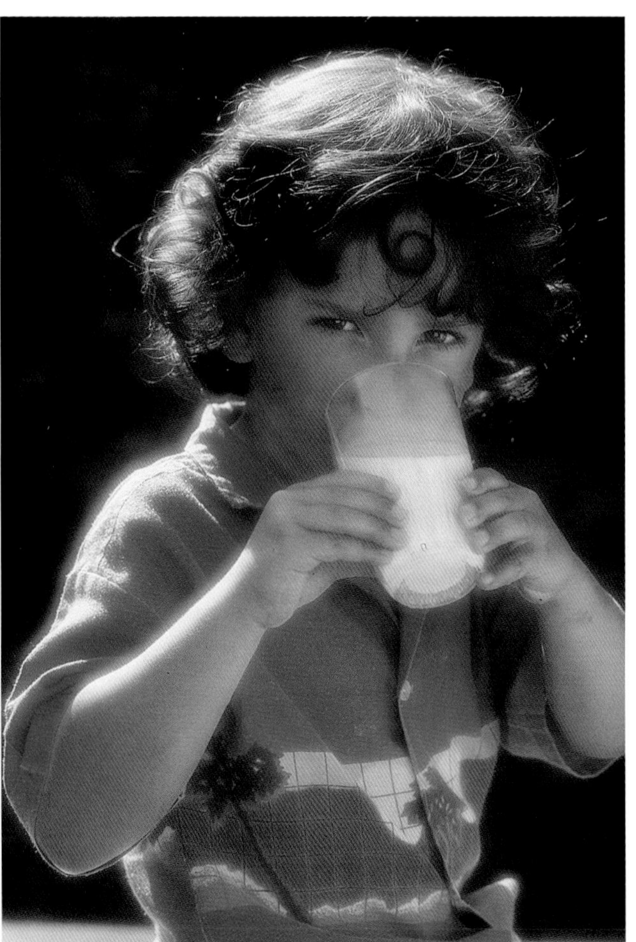

FOODS FOR PRESCHOOLERS	
EAT PLENTY OF	**EAT LESS OF**
Full-fat dairy products Red meat Fruit and vegetables	High-fiber cereal, whole-grain breads and cereals Reduced-fat products

SMOKERS

All smokers know the health risks they take. Each puff of smoke contains literally billions of free radicals–unstable molecules that attack and oxidize body cells–and the only way to stop the damage they cause is to quit completely.

In the meantime, smokers have increased nutritional needs, particularly for vitamin C and other nutritional anti-oxidants that offset the damaging effects of free radicals. Including a wide range of fresh fruits and vegetables in the diet is the best way to meet this increased anti-oxidant need. Most authorities say smokers need 80–100 extra milligrams of vitamin C a day just to keep their blood levels the same as nonsmokers. That is the amount contained in one large orange or about half a bell pepper.

ATHLETES

Keen athletes have a greater need for energy and a wide range of nutrients than sedentary individuals. In particular, athletes may need more B complex vitamins to aid energy release in cells and more anti-oxidant nutrients (vitamins C, E, selenium and beta-carotene) to mop up the rogue oxygen molecules produced by large amounts of aerobic exercise.

For athletes, carbohydrate foods, such as pasta, bread, rice and potatoes also assume greater importance. Eating these foods regularly helps build a supply of glycogen (stored energy) in the muscles, to be used for muscular activity when needed. Very large quantities of protein used to be hailed as the best way to enhance performance, but it is now known that loading the system with protein is not necessary. Strength and endurance athletes may need to increase their protein intake a little, and all athletes should ensure adequate dietary levels.

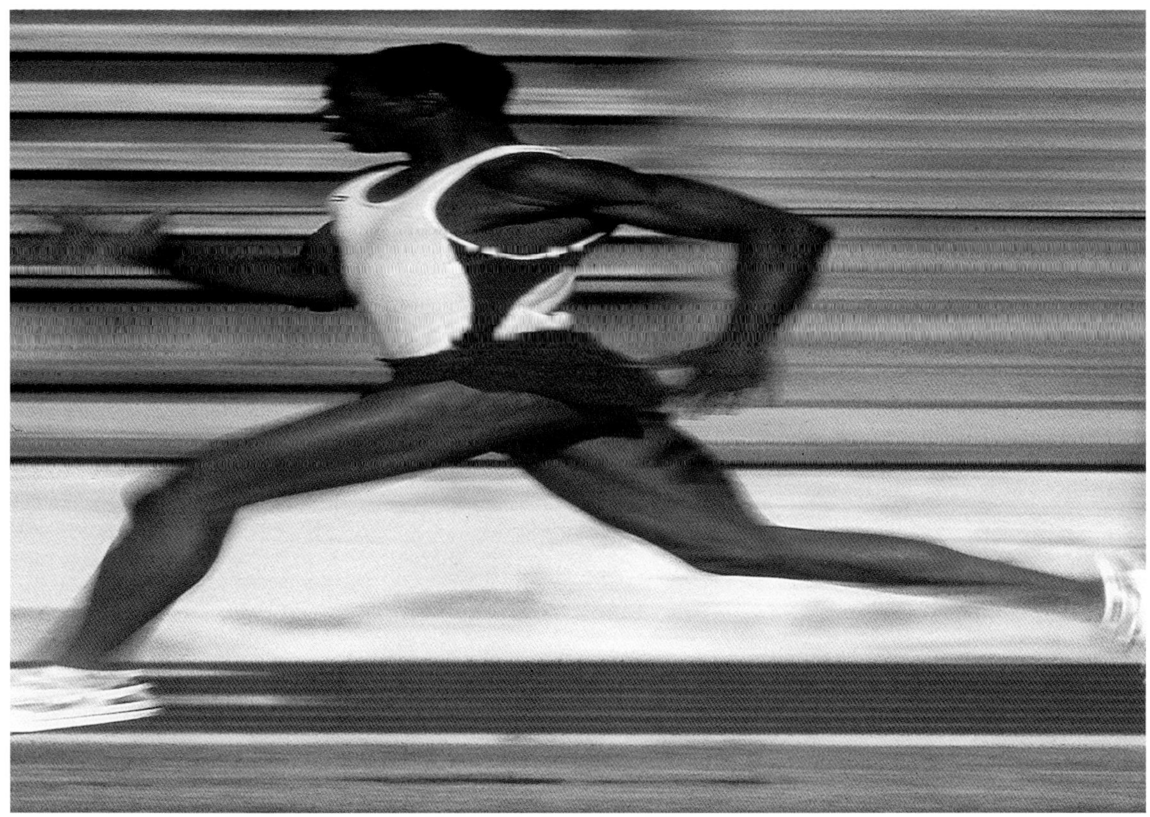

▲ *Athletes have increased nutritional needs and must eat more of certain foods for the very best performance.*

FOOD FOR ATHLETES	
EAT PLENTY OF	**EAT LESS OF**
Starchy carbohydrates, (e.g. pasta, bread, rice, potatoes)	Sugary foods
Fruit and vegetables	Foods with saturated fats
Lean meat, poultry, fish	

VEGETARIANS AND VEGANS

Most nutrients can be supplied adequately by a vegetarian diet, but intake of those which occur naturally only in animal food—such as vitamin D (for strong bones) and B_{12} (for a healthy nervous system)—may be marginal. Vitamin B_{12} can normally be obtained in sufficient amounts from dairy products, but vegans (who avoid dairy products and eggs) may need to take supplements and eat plenty of foods such as yeast extract, fortified cereals and soy milk. Vitamin D can be found in vegetable margarines and fortified breakfast cereals and can be made in sun-exposed skin.

Contrary to popular belief, most vegetarians and vegans actually consume adequate amounts of iron in their diets. However, absorption of the mineral from vegetable sources is very much poorer than from meat. In practice, vegetarians and vegans adapt to their diet by acquiring an increased ability to absorb iron, and their higher intake of vitamin C is also useful as this vitamin markedly enhances the uptake of iron from non-meat sources. However, vegetarians and vegans should avoid drinking tea with meals, as the tannins in the drink can have an adverse effect on iron absorption from plant sources.

Dietary intakes of bone-strengthening calcium are generally no lower in vegetarians than in meat eaters as both groups include dairy products in their diet. Vegans need to increase consumption of calcium-rich vegetable foods (for example broccoli and calcium-enriched soy milk) to compensate for the lack of dairy sources.

Another mineral of concern is iodine, which plays an important role in regulating metabolism. Vegetarians who regularly drink milk can obtain enough iodine, but vegans need to include fortified foods or seaweeds in their diets to ensure an adequate supply.

Weight Control

Most people can carry a little extra weight without too much detriment to their health. But people who are 20 percent over their healthy weight risk joint problems, high blood pressure and diabetes.

ARE YOU OVERWEIGHT?

The degree to which you are overweight can be determined by dividing your weight in kilograms (kg) by your height in meters squared (W ÷ H × H) to arrive at your Body Mass Index (BMI). If your calculated BMI is between 19 and 25, you are of an acceptable weight; between 25 and 30 indicates a degree of overweight; and over 30 indicates obesity. For example, a woman weighs 154 pounds (70 kg) and is 5 ft $2\frac{1}{2}$ in (1.6 meters) tall. Her BMI = 70 kg ÷ (1.6 m × 1.6 m) = 27.3; so she is overweight.

To arrive at your BMI using pounds and inches, multiply your weight in pounds by 700. Divide the result by your height in inches squared. That is, BMI = (154 pounds × 700 ÷ 62.5 in × 62.5 in) = 27.5.

REGAINING CONTROL

Regaining control of your weight is simple in theory but hard in practice. There is no magic formula: Whether you lose or gain weight is a simple balancing act between the amount of energy (calories) ingested and the amount used up in daily activity and exercise. To lose weight, you need to reduce the number of calories you eat while ideally also increasing your amount of exercise.

Whatever your method of weight control, don't expect to lose more than 2 lb (1 kg) a week, and never go on crash diets as they inevitably lead to weight regain.

The following tips should also help in shedding the weight:

- **Always eat breakfast.** Studies show that people eat more calories in total if they skip the first meal of the day.
- **Use smaller plates.** Psychology plays a role in weight loss. Fool yourself into thinking you are eating a bigger meal by putting it on a smaller plate.
- **Graze, don't gorge.** Some people lose weight better by spreading their calorie intake throughout the day and eating little and often. But you must be sure not to eat full meals *and* snacks!
- **Chew, chew, chew.** If you eat too quickly, your "fullness" sensors may not be able to react in time, and you could easily end up overeating. So take your time and chew every morsel well.

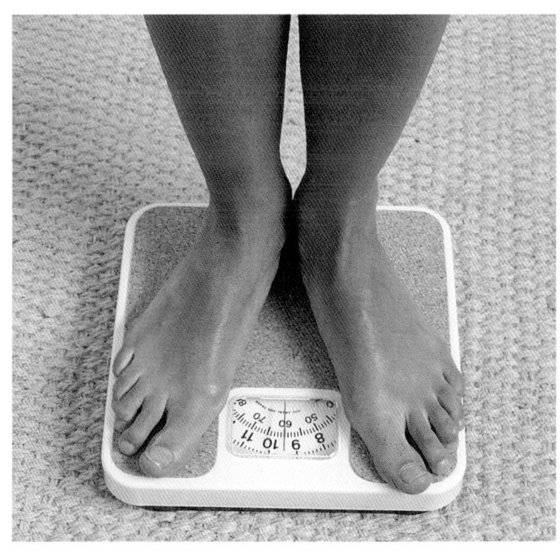

▲ *How you look is more important than what the scales say, but your weight is still important.*

Looking and Feeling Good

Looking and feeling your best involve more than just being free from disease. They mean having loads of energy, clear skin and shiny hair. If this level of vitality eludes you, read on . . .

ENERGY AND STAMINA

Even if all we appear to do is sit at a computer all day, our hearts are pumping, synapses in the brain are firing repeatedly, our lungs are working and our muscles are holding us erect. In order to make it through the day without flagging, we need to ensure we have a good, steady source of energy for our bodies.

Carbohydrate foods are one of the best ways to raise our blood sugar (glucose) levels and to ensure that we are offering our bodies the energy they need. It was once thought that the speed at which a food raises blood sugar levels was determined by whether carbohydrates were simple (sugars) or complex (starches). But it is now believed to depend on the exact type of starch or sugar, the degree of processing it has received and how quickly it can be emptied from the stomach. In fact, complex carbohydrates such as bread and potatoes cause a quick blood glucose "high," while simple carbohydrates (sugars) such as fruit cause a slower response. Accompanying fat, fiber and protein, however, slow down the emptying of the stomach, so the quick "high" can be slowed down if, for example, you eat cheese with your bread or butter with your potato.

Use the following lists to help you choose foods that will keep your energy levels high throughout the day:

FOODS FOR ENERGY	
FOR A QUICK BOOST	**FOR A LONGER LIFT**
Bread, rice and potatoes	Beans and lentils
Raisins	Apples and cherries
Bananas	Yogurt
Orange juice	Whole-wheat pasta
Rice cakes	Oats
Cornflakes	Oranges
	Grapes

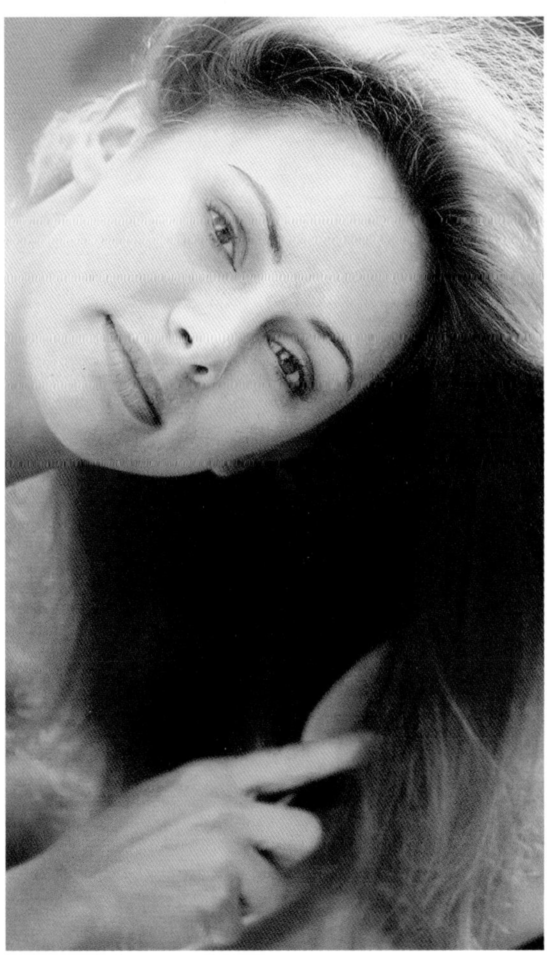

▲ *Skin, hair and nails reflect the state of your inner health and nutritional status.*

SKIN, HAIR AND NAILS

It is often said that you can see a person's state of health reflected in the condition of his or her skin, hair and nails, which are all affected by diet.

All tissues, including skin, hair and nails, are basically made up of protein and water, so including plenty of fluids and good sources of protein in the diet will help to keep them healthy. Small quantities of nuts, seeds and vegetable oils are also important as they contain essential fatty acids that keep the skin moisturized and waterproof. Zinc and vitamin A help combat dryness and pimples, and zinc also affects nail health. White flecks on the nails can indicate a deficiency of this important mineral.

Skin Aging

Anti-oxidant nutrients help to prevent the skin from aging prematurely. Some evidence suggests that the brightly colored carotenoid family of anti-oxidants may be particularly helpful in protecting the skin against sun damage. Flavonoids, found in the pithy parts of citrus fruits, may also be important in maintaining young-looking skin as they help maintain its firm collagen structure.

Hair Health

Healthy hair depends on various nutrients, including protein and B vitamins. An iron deficiency can lead to hair loss but is not usually the primary cause. Hormonal imbalance, stress and medication are often other important factors.

EATING FOR HEALTHY HAIR, SKIN AND NAILS	
EAT PLENTY OF	**EAT LESS OF**
Fruits and vegetables	Sugary foods
Nuts and seeds	Fatty foods
Fish, poultry and lean red meat	
Whole-grain bread and cereals	
AND DRINK	
Plenty of water	

Your Healthy Body

Your body has many different systems that, in times of good health, interrelate in perfect harmony. For example, the heart and lungs work together to oxygenate the body, while a part of the nervous system sends messages to the heart telling it to beat. The digestive system breaks down and digests foods to make them ready for absorption by the body, and hormones act on the digestive tract and affect the amount of certain minerals absorbed. The nervous system may also affect the immune system and hormone balance.

Although many factors can affect body systems (for example, smoking, stress, exercise, body weight), diet is also an important factor in determining how well these systems function. Understanding this can help to keep you well.

In this section we examine the different body systems and which foods or nutrients are important to help them function optimally. Understanding the delicate relationship between nutrition and body systems also helps if things go wrong.

▼ *Yogurt and garlic can help improve the balance of friendly bacteria in your digestive system. This can boost your resistance to intestinal infections.*

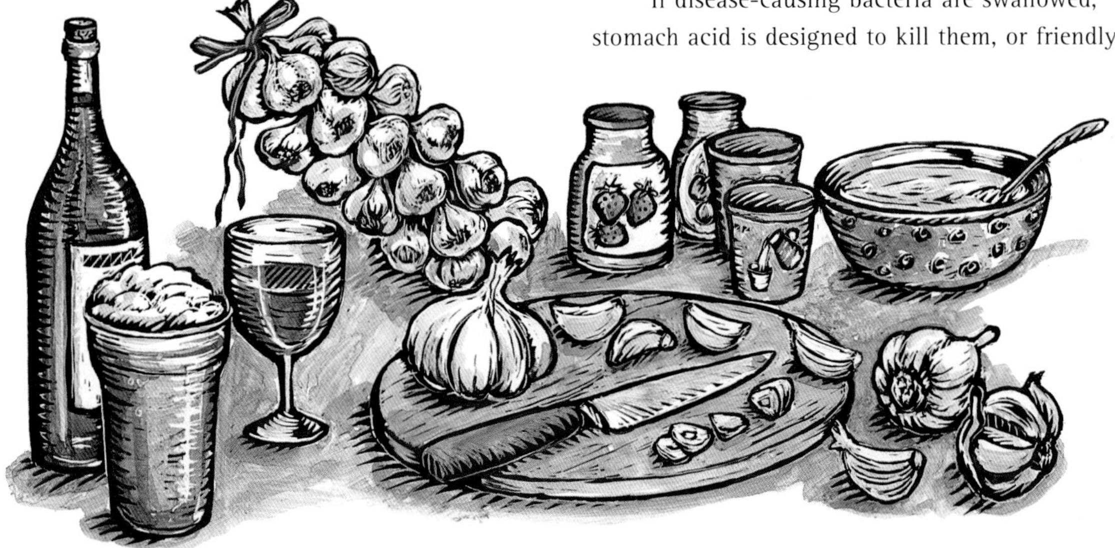

The Immune System

Eating a healthy, balanced diet will help ensure that your immune system functions optimally. Of course, having the perfect diet won't always stop you from catching a cold or coming down with flu, but it will mean you suffer less severely and bounce back more quickly from illness.

A diverse collection of cells, tissues and organs makes up the immune system. Skin is actually part of our immune system, acting as a barrier to dirt and bacteria. The mucous membranes in the nose, throat and respiratory passages act as primary protection against infectious micro-organisms, and we need vitamin A to keep these passages healthy.

If disease-causing bacteria are swallowed, stomach acid is designed to kill them, or friendly "bugs" in the intestines crowd them out. Yogurt, especially if it contains special cultures, can enhance the action of friendly gut flora against harmful bacteria. Garlic contains sulfur compounds, which also boost the immune system.

Inside the bloodstream, a whole range of immune-specific cells get to work to destroy any invaders that have passed the primary defenses. These require certain vitamins and minerals to work effectively, including vitamin C, B complex, vitamin E, zinc and selenium.

A little alcohol can boost the immune system, but always keep well within safe limits. Sufficient sleep relaxes the body and allows the immune system to rejuvenate, while moderate exercise stimulates the circulation, increasing the efficiency of immune cells. On the other hand, smoking and excess alcohol load the body with toxins that tax the immune system; excess fat makes immune cell circulation sluggish, and too much sugar can also affect immunity.

EATING FOR BETTER IMMUNITY	
EAT PLENTY OF	**EAT LESS OF**
Fruits and vegetables	Sugary foods
Yogurt	Fatty foods
Garlic	
Nuts, seeds and grains	
AND DRINK	
Orange juice	

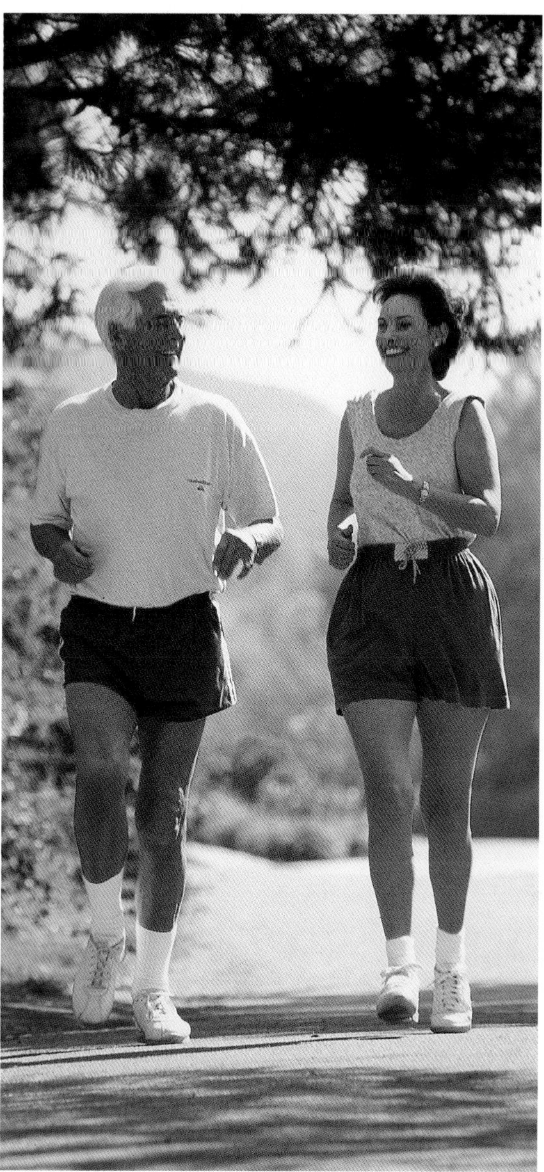

▲ *Keeping fit is essential to health. Movement of the joints through walking or jogging encourages strong bones—although care should be taken not to injure the joints.*

The Bones and Joints

Strong, healthy skeletons are essential to carry us through life. Bones may seem like "dead" structures, but they are in fact made of living tissue, which is constantly being remodeled. Eating a calcium-rich diet helps maintain bone strength and is particularly important before the age of 30, when peak bone mass is achieved. Regular weight-bearing exercise (for example, walking, jogging, skipping) also encourages strong bones, as do other nutrients including vitamin D, zinc, magnesium and copper. High-fiber diets may reduce the absorption of minerals important for healthy bones, so it may be wise to avoid added bran.

Joints exist where two bones join together and, naturally, after many years of bending, walking and stretching, they can suffer from wear and tear. However, the cartilage and lubricating fluid surrounding the joints can be protected by consuming a diet rich in vitamin C—found in citrus fruits, bell peppers and blackcurrants—and the mineral manganese—found in foods such as whole-wheat bread, legumes, hazelnuts and tea. Inflammation around joints can be kept at bay by including oily fish in the diet and reducing the intake of saturated fats.

Muscles attach to the bones via tendons, and are made up predominantly of protein. With

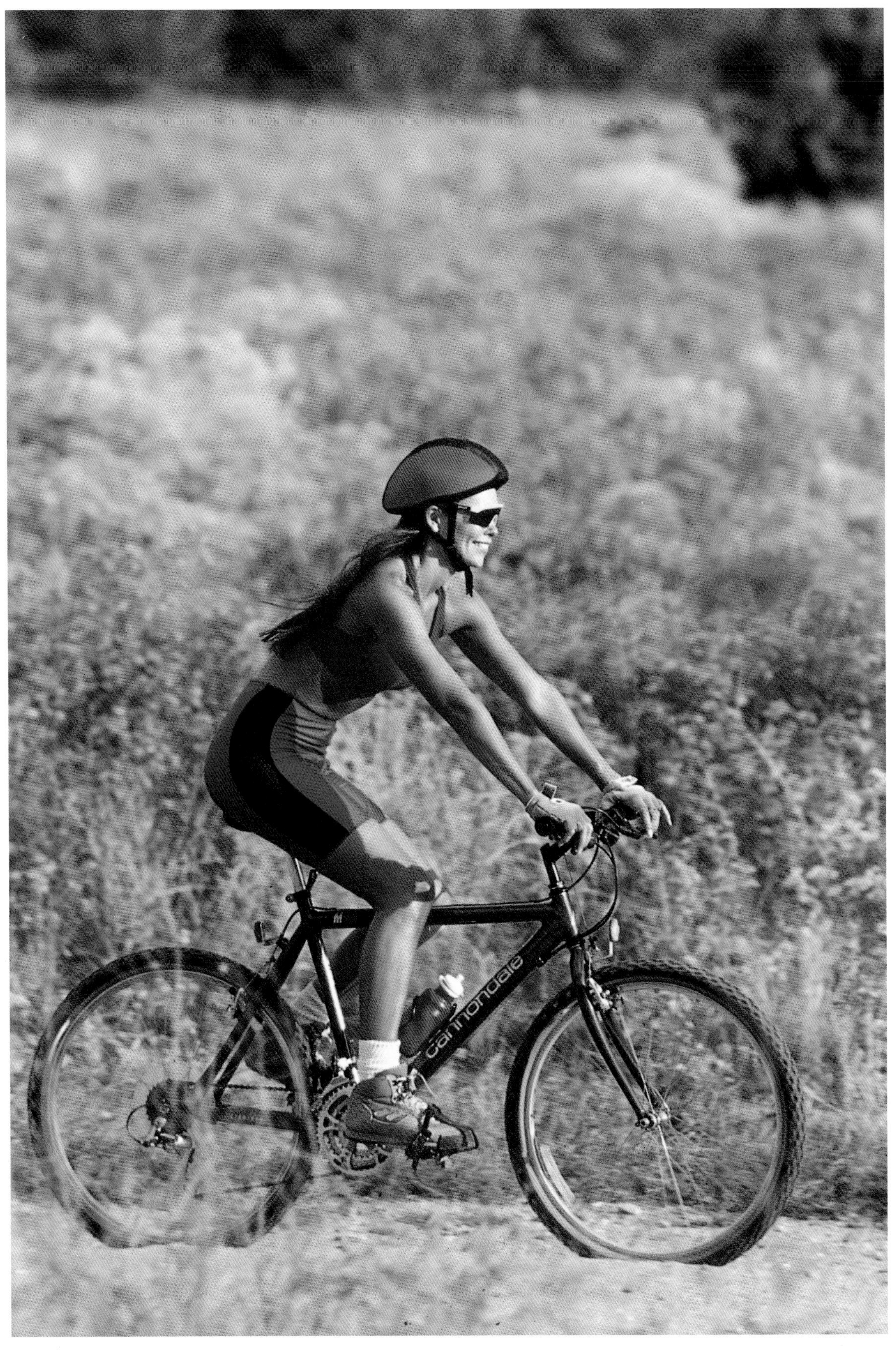

▲ *A healthy diet combined with regular exercise is the ideal combination for a strong heart and lungs.*

every movement, muscles are required to contract or relax; the energy for this process is supplied by carbohydrates. Calcium and magnesium are also essential for muscles to function correctly.

EATING FOR HEALTHY BONES AND JOINTS	
EAT PLENTY OF	**EAT LESS OF**
Reduced-fat dairy foods Oily fish, (especially canned fish with bones) Green vegetables Nuts, seeds and grains	Added bran Saturated fats (fatty meats, cookies [biscuits], pastries, and so on)

The Heart and Lungs

The heart circulates blood carrying oxygen and nutrients around the body. The left-hand side of the heart pumps oxygenated blood from the lungs to the tissues, and the right-hand side pumps low-oxygen blood back from the tissues to the lungs. To maintain a regular beat, the heart requires the right balance of minerals including potassium and magnesium. Aerobic exercise (exercise which utilizes oxygen) strengthens the heart muscle and helps it beat more efficiently. Being overweight and consuming too much saturated fat and salt tend to raise blood pressure and cholesterol—risk factors for heart disease. Diets rich in oats, fish oils, vitamin E and garlic are believed to reduce the risk of heart disease.

The lungs completely fill the thoracic cavity, and breathing is brought about by increasing and decreasing the size of this cavity. Pollutants such as cigarette smoke can markedly reduce the efficiency of the lungs. Antioxidant nutrients, such as vitamin C and beta-carotene help protect lung function.

EATING FOR A HEALTHY HEART AND LUNGS	
EAT PLENTY OF	**EAT LESS OF**
Fruit and vegetables Garlic Oily fish Avocados, wheat germ, nuts and vegetable oils Oatmeal (porridge)	Salty foods Saturated fats (fatty meats, cookies [biscuits], pastries, and so on)

The Reproductive System

Nutrition is important in maintaining a healthy reproductive system in both men and women. In particular, the mineral zinc is vital for maintaining fertility. This mineral is found in grains, meat and nuts and is particularly plentiful in oysters.

Antioxidants help maintain the integrity of male sperm, and some studies have shown that increasing the intake of vitamin E (found in avocados, wheat germ, nuts and vegetable oils) can increase the number of undamaged sperm and increase their mobility.

EATING FOR A HEALTHY REPRODUCTIVE SYSTEM	
EAT PLENTY OF	**EAT LESS OF**
Seafood (especially oysters) Citrus fruits Avocados, wheat germ, nuts and vegetable oils	Sugary foods Foods with saturated fats

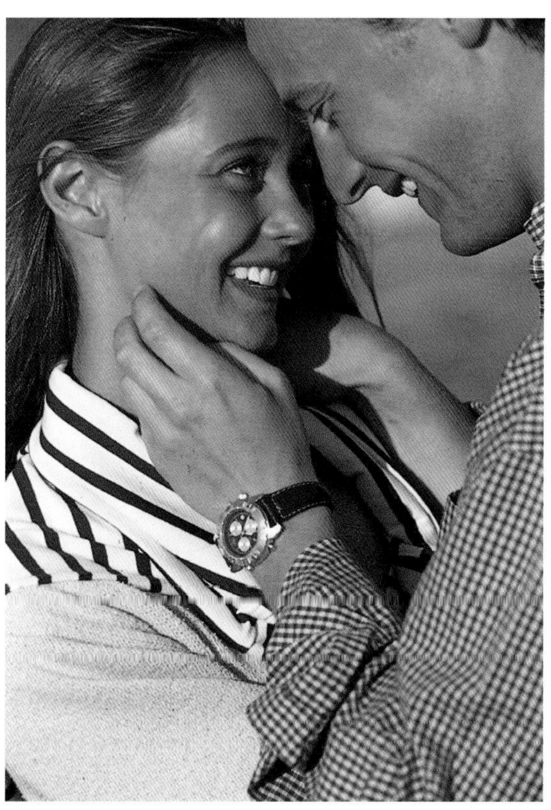

▲ *A healthy diet and lifestyle can enhance your love life and improve fertility.*

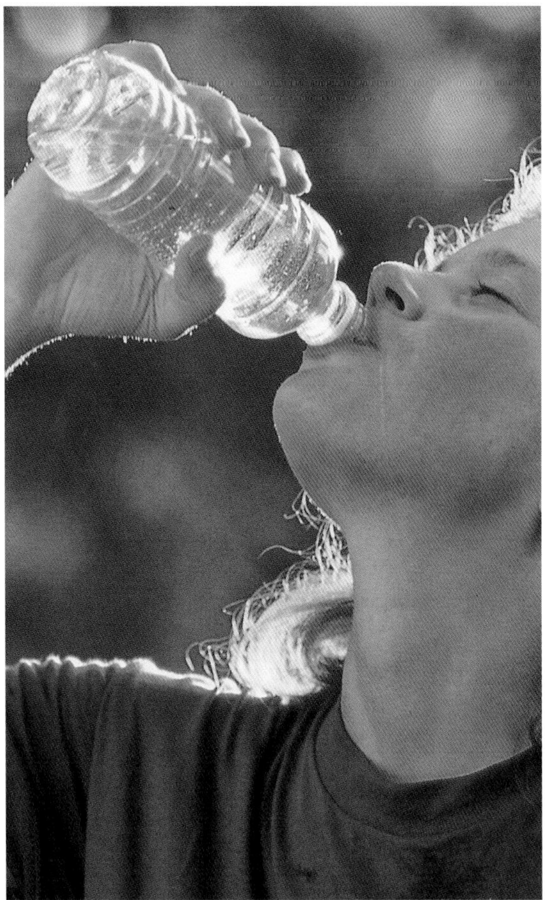

▲ *Drinking plenty of fluid (around eight glasses of water every day) keeps our kidneys functioning correctly and removes toxins from the body.*

The Digestive and Urinary Systems

The digestive tract consists of the mouth, esophagus, stomach, small intestines and bowel (large intestines), and its purpose is to break down food into smaller and smaller parts, which are then absorbed by the body.

Fiber in foods such as fruit, vegetables and whole-grain cereals is very important for a healthy digestive system because it adds bulk to the feces and enables toxins to pass more quickly out of the body. Fiber also has the ability to bind small amounts of fat and cholesterol and remove them from the body.

Adequate fluids are necessary for the fiber to do its work as a bulking agent. Water is also vital for a healthy urinary system. It flushes toxins from the kidneys and reduces the risk of bladder infection.

EATING FOR HEALTHY DIGESTIVE AND URINARY SYSTEMS	
EAT PLENTY OF	**EAT LESS OF**
Whole-wheat bread, pasta and rice Fruits and vegetables Beans and legumes **AND DRINK** Plenty of water	Sugary foods Saturated fats

The Nervous System and Hormones

The nervous system is made up of a very large number of nerve cells that transfer electrical messages from touch or pain sensors in the skin to the brain, and from the brain to the muscles. Electrical stimulation of nerves depends on the interchanges between various minerals in the body, particularly potassium (abundant in dried fruits and bananas) and sodium. Messages passing from nerve to nerve or from nerve to muscle do so via neurotransmitters, and good nutrition can ensure proper production of these chemical messengers. For example, one common neurotransmitter requires choline for its formation, and this is found plentifully in egg yolks, wheat germ, soy and liver. Other neurotransmitters require B vitamins to function properly.

Hormones also act as chemical messengers, but they originate in one part of the body and travel round the bloodstream to have an effect on another part. For example, parathyroid hormone is produced by a gland in the neck, but it acts on the digestive tract, stimulating the absorption of calcium. To maintain a healthy hormone balance, a wide range of nutrients is required.

EATING FOR A HEALTHY NERVOUS SYSTEM AND HORMONES	
EAT PLENTY OF	**EAT LESS OF**
Whole grains, whole-wheat bread and pasta, and brown rice Lean meat, poulty, liver and eggs Dried fruits and bananas Fruits and vegetables	Highly refined and processed food

Your Unhealthy Body

The body can all too easily become diseased, and when major body systems are attacked, the effects can be devastating (for example, the bones and joints in arthritis). The two commonest major illnesses that affect Western societies are heart disease and cancer. The good news is that in both cases, eating the proper diet can significantly reduce a person's risk of developing them.

Heart Disease

Poor dietary habits, lack of exercise and certain "lifestyle choices" have a great deal to do with how vigorously your blood flows, your heart beats and your entire circulatory system operates. Heredity plays a part, too; some families have histories of high blood pressure, raised cholesterol, heart attacks and strokes. To maintain the best overall cardiovascular health you need to adopt a diet that is high in fruits and vegetables (eat at least five portions a day) and low in saturated fats. Cut back on fatty red meats and learn to prefer meals based on fish. A vegetarian diet, as long as it is not heavy on fatty foods such as cheeses and eggs, may be a helpful choice for some people.

HIGH CHOLESTEROL

Cholesterol is a fatty substance made by the body and found in foods. As cholesterol deposits build up on the interior of arteries, the flow of blood is restricted and eventually blocked. The blockages prevent blood flow to the heart or brain and may lead to permanent damage and heart attacks or strokes (particularly for those with an inherited tendency towards high cholesterol levels). For most people, the amount of cholesterol consumed bears little relation to cholesterol levels in the bloodstream. This is because the liver can reduce its production of cholesterol in response to high levels ingested in food. What does raise blood cholesterol, however, is saturated fat: Avoid cookies (biscuits), cakes, cream, pastry and fatty meats. Increasing your intake of antioxidants in vegetables and fruits stops cholesterol from becoming oxidized, which is the precursor to narrowing of the arteries.

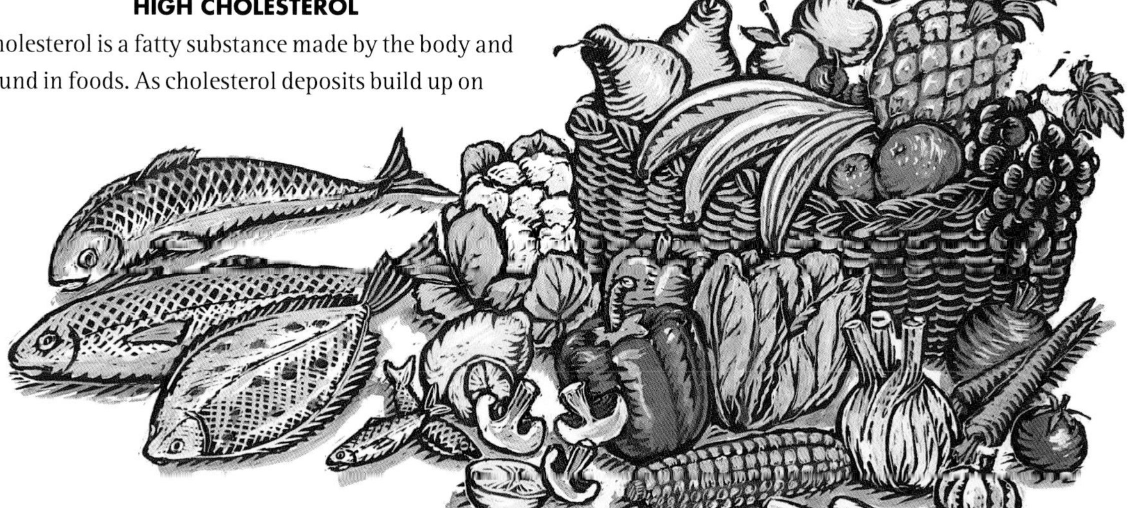

HIGH BLOOD PRESSURE (HYPERTENSION)

While very common, high blood pressure is undesirable because it can lead to heart attack or stroke if unchecked. Some individuals suffer from stress-induced high blood pressure; others suffer from it as a result of being overweight or having diets that are too high in sodium. There may also be an inherited tendency to have high blood pressure.

Help to keep your blood pressure normal by cutting down on salt in food. About 25 percent of our sodium comes from the salt we add at the table, so resist the temptation to shake before you taste. Processed and "fast" foods, however, are by far the biggest source of sodium in our diets. Try to eat less of these and to concentrate on potassium-rich foods instead, especially fruits and vegetables. Eating more oily fish and garlic and keeping your weight within normal limits will also help to keep blood pressure from rising.

Avoiding a Heart Attack

Following the dietary tips in the previous two subsections will do much to reduce your risk of suffering a heart attack. It is particularly beneficial to incorporate oily fish into your diet, as this provides important omega-3 fatty acids, which reduce the stickiness of the blood and improve its flow. Researchers believe that two or three servings a week will reduce the risk of heart attack. In people who already have a degree of heart disease, a daily 400 i.u. vitamin E supplement is also beneficial and may reduce the risk of a nonfatal heart attack by as much as 75 percent.

A pleasurable component of a diet that aims to reduce the risk of heart disease is red wine. The flavonoids it contains act as anti-oxidants and stop platelets in the blood clumping together. Try not to exceed two glasses a day.

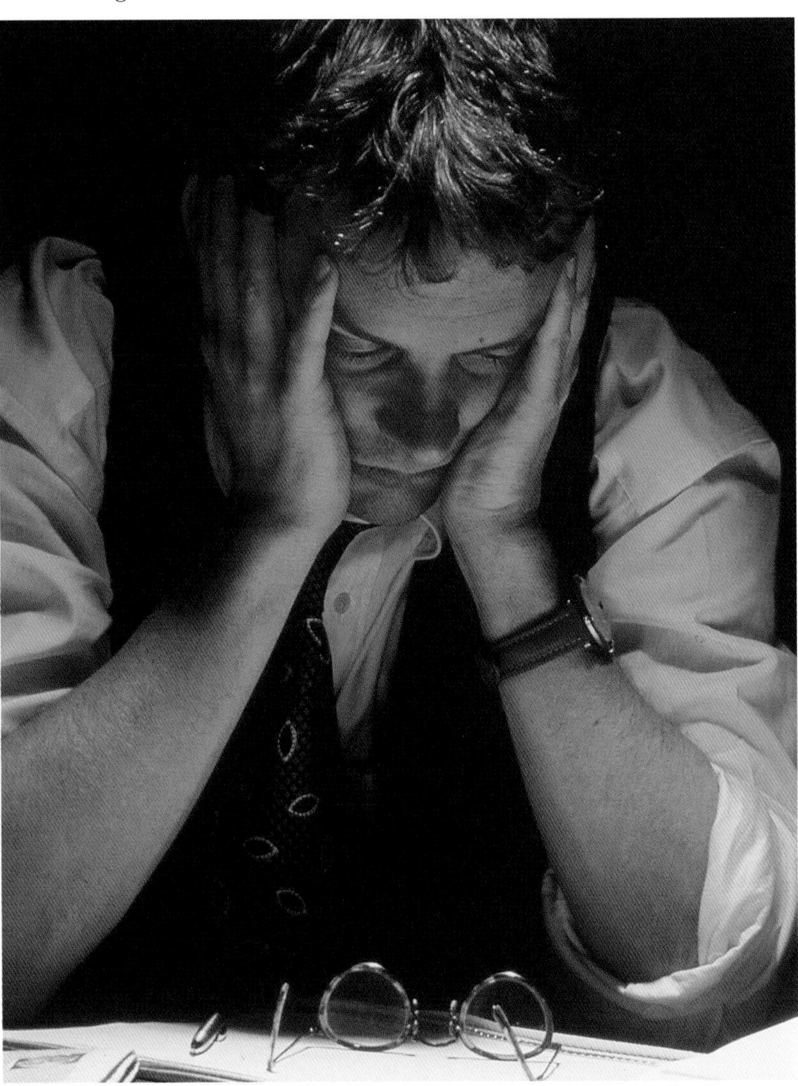

▶ *Stress is a major factor in raising blood pressure and increasing the risk of heart attack. A healthy diet will help offset some of the effects of stress, but you should take time to relax too.*

Cancer

Science is still working to unravel many mysteries associated with cancer. Hereditary factors mean some individuals are affected, while others are not. Cancers are typically slow to develop, so early detection and treatment are valuable in preventing death.

Environmental factors, such as toxins in polluted air, industrial wastes and radiation are thought to be linked with cancer. Smoking is by far the leading cause of lung cancer, and a stressful lifestyle may also be a factor in some forms of the disease.

You may not be able to change your environment or genetics, but you can stop smoking and change your diet. As many as 35 percent of cancers are diet related, so eating correctly is a very positive step in cutting your cancer risk. We still need to learn a lot about diet and cancer, but below are some known steps you can take to reduce your chances of contracting the disease:

1. Maintain a healthy body weight.
2. Moderate the amount of smoked, pickled and nitrate-cured foods you consume (bacon, ham, smoked fish, corned beef) as these contain carcinogens (cancer promoting agents). Avoid burnt foods for the same reason.
3. Limit your intake of all fats. This may be especially important for women with a history of breast cancer in their family.
4. Eat a variety of foods that are rich in fiber (apples, oranges, beets [beetroot], tomatoes, oats, wheat, rice, beans, carrots, celery, pasta and corn, for instance).
5. Concentrate on including five servings each day of fresh fruits and vegetables. These foods are typically high in fiber and anti-oxidants. If possible, try to choose foods that are organically grown.
6. Include foods rich in vitamins A and C such as carrots, spinach, sweet potatoes, peaches, apricots, strawberries, potatoes and all varieties of citrus fruit.
7. Eat at least one serving each day of vegetables in the cabbage family: red, green, savoy or other cabbages, plus kohlrabi, broccoli, cauliflower or Brussels sprouts.

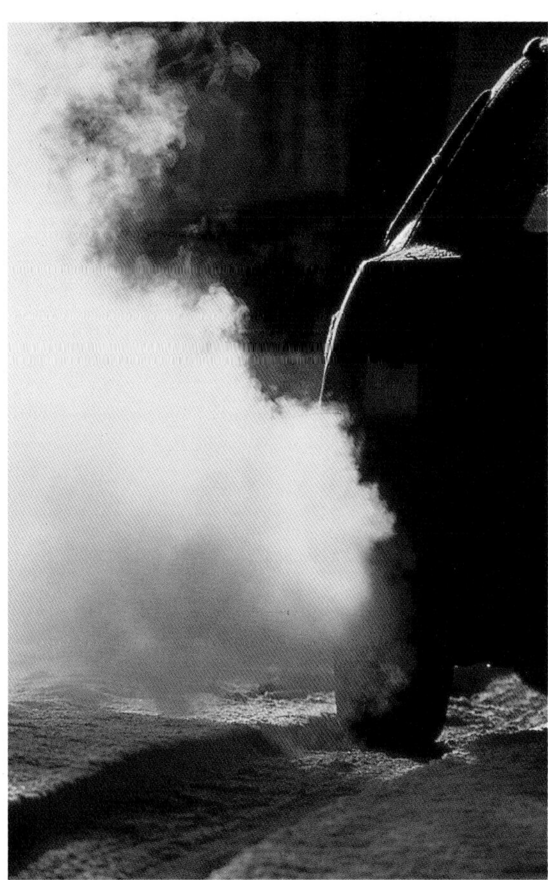

▲ *Cancer has many causes. Help protect yourself by eating a diet rich in antioxidant nutrients (such as fruit and vegetables).*

8. Women may want to increase their consumption of soy foods which some believe may reduce the risk of breast cancer.
9. Incorporate Brazil nuts in your diet. They are very rich in selenium, which is an anti-oxidant lacking in very many soils and which may protect against cancer.

Unfortunately, some of the treatments for cancer, such as chemotherapy and radiation, are very debilitating, sometimes producing unpleasant side effects. Vomiting, diarrhea, hair loss, weight loss and lack of appetite are common. Find foods that provide adequate nourishment in the most palatable form possible. Several small meals over the course of a day may be easier to handle than traditional large meals. Don't forget that food should be a pleasure, even while noting any possible interactions with medications being taken as part of the treatment.

Directory of Ailments

Ailments and health conditions, whether minor or chronic, can sometimes respond to special modifications in the diet. Of course, it is important to be diagnosed and treated medically too, but you will be surprised how healing the right nutrition can be.

The Immune System

FOOD ALLERGIES

Food allergies arise when the immune system reacts against a harmless food or other edible substances as if it were a poison. Food intolerance is less serious but still causes an upset stomach or vomiting.

Eat more fruits and vegetables for a healthy immune system.

Eat fewer foods that trigger the allergy or intolerance. Common culprits include milk, wheat, eggs, fish, shellfish, nuts, soybeans and additives.

COLDS

Everyone gets colds, but frequent suffering may indicate that the immune stem is overstressed.

Eat more zinc-rich foods, such as oysters, grains, meat and fish, or suck zinc lozenges which help stop cold viruses from replicating. Increase the intake of vitamin C (found in citrus fruits and juices) and colorful, beta-carotene-rich vegetables, both of which boost the immune system.

Eat less sugar and fat, which make the immune system sluggish.

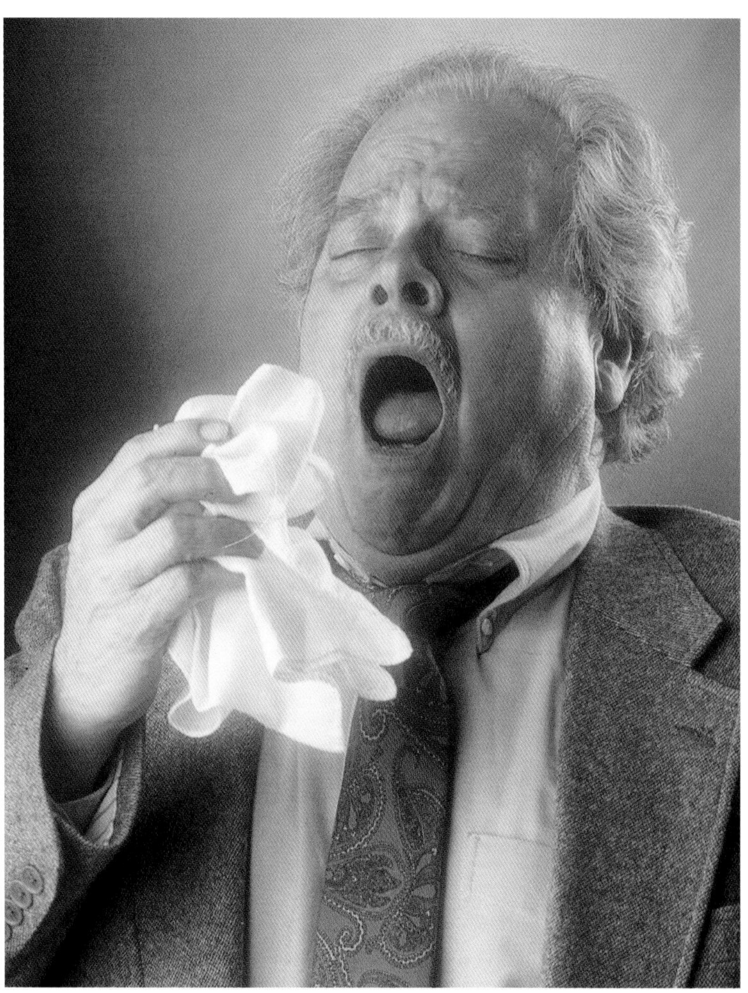

▲ *Hay fever and colds are both signs that something is wrong with the immune system. Help protect yourself by increasing your intake of vitamin C.*

"ALLERGIC RHINITIS"

This is an allergy to pollen, molds, dust or animal dander, that causes a runny nose, itchy eyes and sneezing.

Eat more vitamin C-rich foods as they have an antihistamine effect on the symptoms.

The Bones and Joints

ARTHRITIS

Rheumatoid arthritis is thought to be an illness of the immune system, whereas osteoarthritis is caused by wear and tear on joints. All types of arthritis result in pain, stiffness and inflammation of the joints.

Eat more oily fish, which encourages anti-inflammatory substances to be produced by the body, as well as fruits and vegetables rich in antioxidants. For osteoarthritis, eat more canned fish, which provides vitamin D for healthy bones.

Eat less fatty red meat and fewer full-fat dairy products and other sources of saturated fats, which may encourage inflammation in the body.

OSTEOPOROSIS

Osteoporosis is a bone-thinning disease that affects one in three women after menopause and an increasing number of elderly men.

Eat more calcium-rich foods including dairy products, broccoli and nuts.

Eat less salt and avoid heavy alcohol consumption—both leach calcium from the bones.

The Heart and Lungs

ASTHMA

Asthma causes constriction of the airways and (sometimes severe) difficulty in breathing. It is often associated with allergic conditions.

Eat more oily fish, which helps improve the balance of anti-inflammatory chemicals in the body. Increase your intake of antioxidant-rich fruits and vegetables, which help mop up harmful free radicals produced as part of the inflammatory process. Eating more magnesium (found in dark-green leafy vegetables) can also relax the airways. If your attacks are stress-related, step up your intake of legumes, grains and lean meat as they supply B vitamins vital for the nervous system.

Eat fewer foods that might provoke an attack. These vary from person to person but can include cows' milk, sulfite additives and wine.

POOR CIRCULATION

Poor circulation can manifest itself in cold hands and feet and may exacerbate symptoms of nerve damage in diabetics.

Eat more garlic and fish oils, which help reduce the stickiness of the blood and ease its flow. A supplement of the herb ginkgo biloba can also help.

Eat fewer saturated fats such as in fatty meats) as they can clog the blood vessels.

The Reproductive System

INFERTILITY

Infertility affects as many as one in six couples. If there is no physical cause, eating more of the right foods may help.

Eat more zinc-rich foods such as seafood, lean meat and grains, which help both the male and female reproductive systems including increasing sperm count. Increase the intake of vegetables and fruits and vitamin E-rich avocados, vegetable oils and nuts; these provide antioxidants to protect sperm function.

IMPOTENCE

Impotence can have many psychological causes but can also be affected by diet.

Eat more zinc-rich foods such as seafood, lean meat and grains, as these help to raise levels of the male sex hormone testosterone.

Drink less tea, coffee and colas as caffeine inhibits blood flow.

MENOPAUSAL PROBLEMS

Menopause can be a stressful time of life for women. As the levels of the hormone estrogen fall, the risk of brittle bones and heart disease increases. Symptoms include hot flushes, irritability, and dry skin.

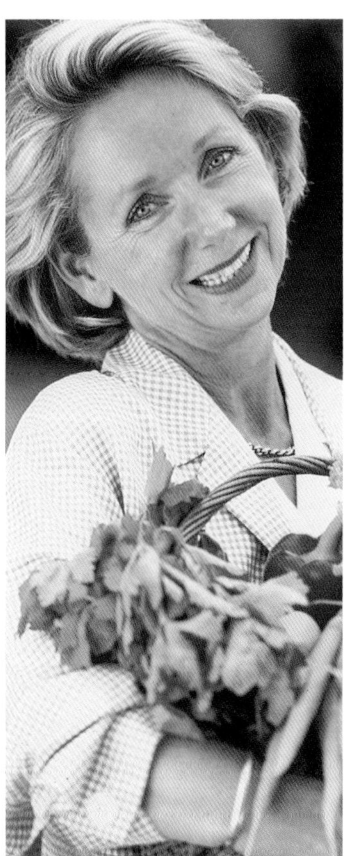

▲ *Women enter a new phase of life at menopause, but staying happy and healthy is within your reach with the right diet and lifestyle choices.*

Eat more low-fat dairy products and oily fish which provide, respectively, calcium and vitamin D for a healthy, strong skeleton. Increase the intake of wheat germ, vegetable oils, nuts, seeds and avocados, which are rich in vitamin E, for a healthy heart.
Drink less tea, coffee and colas as caffeine can exacerbate hot flushes.

PREMENSTRUAL SYNDROME

Premenstrual syndrome (PMS) is a collection of physical and emotional symptoms suffered by many women in the days before a menstrual period.
Eat more regular meals rich in carbohydrates, vitamin B_6 and magnesium (good choices include bananas, dried fruits and nuts). These help keep blood sugar levels steady and feed the nervous system.

The Digestive and Urinary Systems

IRRITABLE BOWEL SYNDROME

As many as one in five people is affected by this condition. Symptoms, which arise because of abnormal spasms of the intestinal wall, include cramps, bloating, gas and alternating bowel movements (constipation and diarrhea).
Eat more foods high in fiber to encourage healthy digestive action. Regular, smaller meals can also help.
Eat fewer foods liable to cause flare-ups, including very hot or cold foods, caffeine and spicy foods. Avoid greasy meals as fat causes strong bowel spasms.

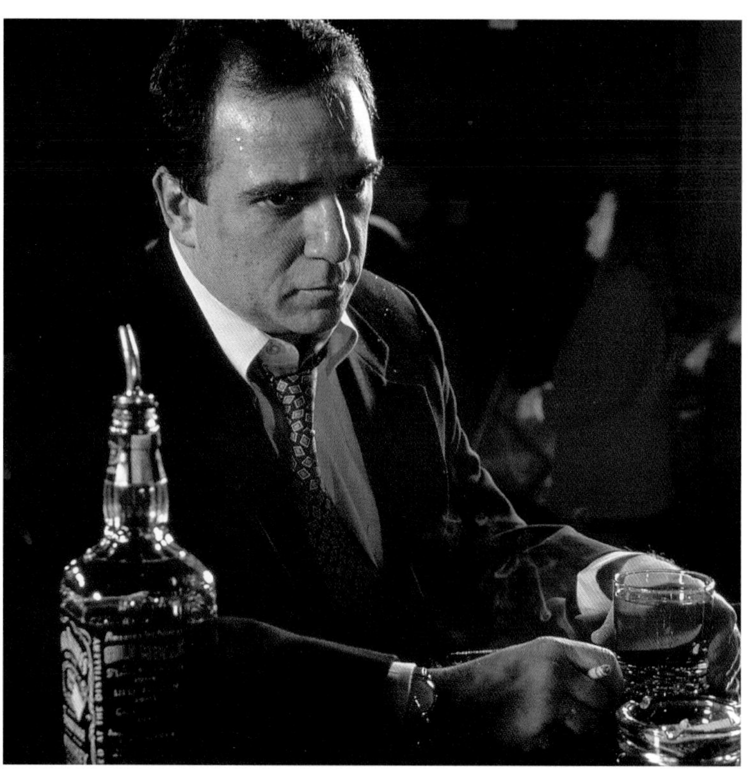

▲ *Stomach ulcers are exacerbated by alcohol, spicy foods and a high-stress lifestyle. Stop smoking and cut back on high risk foods.*

CYSTITIS

Cystitis is a painful bladder infection that causes a burning sensation during urination.
Eat more cranberries and drink cranberry juice. Cranberries contain a component that stops bacteria from adhering to the walls of the bladder. Drink plenty of water and fluids in general to help flush the bacteria from the system.
Eat fewer hot and spicy foods as they may exacerbate the condition.

ENLARGED PROSTATE

Lots of men develop enlarged prostates as they get older. Men who experience difficulty with urination should see a doctor, but eating more of the right foods can also help.
Eat more zinc-rich foods, for example, oysters, seafood, lean meat and grain to nourish the prostate. Increase the intake of processed tomato products (soup, pizza, baked beans), which supply an antioxidant called lycopene that may protect against prostate cancer. Supplements of the herb saw palmetto may also help.

ULCERS

Peptic (stomach) and duodenal ulcers have many causes, including bad diet, stress or infection with a bacteria called *helicobacter pylori*.
Eat more chili peppers! As long as you can tolerate them, chilies actually ease, ulcers.
Drink less milk – it may soothe an ulcer immediately but can lead to increased acidity of the stomach over the long term. Alcohol and spicy foods can also exacerbate stomach ulcers.

KIDNEY STONES

Kidney stones are caused by the painful crystalization of oxalic acid in the kidney.

Eat more calcium-rich foods such as dairy products. Contrary to popular opinion, these actually reduce the risk of developing kidney stones. Green vegetables, and grains that contain magnesium can also reduce the risk of stone formation. Drink plenty of water to dissolve the stone.

Eat fewer foods rich in oxalic acid, such as chocolate and spinach. Avoid high-dose vitamin C and calcium supplements if you are at high risk of kidney stones as these increase the level of calcium and oxalic acid passing through the kidney.

THRUSH

Thrush is caused by an excess growth of the *Candida albicans* yeast in the vagina—it causes itching and discharge. Thrush can also be present in the mouth where it causes a white growth.

Eat more live yogurt and garlic, which fight infection and encourage friendly bacteria to flourish.

Eat less sugar as it encourages the *Candida* yeast to grow.

The Nervous System

STRESS

A little stress can be very valuable, but too much can cause high blood pressure, muscular pains and depression.

Eat more Vitamin B rich foods, such as legumes, grains, lean meats and liver, which help to nourish the nervous system.

Eat less refined foods and avoid too much sugar as it depletes vitamin B_1 (thiamin).

DEPRESSION

Eat more carbohydrate-rich snacks, which raise the levels of the antidepressive chemical serotonin in the brain. Good choices include dried fruits, bananas and bread. Bananas and nuts include vitamin B_6, which can help PMS-related depression.

MIGRAINES

Migraines can have many causes, but certain foods are known to trigger them.

Eat more magnesium-rich foods, such as green vegetables, dried fruits, and grains, which help relax the muscles in the head.

Eat fewer trigger foods containing substances called tyramines, such as cheese, coffee and red wine.

General

FATIGUE

Factors ranging from too many late nights to hormonal changes or anemia may be responsible for fatigue.

Eat more lean red meat and liver to provide anemia-preventive iron and B vitamins. Vegetarians should increase their intake of dark-colored green vegetables.

Eat less refined sugar in sweet snacks as it can lead to fluctuating blood sugar levels.

SKIN DISORDERS

Skin disorders can range from occasional pimples to chronic psoriasis in which the skin reddens and flakes.

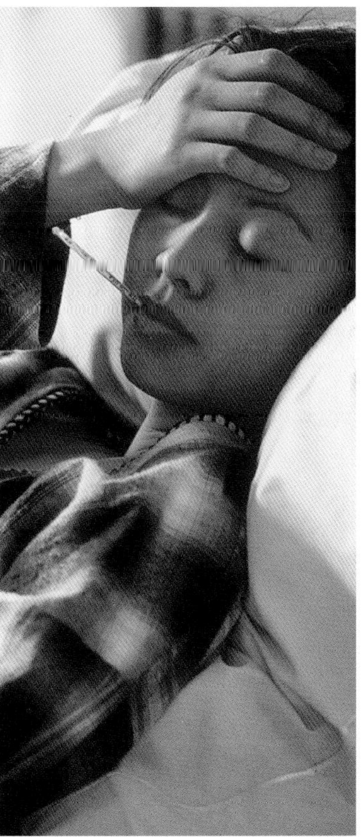

▲ *Fatigue can have many causes, so see your doctor. Eat a diet rich in iron and B vitamins. Avoid sugary foods that ultimately make you more tired.*

Eat more fruits and vegetables containing anti-oxidant vitamins and increase the intake of vitamin A (in foods such as liver and deep orange fruits and vegetables) and zinc to help improve acne. Eczema may respond to zinc and evening primrose oil. Oily fish may reduce inflammation in psoriasis.

Eat less full-fat dairy products and red meats.

CRAMP

Cramp is a condition in which muscles go into painful spasms.

Eat more calcium- and magnesium-rich foods (dairy products, grains, vegetables and nuts) which help muscles to function normally.

Glossary

Aerobic exercise Exercise such as walking or running that uses oxygen. After around 20 minutes of aerobic exercise, the body begins to burn fat significantly.

Amino acid Protein building block. There are eight essential amino acids that are not manufactured by the body and must be supplied by the diet.

Anaerobic exercise Energy expenditure that takes place without using oxygen. Anaerobic exercise includes sprinting, weight lifting and other short bursts of activity.

Antioxidant A dietary element or internally produced factor that protects body cells from becoming oxidized (rancid).

Atherosclerosis Narrowing of the arteries mainly through blockage with cholesterol and fats; a common precursor to angina or a heart attack.

Body Mass Index (BMI) A body mass measure that can be used to determine overweight or obesity; calculated by dividing your weight in kilograms by the square of your height in meters.

Bioavailability Ability of a nutrient to be available for use in the body. For example, iron from meat is more bioavailable than iron from vegetable sources.

EXPLANATIONS OF NUTRITIONAL SHORTHAND TERMS		
Used in analysis charts on pages 24 –103 and 107–129		
Ca	=	Calcium
CHO	=	Carbohydrate
CHOL	=	Cholesterol
Cu	=	Copper
Fe	=	Iron
Folat	=	Folic acid
I	=	Iodine
K	=	Potassium
Mg	=	Magnesium
MUFA	=	Monosaturated fat
Na	=	Sodium
NAeq	=	Niacin (vitamin B_3)
NSP	=	Fiber
P	=	Phosphorus
PRO	=	Protein
PUFA	=	Polyunsaturated fat
Se	=	Selenium
SFA	=	Saturated fats
Zn	=	Zinc

Calorie The basic unit in which the energy value of food is measured.

Carbohydrate The body's preferred source of dietary energy, found in foods such as sugar, flour, potatoes and so on.

Carotenoids Important dietary antioxidants the most well-known of which is beta-carotene, also a precursor to vitamin A.

Cholesterol A fat-like substance made naturally by the liver. Although it is vital for the synthesis of certain hormones, in excess it can clog arteries; leading to heart disease.

Collagen Intercellular "cement" that binds together skin cells and other body structures including joint cartilage.

Fiber Non-digestible parts of food, such as, grains, vegetables and fruits, that improve digestive action and help to prevent constipation. Some types (soluble fiber) can be fermented in the digestive tract and may help to lower blood cholesterol levels.

Free radicals Chemically reactive molecules that play a part in oxidizing and damaging body cells and tissues.

Flavonoids Chemical components found especially in fruits, vegetables, red wine and tea. May act as protective antioxidants in the body.

Glycogen Storage form of carbohydrate found in muscles. It acts as a major source of energy for muscular activity.

Hydrogenation A chemical process that solidifies oils and effectively turns polyunsaturated fats into saturated fats.

Hypertension The medical term for high blood pressure. Hypertension is one of the major risk factors for heart disease.

Indispensable, or Essential, fatty acids Polyunsaturated fatty acids that can't be made in our bodies and have to be provided from dietary sources. Essential fatty acids maintain cell membranes and are needed to make important hormone-like substances that regulate many body functions such as the menstrual cycle, blood pressure and so on.

Legumes The edible seeds of any member of the pea family (including chickpeas, soybeans and lentils).

Listeria A bacteria which, while harmless to most people, can increase the risk of miscarriage in

MEASUREMENT CONVERSION CHART

	U.S./U.K. Imperial		metric
Weight			
	1 ounce (oz)	=	28.35 grams (g)
	1 pound (lb)	=	453.6 grams (g)
	2.2 pounds (lb)	=	1 kilogram (kg)
Volume			
	1 fluid ounce (fl oz)	=	28.4 milliliters (ml)
	1.76 pints (pt)	=	1 liter (l)
	1 teaspoon (tsp)	=	5 milliliters (ml)
	1 tablespoon (tbl sp)	=	15 milliliters

Note: some U.S. and U.K. volume measurements differ; below are some typical examples:

		U.K. **fluid ounces (fl oz.)**	U.S. **fluid ounces (fl oz.)**
1 pint	=	20	16
1 quart	=	–	32
1 cup	=	10	8

pregnant women. May occur in blue-veined and unpasteurized soft cheeses, as well as patés.

Metabolism A term which describes all the chemical processes that take place in the body to keep it alive and functioning.

Microgram (mcg) A weight equivalent to one millionth of a gram (one thousandth of a milligram).

Micronutrient Vitamins and minerals that are essential to health but are needed by the body only in tiny amounts.

Milligram (mg) One-thousandth of a gram or 1,000 micrograms.

Monounsaturated fats Fatty acids (components of fat) which help to lower total cholesterol and improve the balance of cholesterol types in the blood. Olive oil is the richest source of monounsaturated fats.

Neurotransmitters Chemicals released in the brain and at the end of nerves to facilitate the passage of messages from one nerve to another.

Nonstarch polysaccharides (NSPs) Technical term for fiber. The desirable intake of fiber measured as NSPs is ½ ounce (18g) per day. (See fiber entry).

Omega-3 fatty acids A group of fatty acids that help to thin the blood and may protect against heart disease. A particularly rich source of these fatty acids are found in oily fish.

Organic meats These are meats from animals which have been raised on a nonchemical ethos, that is, they have not been treated with chemical growth stimulants, antibiotics or pesticides.

Oxalic acid A chemical that is toxic in high amounts and that in smaller amounts inhibits the body's absorption of minerals such as calcium and iron. Small amounts of the chemical are present in spinach, rhubarb and chocolate.

Polyunsaturated fats Fatty acids (components of fat) that help to lower total cholesterol but that are susceptible to becoming oxidized (rancid) in the body. Polyunsaturated fats are generally liquid at room temperature (for example, vegetable oil).

Protein Important dietary component that is vital for healthy skin, body tissue and muscles. Good sources are meat, fish and poultry.

Refined foods Foods such as white sugar, white flour and polished rice, all of which have been processed for better taste or more convenient use, usually with the result that some nutrients have been removed.

Saturated fats Fatty acids (components of fat) that contribute to raised blood cholesterol levels. Saturated fats have an inflexible chemical structure which makes them solid, even at room temperature (for example, butter).

Sodium Component of salt that may contribute to raised blood pressure.

Soluble fiber This is fiber that is partly broken down by bacteria in the intestines and may help in reducing cholesterol levels.

Starch (Complex carbohydrates) The major form in which energy is stored in plants. Bread, potatoes, pasta and rice are all good sources of starch.

Sulfites/Sulphites Compounds of sulfur used as additives in food. Mixed with acid, they form the gas sulfur dioxide used in wine making to kill yeast. In sensitive individuals, sulfites and sulfur dioxide may trigger asthma-type symptoms.

Tubers The underground stems of certain plants, such as the potato.

Toxic Poisonous or harmful to the body. A toxic compound is also described as a "toxin" and can be described as having "toxicity."

Vegetarian/Vegan A vegetarian is someone who does not eat the flesh of animals of fish. A vegan eats no animal products at all.

Index

Credits

Quarto would like to acknowledge and thank the following for providing pictures used in this book. While every effort has been made to acknowledge copyright holders we would like to apologize should there have been any omissions.

Ace Photo Agency p.137, p.138, p.139, p.141; **The Image Bank** p12, p.19, p.132, p.133, p.144, p.145, p.149, p.151, p.153; **Pictor International** p.136, p.146, p.148, p.150, p.152; **Powerstock** p.17, p.143; **Tony Stone Images** p.135.

Quarto Publishing acknowledgements:
Senior Editor Gerrie Purcell
Text Editors Alison Leach, Trish Burgess
Senior Art Editor Penny Cobb, Catherine Shearman
Designer Neville Graham
Photographers Anna Hodgson, Paul Forrester, Laura Wickenden
Illustrator Valerie Hill
Picture Researcher Zoë Holtermann
Editorial Director Pippa Rubinstein
Art Director Moira Clinch